THE LONGEVITY LIST

About the author

Merlin Thomas MBChB, PhD, FRACP is Professor of Medicine at Monash University, Melbourne. Professor Thomas is both a physician and a research scientist. His research primarily focuses on diabetes and its complications, and finding practical means for their control, but he has a broader interest in all aspects of preventive medicine and ageing. He has published over 300 articles in many of the world's leading medical journals, as well as several books, including *Understanding Type 2 Diabetes* and *Fast Living, Slow Ageing*. He is internationally recognized as a speaker, opinion-leader, teacher and medical storyteller.

THE LONGEVITY LIST

PROFESSOR MERLIN THOMAS

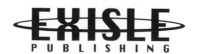
EXISLE
PUBLISHING

First published 2017

Exisle Publishing Pty Ltd
PO Box 864, Chatswood, NSW 2057, Australia
226 High Street, Dunedin, 9016, New Zealand
www.exislepublishing.com

A CiP record for this book is available from the National Library of Australia.

ISBN 978-1-921966-73-6

Designed by Nada Backovic
Typeset in Sabon 11/14pt
Printed in China

This book uses paper sourced under ISO 14001 guidelines from well-managed forests and other controlled sources.

10 9 8 7 6 5 4 3 2 1

Disclaimer
This book is a general guide only and should never be a substitute for the skill, knowledge and experience of a qualified medical professional dealing with the facts, circumstances and symptoms of a particular case. The nutritional, medical and health information presented in this book is based on the research, training and professional experience of the author, and is true and complete to the best of their knowledge. However, this book is intended only as an informative guide; it is not intended to replace or countermand the advice given by the reader's personal physician. Because each person and situation is unique, the author and the publisher urge the reader to check with a qualified healthcare professional before using any procedure where there is a question as to its appropriateness. The author, publisher and their distributors are not responsible for any adverse effects or consequences resulting from the use of the information in this book. It is the responsibility of the reader to consult a physician or other qualified healthcare professional regarding their personal care. This book contains references to products that may not be available everywhere. The intent of the information provided is to be helpful; however, there is no guarantee of results associated with the information provided. Use of drug brand names is for educational purposes only and does not imply endorsement.

Contents

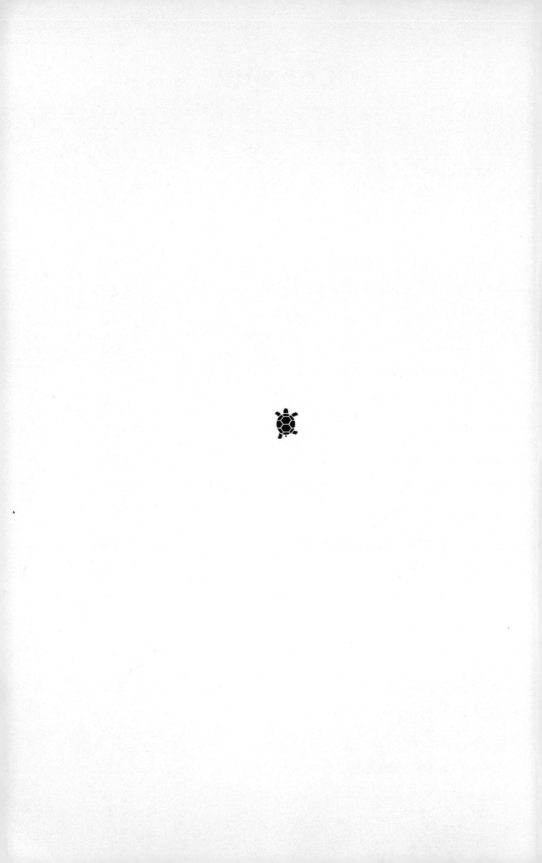

Introduction

Many years ago I used to play cricket. In this complicated game the pinnacle of success is to score a hundred runs in a single innings. It was something I never achieved. Actually, I never even came close and seldom troubled the scorers when it came my turn to bat.

It was not that I was reckless or didn't care. In fact, I cared a great deal. I was desperate not to get out. I practised hard. I read the histories of all the great century makers, the ones who could score a hundred almost at will, time after time. I copied their choices: what to go for, what to avoid. I visualized my success as if I were them. In my mind I reached every milestone with ease and enjoyed the accolades of my peers. I had the best intentions. Yet every time I went out to bat, I was duly sent back to the pavilion well before my time in the sun.

Perhaps the game was simply unfair. Perhaps I could blame my parents or my grandparents. My teammates were endowed with the cumulative prowess of generations past (and often reminded me of this fact). It was in their blood. It was in their genes. How could I possibly compete?

Once dismissed, I usually argued that the opposition was so exceedingly strong that even the mighty would fall. Or I was simply unlucky to receive a delivery of such potency that none could have withstood it, not without the direct intervention of God. What are the chances? Perhaps God rooted for the other team?

I blamed fate. I blamed karma. I blamed bad luck. I blamed the unassailable triumvirate of all of them at once that conspired against me.

And yet, despite my best efforts, our team was extraordinarily successful. We swept all before us in the junior competition and easily won the season-ending final.

The secret to our success was a batsman of singular talent. He was fearless, extravagant and calm under pressure, riding his luck. His extraordinary scoring ability remains unmatched to this present day. I had no idea how he did it.

I recall coming in to bat late on the first day of the final. We had lost nine wickets and one more out would trigger the end of the innings for our illustrious team.

At the other end of the pitch was my famous partner. His tally had already reached into the nineties and he was batting like he could easily reach a thousand before stumps.

As I came into the middle of the field we conferred, or rather, he told me the most important piece of advice that I have ever been told by anyone. He asked me: 'Do you know what the secret to scoring a hundred is?'

Having read every book on the subject in the vain attempt to solve this conundrum, I was immediately ready with my answer. 'The secret to scoring a hundred is not getting out,' I replied assuredly.

'That's right,' he scowled, 'the secret to *me* getting to a hundred is *you* not getting out.'

We should all score a century. I'd still like to help if I can.

Fate, karma and bad luck

We often think of our prospects for a long innings in exactly these terms.

Sometimes we wonder if we are simply prisoners of our fate; that through no fault of our own, a chain of events is set in motion. And given a particular set of conditions, only one thing can happen. While it may seem like we have a choice, all paths ultimately lead to the same point. It is inevitable. It is our destiny.

For example, most people think of their genetics fatalistically, as a form of irreversible destiny that can't be shrugged off no matter how hard we try. Our genes made this happen. We can't choose our parents. The upshot of this is the idea that if we only had the tools to sequence every inch of our DNA we would be able to read our future, just like in the movies. Moreover, if we understood our fate early enough we could even do something about it pre-emptively, like a double mastectomy for a woman who has all the bad genes for breast cancer.

But while genes can significantly bias the course of our life, and genetic fate may be partly true for some rare genetic conditions, by and large it is not our genes that matter but what we *do* with them that *is* important. There is almost always substantial wriggle room, meaning that even with the bad genes, good outcomes can still occur. Equally, with all the good genes, things can still go horribly wrong.

Before the time of genetics (and other internal forces that set us down one path), the most important source of fate was God and, more specifically, that God had predetermined which events should or should not occur. Any significant problems that appeared completely out of our control, like illness and accidents, were attributed as an 'Act of God' in much the same way that our genes are often blamed today.

Yet in other situations, what happens to us seems to be the direct result of the things we have done or not done. There is justice in the universe. We reap what we sow. This is often called karma and each individual is said to be responsible for their own karma and its ultimate fruits. In this view everything we do or think has consequences or, in other words, all consequences have a cause (if we were smart enough or had the technology to see). Was it something I did wrong, doctor? Was it something I didn't do? Is illness and ageing simply the accumulated consequences of bad karma; the modern equivalent of a curse for all the bad things we have done or the good things we didn't do?

Critically, karma is not simply a dynamic form of fate (i.e. once we start the ball rolling it's inevitably going to fall). Karma can be mitigated or unwound by other actions or intensions, especially efforts of self-control and austerity. Medicines are often viewed in this light — in order to restore our health we have to swallow the bitter pill, follow the punitive diet or exercise regime, lead an austere life devoid of chocolate, sugar and other pleasures, as though our punishment (puja) could counteract the bad karma of our past misdemeanours.

Finally, some things that happen to us feel like just dumb luck, like being struck on the head by a falling roof tile. Gee, that was unlucky! To be walking down the street at exactly the same time that the tile came loose and hit you on the head. What are the chances?

All luck works in this way, the random intersection of different causal pathways. All it took was for you to be there at that time. And then a second event, the tile falling off the roof, intersecting with your path. This is why luck is also often literally called **coincidence** — the common incidence of very different events at the same time and place. Because it only seems to happen very rarely (I mean, how common is it for people to be hit on the head by a falling tile?), coincidence seems remarkable. So we call it luck and attribute it some importance. But it is just as likely that if the tile fell at some other time when we weren't around, we would have never known or even cared.

Without luck nothing comes together, and coincidence never happens without luck. However, it was inevitable that the faulty tile should fall off the roof someday. That was its fate. It was built that way. And of course the builder who incorrectly installed the tile on the roof in the first place is now in big trouble. He'll be the one held to blame, rather than it being your fault for walking along the street at that time. But it was randomness or bad luck that the tile actually hit you.

People often feel unlucky to get sick. And for good reason! They've eaten all the right things, done their exercise and looked after their mind. They've walked down the sunny side of the street. And now they fall unwell. How unlucky! And it's true, no matter what the doctors say, most disease is random and largely unpredictable when or if it strikes us.

But just because it is a random coincidence does not mean that it doesn't have a cause or there's nothing that could have been done to prevent it. The worker who laid the tiles on the roof could have done a better job, and that might have saved your head. Equally, heavy smokers have only a one in ten chance of getting lung cancer. It's still their smoking that is to blame. But there is a random play of luck that eventually leads to them getting cancer.

The element of luck is seldom part of any discussion when doctors talk to their patients. Imagine a doctor telling a smoker with cancer, 'Oh you were just unlucky.' Luck is not part of the discussion because most people think of luck as a poor excuse for not understanding, like superstition. However, luck is real. It's random but it's real. And it is as important a reason for staying in or getting out as skill or destiny.

But is also possible to change our luck. The more tiles the tiler messed up, the greater the chances one would have fallen on someone's head. The same with a smoker. The more cigarettes they smoke, the greater the chances they will get lung cancer. So even though coincidence happens randomly, karma and fate provide the causal substrate upon which luck can play out. In this way, we can all make our own luck on our way to a hundred not out.

The checklist

The way we often start doing what needs to be done is by making a list. I did.

Our brain loves lists. Lists are like an easy, ready-made meal; they require little preparation before our brain can consume and digest them without much chewing over their contents. The information they convey is already organized, easy to remember, succinct, to the (bullet) point. They have a beginning and (thankfully) a finite end.

The whole point of lists is to distil a lot of ideas into the semblance of a plan downloaded onto a piece of paper the size of a paper napkin. Each dot point is a door into an entirely different universe of thought now neatly separated from other notions.

There are many different ways human beings can shorten their lives. By and large we take very few of them. For example, while researching this book, the only really useful thing I did was make this list.

It's not rocket science. Everyone I spoke to had a list very similar. Even the World Health Organization has a list of the most important things we should probably all be doing to improve our health prospects.

There are a million other things we might think of doing for our health and wellbeing. However, for the most part, there are just a few things we currently think are really important, or at least important enough to warrant listing them or telling them with conviction to others, like our children. Your order of priorities will almost certainly be different to mine. So you can make your own list and dip into this book where you want.

Each chapter is dedicated to understanding why a few elements have become so important to our health that we are prepared to list them as priorities. And why, when we go against them, we feel guilty, as if we have probably done something bad and half expect there will be consequences.

This book can tell you the why or why not, but not how. How we can ever achieve any of the things on our lists is up to the individual. There is no generic solution, no panacea or universal remedy. We are all good at different things and bad at others.

No matter what the advertising says, one size never fits all. This doesn't mean that nothing ever fits properly. It's just that we need to take a bit of time finding out what fits well and feels good and what doesn't. Making a checklist is as good a place as any to start.

Do I really have to ...

#1

Cut out the chocolate?

Q: Why is chocolate a bad thing?
A: It isn't (except for dogs).

Q: Is dark chocolate better than white?
A: White chocolate isn't really chocolate.

Q: Isn't chocolate just fat and sugar?
A: No, it's so much more.

Q: Can chocolate ever be good?
A: Chocolate is always good. It's us who are sometimes bad.

Q: Why does it make me feel so much better?
A: Because it's chocolate!

Q: Can chocolate improve my sex life?
A: Depends on who you are giving it to, as well as when and why.

There is nothing like chocolate. When it comes to exclusive luxury and hedonic appeal, its taste, texture, aroma and presentation are hard to beat.

On average, we consume around 4.5 kilograms (10 pounds) of chocolate per person, every year. And often even more. After we eat our chocolate Easter eggs, then there's Mother's Day, Father's Day, Halloween and Christmas, not to mention Valentine's Day. We know we eat too much of everything! But why is it that when we think about all the things we might have to do away with to improve our health, our chocolate fix is always first on the chopping block when the health revolution comes?

A slice of heaven

Chocolate is made from the seeds of the cacao tree. These are usually called **cocoa beans**. But while they may look a little like beans and come from a pod, they are not beans. They are actually seeds.

For millennia, products made from cocoa have been considered a valuable and exclusive item. So much so that cocoa seeds were used as a form of currency by the ancient Aztecs. They also spent them to make a hot beverage, so were literally drinking their money away if they had some to spare.

Carl Linnaeus, the Swedish botanist and physicist who provided the scientific names for so many things, named the cocoa tree *Theobroma cacao*, which comes from the Greek words *theo* (meaning god) and *broma* (meaning drink, as in brew) i.e. the gods drink cocoa. Across Central America, the Mayan people believed that hot chocolate was the drink of choice for their gods, just like soma was for the gods of Hindu mythology and ambrosia for the Greek deities. However, unlike these other mythical beverages, which were kept strictly top-secret and beyond the reach of mortal men, the classified recipe for cocoa was leaked to the Mayan people by Quetzalcoatl.

Forbidden fruit

 Quetzalcoatl was the infamous feathered serpent god of Aztec mythology. He was part bird and part rattlesnake. But he was also the god of learning and knowledge.

On one of his visits from Heaven he gave mortal humans the knowledge of how to make chocolate. Not surprisingly, the other gods were upset about this. They felt that the great unwashed masses were far too plebeian to appreciate this slice of heaven.

As in the Garden of Eden, the half-serpent was ridiculed and punished for letting the intelligence slip and giving away forbidden fruits that had previously been exclusively for gods.

In deference to the gods, humans found an acceptable compromise. They agreed that only the 'god-like' royalty and the upper classes were allowed to drink chocolate, and only on special festive occasions. Not too much has changed.

~~~~~~

The allure of exotic mystery, its supernatural origins, fashion and exclusivity all partly explain why the West — and subsequently the entire world — fell in love with chocolate.

Cocoa first reached Europe in the 17th century. It became the first beverage stimulant with mass appeal, a mantle only later supplanted by coffee and tea. Because it only came in very limited supply from imposingly distant places, it was also imposingly pricey. After gold, cacao was the next most precious commodity imported into Europe from the New World.

Not surprisingly, given its super-exclusive status, chocolate quickly became the vogue drink of the curious and worldly aristocracy. Anyone who could afford chocolate wanted a piece of the action, even though it was almost undrinkable by today's standards. At least initially it was all about the show, a status symbol like diamonds or a fancy car. Giving chocolates became a way of saying that we'd wish to treat her like a princess, because any good princess was eating chocolates or at least expected her prince to have enough money to buy them for her.

Not wishing to miss out on a heavenly good party, the clergy also became fascinated by chocolate. But when periods of strict fasting were prescribed, chocolate made it harder to comply. We all know the feeling. To fix this dilemma, the Bishop of Rome made a dispensation that taking chocolate did not mean that the devout had broken their fast. At least officially, chocolate was not sinful.

At the same time, Europe was changing. Gone were the dark days of frugal subsistence. A growing middle class of people emerged with a disposable income and appetite to bridge the social divide. The consumer revolution rolled like a tsunami across the countryside. Drinking chocolate really took off, along with other, newly fashionable and formerly exclusive products such as sugar, tobacco, tea and coffee in the vanguard. Chocolate consumption became an indulgent attempt by some to rise above their station in fashionable society.

Café culture

 Since the origins of civilization, there have always been sites of public gathering, gossip and communal eating and drinking. These were public houses, and so called 'pubs' for short.

But the advent of a new beverage (chocolate), and a far better clientele, required a new kind of public house. And so the Chocolate House was born. All the bigwigs, dukes, earls and lords now had a place to hang out together. Not unlike modern bars, the original chocolate houses were centres of debauched glory, smoking, plotting, scandal, gambling, politics and business. They were a great place to work off your hangover. And there were no women allowed.

But even if drinking chocolate made us look and feel fashionable in the 17th century, why would it still have the same allure today? Fashions like wigs, hats and pantyhose have come and gone, and come and gone again. But chocolate has been a constant companion, even though the advent of mass production means it is now accessible to almost every run of the mill human being on the planet. If everyone can get some chocolate whenever they like, there must be more to its appeal than the enduring placebo of fashion and luxury.

The hot pleasure of chocolate

Another obvious reason why chocolate has become so popular is simply the pursuit of pleasure (known as **hedonism**). And drinking and eating chocolate is certainly physically and mentally pleasurable.

Cocoa probably wasn't that tasty in the beginning. The combination of ingredients that we call chocolate today is a far cry from the acrid cacao beverage drunk in 17th-century Europe. A typical mug of chocolate was likely a far worse prospect than any instant coffee available today.

But it was hot. And in a world without central heating, it felt nice to be warmed from the inside. It was also frothy. The froth has long been considered the best part. Even the Mayans made sure that their chocolate drink had a deliciously sensual foam, as they poured the brew back and forth from cup to pot.

As more and more people began to drink it, the acrid chocolate brew slowly evolved into something more than simply palatable. Cinnamon, vanilla, chilli and other spices were occasionally added. And then came sugar. The Mayans had sometimes used honey, but the addition of cane sugar really transformed cocoa into the chocolate superstar it is today.

It turns out that chocolate is a highly versatile delivery system for sugar. As discussed in later chapters, it's universal to the human condition to enjoy something sweet. But not too sweet. And this is why chocolate is almost perfect. Most modern chocolates are really just a thin coating of chocolate over a generous sugar filling. But because chocolate contains some very bitter chemicals, it is possible to disguise an intensely sweet substance like malted milk with dark chocolate. Suddenly almost everyone can enjoy Maltesers (similar to American Whoppers) with or without a sweet tooth. By contrast, the sweet filling inside on its own would have very few takers.

The next breakthrough came when cocoa engineers discovered ways to make solid chocolate suitable for storage and mass production and yet, at the same time, still soft enough so that it readily melted in the mouth.

Getting hard

 Cocoa beans are fermented and roasted like coffee. They are then left hanging in big bags in a hot room, which allows white cocoa butter to melt and drip off the beans. The solids left behind in the bags are then dried and crushed into cocoa powder, also known simply as cocoa.

Most of the chemicals, antioxidants and bitter taste are in the cocoa powder. This was used to make the original hot drink. The cocoa butter was historically considered a tasteless waste product.

However, cocoa butter had some interesting properties. It could be stored for over a year and didn't become rancid. It was velvety smooth and smelled quite pleasant. At room temperature, it even became solid, taking the shape of whatever it was collected in. But it could be made liquid by heating it slightly above body temperature.

In retrospect it seems obvious what to do with it. But it wasn't until 1847 that Joseph Fry conceived of reuniting extracted cocoa butter and cocoa powder. He added some sugar for taste, and the chocolate bar was born.

Whether he was visionary or simply thrifty is unclear. However, his revolutionary contribution to the culinary arts is probably the most important to ever come out of England, exceeding even fish and chips or cheddar cheese.

This perfect chemistry comes about from the way the fat molecules in chocolate are densely packed. This keeps chocolate solid at room temperature, like butter. And like butter, chocolate melts as it is warmed up. But this happens only very slowly, and over a temperature range close to body temperature (between 34°C and 38°C, or 93°F and 100°F). This allows chocolate to slowly soften and not immediately become liquid, creating a lovely melting sensation that only fat can achieve as it warms towards body temperature in our mouth. It also keeps our fingers clean for the few seconds it takes to transfer a chocolate to our lips. This is very different to ice, which at one moment is frozen solid and the next is a puddle. Sucking on ice is a wholly different experience to the wonderfully pleasurable warm soft sensation of letting chocolate melt in our mouth.

By melting and/or solidifying so easily, it means that we can pour chocolate into moulds of almost any shape (even a hollow egg) and have it set hard, at least until it reaches our lips. We can have a fountain of liquid chocolate or a castle of solid chocolate, which would never be possible with almost any other cooking ingredient. Even melted butter never perfectly returns to its original form.

Smarties

 Melting chocolate only became a big issue on really hot days or if you had some sitting in your pocket. The smart solution was to insulate the chocolate in a crispy thin layer of sugar (which doesn't melt easily but quickly dissolves when mixed with the moisture of your mouth).

These became known as Smarties.

Their success was revolutionary. Even soldiers could now carry chocolates without getting their rifle or their trigger finger sticky.

But Forrest Mars Sr was the real chocolate smarty. While working for England in the 1930s he had invented Maltesers, a ball of malted milk coated with chocolate. However, during the Spanish Civil War he saw soldiers eating Smarties, with chocolate safely on the inside of the candy. On his return to America, he quickly patented his own process and in 1941 the first M&Ms began to be produced.

The first 'M' stood for Mars himself. The second stood for Bruce Murrie, son of the head of Hershey chocolates. There was a war on in Europe at the time, so only Hershey's had an assured supply of chocolate. Soon the heat-resistant, easy-to-transport chocolate was included in American soldiers' rations. And the rest is history.

Through ongoing experimentation, Lindt, Cadbury, Nestlé and a host of other chocolate entrepreneurs discovered new ways to make cocoa powder less bitter, by adding more sugar or evaporated milk, or simply alkalinizing it to take out the bitter bits (known as **dutching** — and hence Dutch chocolate). And by progressively getting rid of any negatives, chocolate became the mouth-watering treat we know and love today.

Chocolate on the brain

Beyond the exclusive luxury and the sweet melt-in-the-mouth pleasures of chocolate, another important reason that it took off in popularity was that it was considered to be an exotic mind-altering drug, and was sold as such.

Some of this effect is clearly psychological. We all feel good after being treated to a little bit of delicious luxury. A little indulgence (or the perception of one) can lift our mood and alter the chemistry of our brain. This is particularly the case for chocolate.

In addition to the psychology, there really are mind-altering chemicals in chocolate that have reproducible effects on our brain and the way it functions. Just as coffee is a drug mule for caffeine (see Chapter 3), chocolate delivers to our brain another potent drug called **theobromine**. Its chemistry is about 98 per cent the same as caffeine.

So theobromine has a similar 'pick-me-up' effect on our brain to a cup of tea or coffee, helping us to focus, lifting our mood and creating a sense of optimism.

In racehorses, both caffeine and theobromine are banned substances because they are both performance enhancing. Most tea and coffee drinkers and chocolate eaters would agree on these performance-enhancing qualities, as the afternoon chocolate bar or cup of tea is only thing that gets them through their three o'clock slump.

Theobromine also shares other characteristics with caffeine. For example, both can cause heartburn in some people, by relaxing the sphincter that keeps acids safely in our stomach, allowing it instead to reflux upward, and producing the characteristic burning deep in our chests (which fortunately has nothing to do with our hearts).

Don't feed dogs chocolate

 Like caffeine, theobromine is highly toxic to dogs. Even a small piece of dark chocolate can lead to serious and potentially fatal symptoms in dogs. This may be considered definitive proof that chocolate really is a mind-altering drug.

The reason why dogs find dark chocolate poisonous is that they don't have the enzyme in their liver that breaks theobromine and caffeine down, so even small doses can rapidly accumulate. Humans, on the other hand, have the enzyme in spades, so less than 10 per cent of the theobromine we eat even reaches our circulation, let alone our brain. So we humans are virtually immune to chocolate poisoning.

Cats also don't have the enzyme. But cats are fussy carnivores, and would rather lick the sweat off your arm than touch chocolate. Dogs, like humans, will eat almost anything they are given. But even if it wasn't toxic to them, why would we waste our good chocolate on our pets?

High levels of theobromine are only found in products made from cocoa powder, with much smaller amounts in the fat-rich cocoa butter. This means that a hot chocolate made with cocoa powder contains more theobromine than one made of drinking chocolate (which is essentially just shredded milk chocolate made with cocoa butter).

Because it is more cocoa than butter, a single bar of dark chocolate usually contains enough theobromine to change our minds. However, even though it looks dark, Dutch chocolate has less theobromine, as the dutching process removes some theobromine along with the bitterness.

Regular milk chocolate has smaller amounts again of theobromine, as it is made of almost four times less cocoa powder (so we'd generally need to eat four times more milk chocolate than dark chocolate to get the same buzz). White chocolate is made exclusively with cocoa butter and has almost no theobromine to speak of. Some theobromine is also found in tea and in the cola nut, hence the buzz from many cola-based soft drinks.

Because of the many similarities between caffeine (in tea and coffee) and theobromine (in chocolate), people who are don't drink tea or coffee are generally more sensitive to the stimulating effects of dark chocolate on their brain. As chocolate arrived in Renaissance Europe before coffee and tea had a foothold, the early buzz surrounding it was therefore hardly surprising.

Chocolate has been historically considered a woman's drink, and coffee a man's. And certainly, women are slightly more sensitive than men to its effects, especially when they are pregnant. Women are also more sensitive to caffeine in coffee and tea. However, coffee is more bitter, even when compared to hot cocoa. And women generally have more of a sweet tooth than men.

Not surprisingly, children also get a greater kick from theobromine than adults. This chocolate buzz is one of many reasons many of us have a soft spot for chocolate, remembering the powerful effects on our mood from when we were young.

As well as the caffeine-like theobromine, chocolate also contains small amounts of the chemical serotonin. Serotonin is naturally found in our brains and is used by brain cells to signal to each other. When brain serotonin levels drop we are more prone to feeling low in our mood or anxious. On the other hand, increased serotonin levels enhance our mood, partly by increasing our sense of satisfaction. Whether the serotonin in chocolate really does anything for us is unclear. Many other foods also contain serotonin, such as bananas. But we can't say we feel the same after eating a banana, when compared to eating chocolate.

Chocolate even contains anandamide, a substance related to the active component of cannabis. However, the kind of amounts needed to get the same effects of cannabis would tax even the most serious chocolate lover.

The real effects of chocolate chemicals on our brain, and their similarity to caffeine, has led many to believe that chocolate is just as addictive. A condition known as **chocolatomania** has been described, especially among women, associated with insatiable cravings for chocolate. And, as with caffeine, some of this may be chemical addiction and some psychological.

It's easy to argue semantics. Our chocolate cravings can't really be an addiction if they don't have major negative consequences to our health, mental state or social life. At worst chocolate is a soft addiction or, more simply, a bad habit. At least that's something we can concede when staring down a chocolate bar. But bad habits are hard to break, and this is especially true of chocolate. It is well known that taking the chocolate away (going cold turkey) makes us crave it and like chocolate even more when it's gone. So it's hard not to fall off the wagon and return to the chocolate bars.

Chocolate, the aphrodisiac

There may be many ways to a woman's heart, but is a box of chocolates really one of them?

Some foods are thought to enhance the sexual desires. These are known as libido enhancers or aphrodisiacs. Many products have acquired an aphrodisiac reputation simply because they were once exotic, exclusive or unfamiliar, which added to their allure and eventually to their reputation. Cigarettes, coffee and even sugar have all had a reputation of being sexual enhancers. Oysters, caviar and bananas have also had their appeal. However, chocolate is the best loved of all.

Long before Richard Cadbury developed the clever marketing ploy of putting chocolate in a heart-shaped box for Valentine's Day, chocolate had been promoted as a libido enhancer. Even in Aztec times, cocoa was touted as Montezuma's secret source of unrivalled virility. Whether it was because he drank it or gave it to his mistresses is unclear.

Media hype

 The medicinal qualities of chocolate were well known in Renaissance Europe. However, it was its dark and exotic effects on libido that were perhaps the most fascinating.

Louis Lemery was the physician to the King of France in the early 18th century. Lemery believed that the key to health was what you ate and drank. So he put together a definitive treatise on the health effects of all the foods and drinkables he could think of. In his book, published in England after his death in 1745, he describes chocolate as 'nourishing enough … apt to repair decayed strength … agrees with cold weather, especially in old people'.

However, he also added an anecdote reported to him by Dr Munday, a ribald London colleague. Dr Munday describes how one of his patients 'was in a miserable condition, but taking to the supping of chocolate, he recovered in a short time; but what is more extraordinary is, that his wife … having also accustomed herself to sup chocolate with him, bore afterwards several children, though she was looked upon before as not capable of having any'.

Not surprisingly, the public response to such an incredible write-up was as predictable as the faked orgasm scene from the movie *When Harry met Sally*. We all want what she's having!

It is tempting to hypothesize that chocolate is actually an aphrodisiac. It is almost believable. But as they say, the trick of the very best advertising is that there is usually some truth in it somewhere. Never as much as they say, but enough to make us believe that it might just be working. This is perfectly true for chocolate. Some studies have even supported the notion that women who eat chocolate have a greater libido than those who don't.

Part of the aura about chocolate as an aphrodisiac is likely sympathetic magic. If two things are alike, then it might be possible to garner the same effects from them. Hence the fallacious appeal of rhino horn! Sex and hot chocolate also have much in common as the warm rewarding buzz and blood-vessel-dilating flavonoids help us relax and flush our skin. Is it love or is it just the hot chocolate?

Of course the other sexy thing about chocolate is its obvious appeal to the senses. In mammals, taste and odour are among the most important determinants of sexual attractiveness and receptiveness. The existence of an equivalent human pheromone remains to be established, but if there was one, it would probably smell and taste like chocolate on Valentine's Day. This, combined with the sensory qualities of creamy chocolate melting in the mouth, may actually be far more stimulating to the brain than any mind-altering chemicals contained therein.

Some of the effect of giving and receiving chocolates is also connotation (i.e. the thought behind the gift). Any gift should imply that you're showing some attention, and an attentive partner always gets more sex. In the same way, men who help with housework also have more and better sex. It's not the cleaning of the toilet or giving the chocolate that are the aphrodisiacs, but the bonding that comes from the act. It isn't what he did, it's the why did he do it that gets the results.

The sexual impact of chocolate is also partly contextual; like on an anniversary or Valentine's Day, traditionally we use chocolates to profess love or fidelity. On such days, an intended partner may be more likely to get the intimate meaning of your gift.

Finally, just knowing that something might have anything to do with sex sows the seed, and our mind does the rest. Aphrodisiacs only work because we want them to. There is no biological reason for chocolate or any other aphrodisiac to work. Sexual desire is all in the mind anyway.

Chocolate as medicine

Another possible reason that chocolate has maintained its popularity is that it hasn't obviously killed millions of people, unlike other chemical vices such as smoking, alcohol, drug taking and other classic vices that we would never think of introducing to our children as we do with chocolate. If anything, chocolate comes out smelling like roses.

The idea of the 'health-giving properties' of chocolate partly comes from the old-fashioned idea that being fat was a sign of robust good health. It's easy to understand why we might have thought this at a time when starving waifs were dying of infection or simply starving. The fats in cocoa butter were a potent source of calories throughout many wars, though they are now unwanted in the modern war against our waistline.

However, even in the overly fat modern world, where everyone slams eating chocolate, a number of studies have linked its consumption with improved health, including lower rates of high blood pressure and heart disease. And stretching the chocolate wrapper even further, it turns out that Nobel Prize winners (during their prize-winning research) consume significantly more chocolate than the population average. In no way does correlation prove causality, but at least it gives scientists something to think about (while they are eating chocolate).

Cocoa itself has long been considered to contain magical chemical elements associated with health-enhancing properties. As discussed earlier, part of this is the buzz from theobromine. However, cocoa powder also has a high content of special, flavoursome chemicals known as flavanols, which appropriately contribute to the magical taste and aroma of chocolate.

A walk down the dark side

 It is often recommended that the darker the chocolate the better it is for our health. After all, like the moon, the original Mayan chocolate drink was all dark, made entirely from cocoa powder.

The key flavanols are almost entirely found in the solid cocoa used to make cocoa powder. Most dark chocolate we eat today is 70 per cent to 80 per cent cocoa solids, so has the highest content of flavanols.

Health-wise, this looks a whole lot better than milk chocolate, which in the US can contain as little as 10 per cent cocoa powder, but in most other countries is more like 20 per cent.

White chocolate on the other hand is based on cocoa butter only. It contains no cocoa solids, and therefore no flavanols. Some people don't consider that white chocolate is even chocolate at all, merely sugar and fat.

Many of these flavoursome flavanols in cocoa have the potential to act not only on our senses but directly in our bodies as well. For example, a trial was conducted where some participants were randomly assigned to receive concentrated dark chocolate in a capsule or an inactive blank or placebo. In this way they had no idea whether they got chocolate or not. Then the different responses were compared. And it turned out that the lucky ones who got the chocolate did slightly better on important things like memory, blood pressure, clotting and the function of blood vessels.

This shows that chocolate's flavanols can have a biological effect. But it does not mean chocolate will actually do this in real life. In most studies the very large doses that are used to demonstrate some kind of biological activity could never be achieved by regular chocolate eaters (or at least without significant detriment to their waistlines). It is possible that everyday doses of chocolate over the long term may accumulate some of the same benefits. But these studies have not been and probably will never be performed outside of Willy Wonka's chocolate factory.

Some scientists claim that chocolate can lower cholesterol levels in the blood. Of course, cocoa butter is plant based, so contains little or no cholesterol (see Chapter 10). Some chocolate flavonols, like epicatechin for example, may actually lower cholesterol levels, but again, only when given in high doses.

It is also true that cocoa butter (i.e. the fat dripped out of cocoa beans and added back into chocolate to help it set) contains significant amounts of monounsaturated fat, especially oleic acid and stearic acid. These are the same fats also associated with some of the cholesterol-lowering and health benefits of the Mediterranean diet, rich in olives and nuts (see Chapter 6).

However, the big problem is that cocoa butter also contains lots of saturated fat, and along with the saturated milk fats added to most milk chocolate, the typical milk chocolate has a far less favourable action on our cholesterol levels and our waistline.

Chocolate as a vice

Most people believe that chocolate is probably bad for them. Not sinful — the Bishop of Rome has seen to that — but at least potentially harmful. This perhaps adds to its allure, giving us the naughty thrill of doing something bad. But how did something as heavenly as chocolate get such a bad reputation?

When hot chocolate first reached Europe it was seen as fascinating, sexy, foreign, exclusive and intoxicating. But as the ardour cooled, reports came of deaths and babies mysteriously born with dark skin. This characterization was partly xenophobia, but it was also well known that chocolate stains were impossible to wash away. People began to wonder if they hadn't been dancing with the devil after all. However, far from dissuading consumers, the mesmeric appeal of choclate's dark side only added to its magic.

In the 1950s, research emerged that American businessmen were dying in droves from heart attacks, which rapidly became their leading cause of death. Curiously, this was not happening in post-war Europe, possibly because there was less to eat. So the inference was clear: the 'American diet' was to blame.

The first and most popular theory of the time was that it was the extra fat in the American diet that was poisoning everybody. These businessmen were eating lots of foods high in saturated fat like butter, lard, eggs, beef and, of course, the cocoa butter in chocolate. So putting two and two together, a public health scheme was hatched to radically change the way people ate. On this basis all fatty foods were vilified, along with smoking and salt, as 'modern evils' and the major preventable causes of death. In this erudite low-fat world, chocolate quickly became a quintessential vice. Whether or not saturated fat is actually the cause of our downfall is discussed elsewhere in this book, but the legacy of this 'fat' premise remains a major reason why we feel a little wicked when having another piece of chocolate.

Other researchers later blamed all the added sugars, or simply the excess food energy (known as calories) as the cause of obesity, diabetes and ultimately heart attacks and strokes. And of course, here again, chocolate, which is also rich in sugar and calories, looked doubly culpable.

Certainly, it *should* be making us fatter. Chocolate provides additional energy that our modern lives simply don't need. The fat and sugar calories contained in a Snickers bar, for example, are similar to those expended by jogging for half an hour. And when we are trying to keep our waists in check, and especially if we are not jogging, every extra calorie counts.

But then again, there are many other things in our diet that provide just as many calories. Many of these fly under the radar. By contrast chocolate wears its calories on its sleeve. Typically there are about 500 calories for every 100 grams (3.5 ounces) of chocolate. It's very obvious that we shouldn't overdo it.

The chocolate paradox

 Nothing is a simple as it appears. Chocolate is full of fat, sugar and calories and yet some studies have shown that people who eat chocolate on a regular basis tend to be thinner than those who do not. This is known as the chocolate paradox.

Most rational people think this heretical conclusion is the work of chocoholic scientists hoping to validate their own extravagance by misinterpreting data, but it has actually been studied.

Overweight people already know that they should eat less, and usually the first things they are told to avoid are high-calorie snacks, like chocolate. Overweight people are less likely to admit they have eaten chocolate, due to feelings of guilt from eating the 'wrong' thing.

And yet it can be argued that the combination of chemicals inside chocolate helps us to feel satisfied sooner, so we would as a natural consequence eat less on average. This could be true of dark chocolate especially, as it is so high in flavanols. In this case, it could be said that if we eat for pleasure, chocolate gets us to climax sooner.

The problem is that everybody knows that that we all have a second stomach into which we can always fit chocolate. This is because the feeling of fullness and the intake of sufficient calories are not the only reasons we eat. Most of us get enough daily nutrients in a single meal, let alone three squares a day. So there must be other reasons why we would persist in eating more than we physically require.

Sometimes it's just habit and routine. It's meal time or break time so we eat. Other times it's the pleasure we get from eating. This is known as hedonic eating. Whether it comes from the food, the company or just the satisfaction of sticking to our habits, eating for pleasure is thought to be a common cause of overeating. Moreover, as we gain weight, the pleasure we get from food often tapers off. This means we may need to eat more and more food to receive the same amount of pleasure. One piece of chocolate cake or one cookie just doesn't do it for us anymore, not because we are still hungry, but because we are still not satisfied.

But sometimes the cause can also be the solution. If it's pleasure we crave, a little chocolate can be a perfect gratification. And if it's the good stuff (not milk chocolate) and is a little exclusive, all the better.

This may partly explain the chocolate paradox, whereby chocolate eaters get the pleasures lacking in other food, so don't need to eat more to get their kicks.

Comfort food

Many of us eat when we are stressed or feeling down. This is seldom a conscious thought, like 'Oh, I'm feeling stressed; I will go and eat something'. But it is something all of us do from time to time, to a greater or lesser extent. And doing something that is pleasurable, positive and rewarding, like eating chocolate, provides a brief but real antidote for an unpleasant, negative and unrewarding day.

Negative stress makes us look for rewarding positives. This is partly the increased motivation to obtain a reward (i.e. the wanting) as well as the anticipated hedonic pleasure that we experience when we get our hands on it (i.e. the liking). These are not always the same thing. Liking usually comes first. But if we like it, then we are more likely to want it and react to cues that tell us to go and get it. Chocolate's inevitably yummy taste and easy availability make it hard to resist as a perfect reward.

There are many plausible theories as to why sweet treats like chocolate have comforting properties.

Sweet soft chocolate may stimulate the palate, leading to the brain chemicals responsible for the feel-good feelings — serotonin and endorphins — being activated. Some of chocolate's flavanols may also have direct effects in the brain. Some studies report that giving chocolate drinks made people calmer, with the greatest effects seen with the highest doses of flavanols and theobromine.

Like water for chocolate

 Once upon a time, scientists tried to prove that chocolate really was comforting. Research volunteers were asked to watch sad film clips, and then they were given a chocolate or a (boring) glass of water.

As we might have guessed, the chocolate immediately improved the volunteers' mood after the sad films significantly more than the water. But interestingly, the chocolate effect only lasted for a few minutes. This means it couldn't actually have been the chemicals in chocolate that were responsible, because they take much longer than a few minutes to be digested and reach our brain. And anyway, the dose was far too small.

Moreover, when the scientists gave the volunteers bitter, dark chocolate (which didn't taste as nice as milk chocolate but still had all those flavonoids) nothing happened. There was no feeling better after the sad movie.

In fact, the scientists found that the mere act of being given a chocolate to eat later was enough to lift the volunteers' mood after the films. They concluded that it was the anticipation of chocolatey pleasure, rather than the chocolate itself, that lifted the mood.

So it seems that it's only the act of pleasure or its anticipation that briefly gives us comfort, not the actual eating of chocolate at all. Like those putative aphrodisiac qualities, comfort food is mostly in the mind. And this is probably a good thing because, after all, it is the mind that needs comforting.

This is also why men prefer to eat savoury foods or drink booze when stressed and women prefer eating sweet things like chocolate and cookies (especially chocolate cookies), because that is what they anticipate to be most palatable and pleasurable. If there really was something in chocolate you'd think even men would have caught on by now!

Chocolate spots

No discussion of chocolate would be complete without considering its effects on our skin. Almost every teenager will have acne at some stage, and about a third of all adults will also be troubled with it from time to time.

Many different factors can also influence how bad acne gets, including whether our siblings and parents had it, smoking, body size and emotional stress. In addition, every teenager knows that chocolate sets off their acne.

It is easy to understand how chocolate might look like the problem. Teenagers usually eat a lot more chocolate than any other age group. Teenagers also get more acne than any other age group. In particular, girls who are under stress or overweight often eat chocolate as comfort food, and they are also the ones most likely to be troubled by the appearance of acne. We have to point our fingers at something, and again (given that we shouldn't be eating so much of it anyway) chocolate is an obvious suspect.

Butter me up

 Dry skin feels awful. It looks awful too. By contrast, increasing the water content of our skin makes it look and feel fuller, softer and more youthful. This is why moisturizers are a core element in all skincare treatments, including creams, cosmetics and soaps.

Some moisturizers work by forming a thin oily film on the surface of the skin. This creates a barrier that reduces the loss of moisture due to evaporation. Other moisturizing creams contain chemicals known as humectants. These attract water into the dry, outer layer of the skin and increase the water-holding capacity of the skin itself.

A third group of moisturizing creams work by filling the gaps and cracks between the skin cells to create a smooth shiny surface. This is known as emoliation and these moisturizers are consequently known as emollients or barrier-repair agents as they help to heal a damaged skin barrier. They are responsible for the 'smooth and supple' feeling of our skin following application of any moisturizer.

One of the most popular emollients is in fact cocoa butter. It is clean, white, velvety smooth, not too greasy and smells nice too. Hardly anyone is allergic to chocolate, so it is seldom irritating.

However, a big issue is that for some people, cocoa butter can lead to a flare-up of their acne as it blocks the skin's pores. So chocolate can cause acne. But only if you put it on your face.

A number of different biological explanations for the link between chocolate and acne have been proposed. Eating milk products like milk chocolate modestly increases acne, but chocolate is hardly a major source of milk. It may be that the rapid absorption of sugar when eating very sweet things raises insulin, a hormone implicated in causing acne. Diets with reduced amounts of rapidly absorbed sugars (as in a chocolate bar) do tend to reduce acne a little. But none of these features is specific to chocolate. This is all circumstantial evidence. None is enough to put chocolate away.

To try and get some definite proof, researchers have even fed chocolate to teenagers to see if they got acne. But they didn't. Chocolate doesn't even seem to make acne worse. However, there have only been very small studies with a relatively small amount of chocolate eaten, so a small effect in a minority of sensitive individuals can't be excluded. But at the very least, an unequivocal link between chocolate and acne would appear to be an urban myth.

The bottom line

It is not unhealthy to love chocolate, but only in moderation. In the context of a healthy diet, the best way to eat less is to thoroughly enjoy what we do eat. And for all its soft, smooth sweet wonder, chocolate is thoroughly enjoyable. There are many more things that offer much less enjoyment that we eat every day, just out of habit. And for what? So don't give up chocolate. Just buy the pure good stuff (which is more expensive so you'll eat less of it anyway) and thoroughly enjoy it.

Do I really have to ...

#2

Cut down on the booze?

Q: Is alcohol bad for me?
A: Depends on how much and what you mix it with.

Q: Why do I get so drunk on champagne?
A: It's a conspiracy of bubbles, ice and a tall glass.

Q: How do I sober up fast?
A: You can't. That ship has sailed.

Q: Can I avoid getting a hangover?
A: Only by not drinking.

*Q: If the world was ending in five minutes, what
would be the best thing to drink?*
A: Ice-cold champagne or gin and tonic.

Q: Does drinking a little every day prolong life?
A: No, but those who do live longer.

Q: Is red wine a health drink?
A: You can drink to your health, not for it.

Since the late Stone Age, people have been drinking alcohol to make them feel better. For the most part, this has been in order to 'remember their misery no more' (*Proverbs 31:6–7*), to loosen up and come to life. But beyond simply drowning our sorrows or having a good time, it's also widely believed alcohol has a range of positively medicinal virtues.

Yet, at the very same time, it is also flamingly obvious that alcohol can be an important cause of miseries and bad memories. Alcohol makes many people feel much worse than they already do. Overall, drinking too much alcohol contributes as much to poor health across the globe as obesity and smoking. Consequently, balancing alcohol in our lives is truly a matter of life and death.

Drink, drunk, drank

Alcohol is a tiny, innocent-looking chemical but it sure packs a punch. We can usually tell when we have had alcohol within a few minutes of taking it, especially when our stomach is empty. Because of its simple chemistry, alcohol is quickly absorbed, starting from the very moment it enters our mouth, from where it diffuses to every part of our body.

It was the mouthwash, Officer!

 It is popular to use a mouthwash to freshen our breath and prevent cavities in our teeth. Mouthwash is supposed to be swished and gargled for about 30 seconds, then spat out. You are not meant to swallow it.

Many mouthwashes contain significant amounts of alcohol. For example, the classic mouthwash brand Listerine has about twice the alcohol concentration of a glass of wine, or about half that of a typical glass of whiskey.

In theory it is possible to fail a driver breathalyzer test after rinsing your mouth with an alcohol-laced mouthwash. This is not because you accidentally swallowed a little mouthwash, but more because some can hang around in the tiny crevasses in your mouth.

If you then blow it back into a breathalyzer it can be enough to make it seem that you are over the limit. But this could happen only immediately after using it. Within 15 minutes or so of using a mouthwash, any alcohol on your breath is safely below the detection limit. So there goes that alibi.

When we have a drink, a little alcohol is first absorbed directly in our mouth and maybe 20 per cent is absorbed across our stomach's lining. However, the majority is absorbed across the intricate convolutions of our intestines, where the enormous surface area is about the size of a tennis court. And a greater surface area equals more surface to absorb alcohol.

Blood alcohol levels reach their peak on average about 30 to 40 minutes after having a single drink. Because the peak alcohol concentration correlates with its maximal effects on our brain, it takes approximately this amount of time to get as drunk as we are going to get on a single glass. Of course, if we take a second and then a third and a fourth glass, each successive wave builds on the last, meaning our blood alcohol levels can still be rising over an hour after our last drink, when we may be thinking of heading home.

Although some people become more gregarious and/or volatile when they drink, alcohol is essentially a sedative. It inhibits the functions of the brain. However, the first parts to become inhibited are the brain cells at the front end whose job it is to think through what we are supposed to be doing. This is the same area of the brain where sleeping tablets also work.

Alcohol initially sedates those particular brain cells whose job it is to inhibit brain activity. And when you inhibit the inhibitory parts and sedate the sedators, the balance of brain activities initially tips towards excitement and euphoria. Woo hoo! This why when we feel tired (when the inhibitory part of our brain is slowing us down), a little alcohol sometimes feels more like a pick-me-up; more like a coffee than a sleeping pill.

But caffeine and alcohol have opposing effects in our brain. Coffee increases memory and focus and stops our mind from wandering. Alcohol, on the other hand, interferes with memory and concentration, but opens doors to let our mind out. Many people regard a little alcohol as a tremendous source of creativity and social lubrication. The jokes turn out better and the ideas seem to flow without the inhibitory restraints of a dulled brain. In fact, creative problem solving and lateral thinking can be modestly enhanced after a single glass, through helping our mind to wander. But then we go too far.

The big problem with booze is that as we take more and more we also progressively lose other inhibitions. Some of these are important for self-control and making safe choices, like dancing on tables or driving home. Broadly, the risk of sustaining an injury at least doubles in the six hours after consuming four bottles of beer or half a bottle of wine in a single sitting. If we drink any more than this, the risks increase exponentially. This is because other areas of our brain now start getting sedated, with further doses leading to disturbed balance, slurred speech, blurred vision, confusion and other symptoms that go with being drunk. Eventually we may just fall over.

Alcohol doesn't just intoxicate our brain. It also has direct effects on our stomach. Everyone will know about feeling sick and possibly throwing up if we drink too much. This is partly because the alcohol slows and ultimately stops the stomach from contracting (and emptying) in a regular coordinated fashion. Drink too much and everything just sits there in our stomach, making us belch, hiccup, feel bloated and ultimately throw up. As they say, it is always the dose that makes the poison.

Food with drink

Everyone knows that the easiest way to get drunk is to drink on an empty stomach. Actually, the easiest way to get drunk is to drink lots of alcohol. But if alcohol is the limiting factor, then an empty stomach will not only allow more of the alcohol to reach our brain, but to reach it faster and achieve higher peak levels than if we had drunk it with or after a meal. So you get more drunk for your dollar on an empty stomach.

This is why we are always told to eat some food while we are out drinking. It works to some extent. The maximal alcohol levels achieved and their maximal effects on our brain *are* actually reduced when we mix wine and cheese, or have a beer with our fish and chips. This is not because the food in our stomach is able to soak up the alcohol. Rather, when we have a meal and our stomach is full, it pours out its contents much more slowly than when it is empty. And so the transit of any alcohol we drink with or after our meal is also slowed. Ultimately though, the same amount of alcohol still gets into our system, albeit at a slower rate.

Nuts to you

 At the start of *The Hitchhiker's Guide to the Galaxy*, the ever-resourceful alien Ford Prefect buys six pints of beer, ostensibly as a relaxant, as the world is about to end. A far better option for Ford would have been gin and tonic, which has a far higher alcohol concentration to facilitate rapid diffusion across the stomach wall, ice-cold tonic bubbles to push it onwards, and quinine to further relax the muscles. However, if the world was ending anyway, choice of beverage is best a matter of taste and immediate availability.

To his beers, Ford Prefect also added several packets of salted peanuts from the bar. Most bars have nuts. Some are also edible. But their true purpose remains shrouded in mystery.

Eating small, protein-rich snacks (like nuts) before take-off in an aeroplane can reduce motion sickness. This may be because protein, more than any other nutrient, triggers regular, slow and smooth stomach contractions. These keep it busy and act to suppress any rapid irregular convulsive contractions of our stomach associated with feeling sick and ultimately vomiting.

At the same time, when we eat, stomach emptying is slowed down due to the presence of food, meaning the rate at which alcohol levels rise is also slightly slower. So it takes slightly longer (and more alcohol purchases) to get drunk when we are also eating nuts.

Adding to the conspiracy theory, some argue that the addictively salty nuts are only there to make us thirsty, so we'll have to buy more drinks. But this is not true. Pound for pound, salty nuts or salty pretzels don't make us drink more than if we ate unsalted ones.

Actually, the conspiracy works in reverse. It seems alcohol promotes snacking. It is no coincidence that most nuts and pretzels are displayed at just an arm's length behind the bar. Given the plentiful calories in most beverages we shouldn't be hungry or need to eat. But with a little disinhibiting alcohol on board, we just can't help ourselves.

It is not only food that slows the emptying of our stomach into our intestines. Smoking has a similar effect. Consequently, many smokers claim that having a smoke while drinking means they get drunk slower than their non-smoking friends, which is probably true.

Bubbly

While food can slow down the absorption of alcohol, drinking sweet, warm or fizzy alcoholic drinks can do the opposite, helping it to bubble along through our stomach and into our bloodstream. This is why alcoholic drinks are more rapidly intoxicating when they are bubbly than when they are served flat. It's part of the charm of beer, gin and tonic, rum and Coke and many other effervescent combinations. But the most famous and intoxicating bubbly of them all is champagne, or sparkling wine.

With the release of the cork, carbon dioxide dissolved in the champagne starts to escape, partly as gas bubbles and partly just wafting away from the surface of the drink. When we drink champagne it is still filled with dissolved gas, and this gas continues to be released inside our stomachs but now at a faster rate as it warms to body temperature and gets shaken about. This is when champagne really fizzes, filling our stomach faster and pushing the alcohol onwards in our intestine and into our blood.

As the champagne fizz fills our stomach, it forces the stomach to empty its alcoholic contents more rapidly, or efficiently, into our intestines, where alcohol absorption is faster because of the bigger surface area. So we get drunk faster on champagne than on the same amount of white wine.

The same intoxicating effect can also be seen when drinking beer, cider or other fizzy drinks, although champagne has much more dissolved gas in it than all the others. This is why champagne bottles are made thicker than the average wine bottle and the cork must be reinforced. Champagne would simply blow a beer bottle apart. Even without shaking it, the pressure of gas inside a champagne bottle is over three times that found in the tyres of a car. And this explains its fizz as well as its reputation for putting us under the table.

Once a bottle is opened the gas starts to escape. The sooner you drink it the more gas there is. Drinking straight from the champagne bottle is impolite, except after winning motor races, but the first glasses poured from the bottle are more bubbly and more intoxicating than the last. The same phenomenon may also be observed with beer, although it is quite acceptable to drink straight from the bottle as soon as the cap is lifted. In this way the drinker gets most of the gas, and consequently drinking that cold beer straight from the bottle is far more intoxicating than a glass of a warm beer from a jug sitting on the table. The counter-argument is that sometimes it's not about the alcohol: the full aroma and the frothy pleasure of beer is best experienced when drinking it from a glass.

The right temperature is also important for champagne to work its magic. The warmer the champagne the more it foams and bubbles in our glass. When we drink it there is less dissolved gas and so less intoxication. By contrast, ice-cold champagne doesn't explode out of the bottle in the same way, doesn't bubble as much or foam over the edge of the glass onto our hand or our clothes. When we drink it, there is much more dissolved gas left to be bubbled up inside us when it heats up to body temperature in our stomach. So on ice-cold champagne we get drunk a little faster.

If we didn't want to get drunk as quickly, we could drink wine or intolerably warm, flat champagne. But a more creative method may be to chase the bubbles from our champagne using a swizzle stick.

Mr Darcy's swizzle stick

 In Regency England, champagne was all the rage. Yet the bubbles were considered a rude imperfection, cherished only by the wicked and depraved, like Lord Byron who extolled the virtues of:

'…champagne with foaming whirls

As white as Cleopatra's melted pearls.' (*Don Juan*, 1821)

Many drank expensive still champagne (known as Sillery) to avoid the dangerous 'spirituous parts'. Furthermore, at balls, it was propitious for men to carry a swizzle stick or bâtonnet (little stick) to swish any importunate bubbles out of a lady's drink.

And it worked. Getting rid of the champagne bubbles slows the punch of the alcohol, so their dance partner would at least make it through the set without it going to her head. Given the tight restrictions of corsets used by both men and women, it was also a good way not to fill up with gas and end up bloated and belching. This trick was later employed by Queen Victoria who stirred her own champagne.

Curiously there appears to be no mention of Darcy's swizzle stick in Jane Austen's novel. Either he didn't use one (in which case he was trying to get Elizabeth drunk), or morality precluded any mention of the one he kept deep in his pocket, which he only pulled out for special occasions.

There are many other tricks used to reduce intoxication from champagne. Because of their greater surface area, the traditional broad flat goblets for drinking champagne let the gas and bubbles, as well as the cold temperature, dissipate more rapidly. This style of flat champagne goblet was putatively modelled on Marie Antoinette's left breast, although it is still debated whether this was criticism or idolatry. And why the left and not the right? Was there a palpable difference? Or was it simply that designers could only choose one?

The modern narrow champagne flutes we use today have a very small surface area on top. This keeps the bubbly 'mousse' — or sparkle of champagne — much better, as well as the cold temperature. But it also means those tall glasses of ice-cold champagne are far more intoxicating at fancy parties or weddings.

Another simple trick is to add a strawberry to the drink. In the movie *Pretty Woman*, Richard Gere stresses the importance of the strawberries when drinking champagne with Julia Roberts. 'It brings out the flavour,' he says. But the only flavour that comes out is that of the strawberries. Strawberries will absorb a tiny amount of alcohol, but not enough to matter, especially if we eat them anyway. But they do provide a willing surface for bubbles to form on, so the recipient of the strawberry-filled champagne glass will get less intoxicated and less bloated (both intrinsic features of a pretty woman). In cross section, strawberries also form the shape of heart, to which lovers have toasted for centuries (kind of pretty too?).

As a last resort, leaving a remnant of detergent from when we last washed our champagne glass will also chase the bubbles away. However, this will also kill the taste!

Break it down

As soon as alcohol is absorbed into our bodies, it starts to be broken down into vinegar, and then to carbon dioxide and water. If we drink moderately, most of the alcohol is so rapidly broken down that only moderate amounts will ever reach our brain. This process is broadly known as **alcohol metabolism**. Metabolism is the process by which chemicals are converted into other chemicals by our body's enzymes.

Why humans possess the specific ability to break down alcohol is probably due to the fact that alcohol (or ethanol) is not a foreign substance to us, but a constant companion. Each day some of the sugars we eat are fermented in our intestines, and this generates our own alcohol. Even for people who never touch a drop in their lives, their intestines deliver the equivalent of several beers every day.

In some people who have major problems with their intestines, the endogenous production of alcohol can sometimes be markedly enhanced, meaning they have detectable blood alcohol levels even without drinking. This is known as the '**auto-brewery syndrome**' and is an established legal defence.

Fortunately, most humans have little or no detectable alcohol in their blood, let alone levels enough to appear drunk. This is because our liver is able to efficiently break down alcohol. At its peak, it can get through about 7 grams per hour. One standard drink contains about 15 grams of alcohol so, on average, our liver can cope with one drink every few hours without the alcohol levels rising steeply in our bloodstream. However, the rate of alcohol metabolism varies significantly from individual to individual. Some can drink more. Some can only drink small amounts before feeling tipsy.

For example, women are usually a little more easily intoxicated than men. This is partly because the metabolism of alcohol by the stomach lining is a little less efficient in women and their stomachs are generally smaller. So women generally experience a faster rise in alcohol levels after a single glass when compared to men. This is one reason why it is usually recommended that women consume a third to half less alcohol than men, in order to remain equally sober.

Taller, heavier people are also generally less easily intoxicated than smaller individuals. As a rule of thumb, twice the weight means half the maximum concentration and half the intoxication. However, this is not due to their metabolism breaking down the alcohol. It is simply because alcohol dissolves equally into all body tissues, so the more body tissue we have the more the alcohol gets diluted across it.

Some of the differences in the rate of alcohol metabolism between different people are due to differences in their genes. In particular, Asian people are more likely to carry genes that allow them to break down alcohol at a much faster rate than Caucasian individuals. This means that not only do they get less buzz from alcohol, they also rapidly generate the by-products of alcohol at a rate too quick for their body to cope. This can lead to flushing of the skin, a racing heart and headaches in about one-third of all Asian people if they ever have a drink.

Undoing the damage

 Once alcohol is in our blood, there is no going back. There is nothing we can do to speed up the rate at which it is broken down. Once it has been imbibed, only time can make alcohol go away.

However, this doesn't stop people from giving it a shot. We try going for a run, sweating it out or taking a hot shower. But resistance is futile; the effects are tiny, at best.

One of the most popular home remedies for sobering is Baker's yeast. Some pubs even sell it over the bar for emergencies. The idea is that yeast is normally used to make alcohol, so it must also have the capacity to un-make it, by reversing the process. So by putting yeast into an alcoholic environment (like our stomach during a party), instead of making alcohol it gets rid of it, like a second liver.

But while Baker's yeast may have the capacity to eat up some of the residual alcohol in our stomach, it has little effect on the alcohol that has already passed into our blood or how rapidly we sober up from it.

Black coffee is another popular alternative. However, coffee does nothing to our metabolism and actually speeds up stomach emptying which, like bubbles, can serve to increase our alcohol levels. At best, caffeine only turns a sleepy drunk into a wide-awake drunk.

Alcohol metabolism by the liver breaks down the alcohol we drink. It gets rid of it so that we don't get so drunk. The best example of how important this is for us is to consider what happens when the capacity for alcohol metabolism is taken away.

For example, the chemical chloral is a potent inhibitor of alcohol metabolism. Drinking a mix of chloral and alcohol, the inadvertent consumer quickly becomes intoxicated and eventually passes out. This devilish cocktail was used to great effect by the Chicago pub owner Michael 'Mickey' Finn to incapacitate and then rob some of his customers. This subsequently became known as 'slipping the mickey'.

Some mushrooms can also inadvertently interfere with alcohol metabolism, causing rapidly unpleasant symptoms for anyone mixing them with booze. These specific mushrooms are justifiably known as 'tippler's bane'. Fortunately, they are not the ones commonly available in supermarkets or used with red wine in our beef stroganoff.

Finally, the common painkiller paracetamol (known as acetaminophen in the United States) also slows the breakdown of alcohol by the liver. Not as much as with a Mickey Finn, but enough for more alcohol to end up in our bloodstream, making it easier to become drunk.

The beer belly

There is an obvious link between drinking and growing fat, especially around our waistline. We all know what this looks like. It is commonly known as a 'beer belly', 'love handles' or even a 'muffin top', a physique curiously resembling how muffins and cupcakes lavishly spill out over the sides of their paper case. It is widely considered to be the best part of muffins. But as we look at ourselves in the mirror, the excess fat spilling over the top of our tight pants is usually the first part we poke.

The size of our waistline is largely explained by the food we over-consume and our lack of regular physical activity. This is discussed in detail in other chapters. But despite knowing this, most people find as their belt or their skirt slowly gets tighter round their waist, they will probably blame their drinking.

After all, we have to blame something. If it is not chocolate then alcohol is next on the list of usual suspects. Not only does it have a long criminal history, but it is also in the right place at the right time, for as we get older we tend not only to get fatter but also to drink more booze. There is more than circumstantial evidence or alcohol's prior record of bad behaviour at play here, though; there is also biology to consider.

All alcoholic drinks contain calories, almost all of which are usually in excess of our physical requirements. Any calories in excess are stored away in the body as fat. The more (calories) we consume as drink or food, the more fat we store. Men are more likely to deposit fat around their waist than women, and so fat (beer) bellies are more common in, though not exclusive to, men. It's not that women are protected from getting fat, but excess calories often go elsewhere first in women (usually to their bums, thighs and breasts).

Some of the calories in our beverages come from the alcohol itself. However, unlike other nutrients in our diet, the calories found in alcohol cannot be stored in the human body. Alcohol is toxic and so must take priority to be burned off, which is what our liver does.

But while our liver is busy burning excess alcohol when we drink, it doesn't have the need to burn fat. So a lovely waist is left behind.

The alcohol itself may be only a small part of the weight problem, if at all. In one enviable study researchers fed participants an excess of calories for two weeks either in the form of milk chocolate or as an equivalent amount of alcohol. Not surprisingly, the chocolate eaters gained 3 kilograms (6.6 pounds). But what was surprising was that the drinkers did not get fatter (at least in the short term), despite the fact that their calorie input was much the same.

Saint Bernard of the Snow

 Crossing the Swiss Alps on foot is not something for the faint-hearted. So in 1049, Bernard of Menthon built a shelter to take care of travellers and provide a rescue base for those who became lost in the snow. Soon dogs were added to the party, and after centuries of breeding, a highly specialized dog for snow rescue was created. These heroic dogs later became known as Saint Bernards, after their founder.

The dogs' keen sense of smell could help detect buried travellers. They would then dig them out and lie on top of them to provide warmth until help arrived. They didn't actually carry a barrel of alcoholic brandy around their neck. This appears to be an artistic fiction, loosely based on what it feels like when we drink spirits.

Alcohol increases the flow of hot blood to our skin, causing it to produce sweat, look a little flushed and feel warm to the touch. Take a swig of spirits — it doesn't take long before we feel a tingling. On a cold night, this cosy feeling feels a bit like being wrapped in a blanket (or smothered by a Saint Bernard). And for the same reason, alcohol often mistakenly makes us feel immune to the cold, snug in our 'brandy blanket'.

The problem is that all the extra heat running to our skin makes our core temperature drop. Our core temperature is what keeps us alive in the cold. So alcohol and extreme cold are a dangerous combination, increasing the risk of hypothermia. Anyone lost in the snow who drank a barrel of brandy would suddenly feel a lot better, but would rapidly succumb to the cold before help arrived.

So if it's not actually the booze that maketh the belly, then maybe it's what comes with it that counts? After all, while beer drinkers have their obvious beer bellies, wine drinkers don't, even after adjusting for the amount of alcohol they consume.

A likely reason for the beer belly is that, along with alcohol, beer usually also comes with plenty of sugar added. For example, an average glass of beer contains as many calories as a can of Coke. We all know what too many soft drinks do to our waistlines. It should come as no surprise that our bellies are dancing.

A glass of red wine also contains about the same number of calories as a glass of beer. White wine has only slightly fewer. However, a beer drinker will generally drink a greater volume of beer than a wine drinker will drink wine. Consequently, for the same amount of alcohol, the extra volume of beer we drink and the calories therein explains the infamous beer belly.

The Hangover (Part I)

We all know that the adverse effects of a night of drinking can carry over into the next day. The unpleasant symptoms of a hangover are as familiar to drinkers as a common cold: feeling moody, lethargic, clumsy, headachey, nauseous and sensitive to bright light and noise. It is classically portrayed in the movies as having bloodshot eyes, wearing dark sunglasses, drinking endless cups of black coffee, and bumping into things. This is not just because we have our sunglasses on inside. In fact, all our brain functions go down when we are hung-over, causing impaired performance, lapses in concentration and errors of judgement. We may not have an ounce of alcohol left in our system, but accidents are significantly more likely to happen when we are hung-over. Some studies even show that driving with a hangover makes you just as impaired as driving (illegally in many countries) with a blood alcohol level of 0.08 per cent! So maybe it really is safer if we stay in bed.

Roughly three out of every four people who drink to the point they are intoxicated will have some degree of hangover the next morning. But even if they drink themselves into a stupor, some lucky sods are spared. Conversely, some unfortunate people can get a hangover after only one or two glasses.

The usual explanation for differences in our sensitivity to excess alcohol is that some people must break down the alcohol they drink less efficiently or differently, leading to the accumulation of toxic chemical by-products in the body that cause the displeasing symptoms associated with a hangover. Drink enough and we all will produce enough of these toxic chemicals to make us feel ill the next morning. But some people might rapidly make enough of them to cause them to feel sick after even a single glass.

The problem with this theory is that by the time our hangover symptoms are at their worst (i.e. the next morning) all of the alcohol and its various chemical metabolites have completely left our body. So having a slow or fast metabolism doesn't explain why some people are feeling fine and others are having a doozy!

Another theory is that hangovers are due to **dehydration**. And certainly, that might be part of it. Alcohol interferes with the signal normally coming from the brain telling the kidneys to conserve water and prevent it from being lost into our urine and down the toilet. By blocking the message, the kidneys instead allow water to spill over into our urine and our bladder. This makes us pee more with an alcoholic drink than we might expect just from the amount of fluid we have drunk.

We normally pee more when we are drinking anything, simply because of the volume of water we are taking in. A typical beer is 96 per cent water and about 4 per cent alcohol. This 4 per cent is eventually turned into about the same mass of water by our liver. Consequently, a glass of beer and a glass of water are about the same in water content in the end.

Besides the amount of water in our drink, for every alcoholic drink we have, the alcohol in it will cause us to lose around half a cup more than if we had drunk the same volume of water. Have four drinks and we may well be down by almost a litre. By the next morning our skin and throat feels dry, our eyes are sunken and our head and body ache as if we had just got off a long-distance flight. In fact, many people describe the same hangover symptoms after travelling long distances in a plane even if they haven't bothered with the drinks cart.

It is often thought that drinking extra glasses of water during a night out will prevent dehydration the next morning. The ancient Romans always added water to wine. But this was not to prevent a hangover. Most likely, the unsanitized water was undrinkable on its own and more palatable and far safer to drink when sterilized with some alcohol in it. As a hangover cure, water will also help, but only a little. Most of the extra water we'd try to drink to compensate for the booze will simply make us pee even more or then have to get up in the night to go to the bathroom. Regardless, we will still end up feeling dry, thirsty and hungover in the morning.

Liquorice sorts all

 One innovative hangover cure is to use natural chemicals to make our kidneys retain more fluid, instead of alcohol causing us to pee it out. One of the most well-known is a chemical naturally found in liquorice (licorice).

Today we mostly know liquorice as a sweet treat. But by far its biggest use is as an additive to tobacco to sweeten its flavour. The chemical that provides liquorice's sweetness also has another string to its bow. At least temporarily, it will trigger our kidneys to make less urine, which is the opposite of what alcohol is doing. So in theory by taking liquorice we'll feel less dehydrated in the morning.

Eating liquorice doesn't work the morning after; by then it's too late. So if you don't mind munching on liquorice between beers it may be worth a shot. Liquorice is also found in a wide variety of drinks, from absinthe and anisette to ouzo and sambuca.

However, like all our favourite panaceas, take too much and there is always a catch. With liquorice, if you eat too much your kidneys can retain so much fluid that your blood pressure goes up. As a consequence of water retention you also lose potassium, which is important for your health.

Purveyors of the perfect hangover cure simply solve this problem by recommending people eat liquorice through the evening and finish the night with a glass of fresh juice, a handful of nuts or a banana, all excellent sources of potassium. This cure is also recommended before long-distance flights for the same reasons (as well as the inconvenience of having to get up, step over other people and get to the cramped toilets).

The Hangover (Part II)

Another important contributor to the hangover is how poorly we have slept when we have been out drinking the previous evening. This is not just because we were late to get to bed, although this doesn't help how we feel the next morning, but also because alcohol itself can impact how well we sleep.

Firstly, the alcohol in grog is a sedative (hence the term groggy). Many people use a little alcohol in the evenings to help them get to sleep. This is commonly known as a 'nightcap'. And it actually works to relax and sedate us, if this is what we want, especially for non-drinkers or people who don't drink too much or too often. Of course, large amounts of alcohol are enough to tranquilize a large elephant.

The problems occur after we fall asleep. Too much alcohol suppresses our dream sleep. This is also known as REM (rapid eye movement) sleep, as our eyes are often rapidly moving during this phase of sleep as if we were watching a dream movie projected onto the inside of our eyelids. We need our REM sleep to feel refreshed in the morning. But the booze takes it away.

At the same time, if we've been drinking, the non-dream, non-REM part of our sleep cycle is longer and deeper. This period of deep sleep is when our body is at its most relaxed and floppy and the time we most often snore (as the muscles holding our airways open are also deeply relaxed). This is why when we are drunk we snore an awful lot more and end up sleeping on the sofa.

Even as the excess alcohol wears off, our sleep is further disrupted in the second half of the night. We are more likely to wake between our sleep cycles and find it harder to get back to sleep. By the time morning comes around, we are still trying to catch up on the missed sleep and are left feeling unrefreshed and hungover for the rest of the day.

Our brain desperately tries to make up for the lost dreams. So, after a night out drinking, the last dream just before we wake up can often be longer, more vivid and more likely to be remembered. Unless, of course, we wake up early because our bladder is full. Then we miss the end of the movie, and are left forever wondering what was going to happen next.

Getting drunk also interferes with our body clock, producing a state akin to jet lag, when our body clock is out of alignment with the actual time in the place we have just landed. We feel like it's night but it's actually midday or vice versa. Something like this also happens in a hangover and some researchers believe they may have similar origins. Consequently, desperate people use many of the same cures for both, including coffee, melatonin, vigorous exercise and, of course, sunglasses. Actually, staying in the dark does really help the unpleasant sensation of a hangover and reduces the recovery time. Whether it helps to synchronize our body clock is a moot point. The light always seems much too bright the following day.

The hair of the dog

 Another theory — the repeatedly drunk often have many theories — is that a hangover is really a kind of drug withdrawal. After all, the unpleasant symptoms only start after the alcohol leaves our system. And you can't really be drunk and hungover at the same time, can you?

Taking this impeccable logic to its obvious conclusion, as with any other withdrawal we must take the thing we are missing, which in the case of a bad hangover means having another drink. This is the rough rationale for starting the morning with what is known as a 'counter-beer' in Germany (as in counter-act), a 'repair beer' in Scandinavia, or a *richiamino* in Italy. In the English-speaking world it is known as taking the 'hair of the dog'.

This striking phrase originates from the idea that the hair of the dog (that bit you) could help heal the wound it had just inflicted. And it is perfectly true that if you are going into alcohol withdrawal, taking the hair of the dog temporarily gets rid of the symptoms. However, alcohol withdrawal and a hangover are definitely not the same beast. Anyone can get a hangover after a single bout of drinking, whereas alcohol withdrawal only happens with chronic alcoholics. Of course, alcoholics can and often do have a hangover too, making the hair of the dog a notable cure-all.

Another hangover theory says that it's something else in the drink other than alcohol that really causes the problem. Some Russians swear that they never get a hangover drinking vodka, while others claim that only red wine is the problem (and not their drinking habit).

Other than pure water, every drink we have is a complex mix of chemicals that contribute to its unique flavour, aroma and appearance. These so-called congeners may also partly determine how the drinks affect our health, and how easily they cause a hangover. For example, some patrons protest that 'pure' drinks like gin and vodka (because they have no colour) are less likely to cause a hangover than more complex colourful brews like wine or whiskey, that have visibly more congeners. Another theory is that some drinks (like brandy, bourbon and whiskey) actually contain small amounts of methanol! Yes, that's right, methanol, the dangerous moonshine chemical that makes us sick and sends us blind.

The problem with the congener theories is that even 100 per cent pure alcohol mixed with 100 per cent pure water can cause a hangover. So even if the congeners or methanol played a small role, the problem is mostly drinking too much alcohol in the first place. Go figure!

The magic of moderation

Temperance is more than a virtue. Many studies have documented that those unique individuals who regularly consume a small amount of alcohol every day (one or two drinks for a man, and half this for a woman) have significantly better health. And not just because they have fewer hangovers. Regular moderate drinkers have a lower risk of all sorts of major diseases, including heart attacks, stroke, diabetes and some cancers. In fact, regular but moderate tipplers even seem to have, on average, a longer lifespan when compared to those who don't drink at all or drink only occasionally.

This almost certainly has nothing to do with the booze. But rather, it is all about the kind of people who can pull this kind of (moderate) drinking off. Getting drunk is very easy. On the other hand, drinking small amounts every day without ever falling off the wagon or going for days without a drink is an art. It takes real self-control, sobriety, discipline and self-awareness. It's hardly surprising that these are exactly the kind of people who have better health and also live longer.

Moderate drinkers are also pretty funny. As Garrison Keillor says, 'There is nothing funnier than a man beginning his second drink.' Maybe it is also the laughter and sociability that is the remedial ingredient for moderate drinkers, and keeps them healthy and long-lived.

A glass before or during the largest meal of the day is often said to be the most beneficial for our health. Possibly because this is precisely what moderate drinkers usually do, this observation may have simply come about because it captures their healthier, angelic parameters. Or it could be the other way round — that moderate drinkers seem to have health benefits simply because they drink at meal times.

Drinking at meal times is certainly less intoxicating, and is easier to regulate and habituate. A little alcohol also helps to slow the emptying of our stomach, which helps to promote a sense of fullness and reduces overeating. The right drink can also add significantly to the experience, flavour and social-bonding aspects of a meal. The sheer pleasure of drinking a nice drop also offsets the hedonistic desires to find pleasure in our food by over-eating.

Another cogent theory surrounding the health effects of regular moderate drinking is that any beneficial effects of alcohol on health are real but only short-lived. Much like any drugs prescribed by a doctor, we might need to take them at the same time every day for us to see any benefit. As the former US Surgeon General once quipped, 'Drugs don't work in people who don't take them.' The same might be true for alcohol. But obviously if we take too many prescription pills or too much alcohol, we open ourselves up to toxicity.

It has long been thought that red wine is the only regular tipple that provides any benefits to human health. This myth is widely promulgated by wine-loving physicians and their vintner colleagues but has little basis in fact. Actually, the overall health outcomes in moderate wine drinkers are much the same as those in moderate beer drinkers or those who have a glass of scotch or gin every night. Equally moderate, equally healthy.

Of course, the lifestyle factors that permit a regular-but-limited intake, or drinking alcohol with meals, may be more common with wine drinkers. So there may be more moderate wine drinkers than moderate whiskey drinkers, for example. This is one obvious reason that wine gets all the kudos for good health. However, in the end it is the people and their behaviour (not the beverage) that allows for moderation.

Wine is not without its problems. The half-empty bottle of wine is so very tempting. So even if wine was good for us in moderation, it may still be bad for us because we are immoderate with it. At least with a beer we can safely finish the bottle.

It's the antioxidants!

 The health benefits of red wine are often attributed to its non-alcoholic components, and especially the antioxidant qualities of its **polyphenols**, including caffeic acid, gallic acid and resveratrol. Each of these chemicals has been shown to have potent effects in experiments, but their medicinal qualities remain controversial, especially in the doses delivered to moderate wine drinkers. Besides, if these antioxidants were so good then drinking much more would be even better for us. And it isn't.

Some physicians reluctantly admit that beer also contains its own unique antioxidants (e.g. isohumulones from hops). Some of these antioxidants may be better absorbed into our body than those found in wine. There are also more B-vitamins in beer.

Desperate to validate their predilections, scientists have performed head-to-head trials, showing that red wine's antioxidants slightly outperform those found in beer for some parameters linked to health outcomes. The difference is small, and at the end of the day, the antioxidants we'd get in our regular use of either are highly comparable. Regrettably, in these doses they are also both totally unimportant for our health.

The dark side of drinking

Before we start thinking that a glass of our favourite beverage might be just what we need right now for our health (cheers), it is literally sobering to remember that binge drinking and excessive chronic intake of alcohol are leading causes of preventable death, particularly in young adults and men, but also, increasingly, in women. Its individual and social costs are even more significant.

In the end, moderation is mostly magical because heavy drinking is so fundamentally bad for our health. Heavy intemperate drinkers have more heart disease, high blood pressure, dementia and some cancers (especially of the breast and the colon). It is little wonder that the one-drink-a-day angels seem like health nuts by comparison.

Even episodic excessive alcohol intake (also known as **binge drinking**, amounting to more than four drinks within a few hours, often with intent of becoming intoxicated) is associated with an increased risk of an early death. Why this should happen is impossible to tease out from the reasons that someone might want to become intoxicated in the first place (e.g. their mood, their stress, their lifestyle, their self-control, etc.). All of these are important determinants of bad health. Mix in some alcohol and you have a dangerous cocktail.

The bottom line

Alcohol is a regular part of many lives. About two-thirds of all adults drink alcohol at least occasionally, two-thirds of whom will have at least one drink every week, mostly on the weekends. Only about 10 per cent of adults will drink every day. These proportions are much the same in men and women, although women will generally drink half as much, and half as often as men, on average.

In essence, alcohol is a test of self-control and self- awareness. For those who pass the test, alcohol can be one of life's shared pleasures, a source of domestic bliss. It's not something we want to or need to give up. It won't make us physically healthier, but that doesn't matter. It can help us to feel happy, relaxed and sociable. And that at least *feels* like good health.

But it is a very delicate balance. A little glass can easily become more, especially if the bottle is already open. Sometimes, it's far healthier for us not to drink at all and to give up the booze than go down this slippery slope.

Do I really have to ...

#3

Cut down on the caffeine?

Q: Are coffee and tea bad for me?
A: Not in the amounts you'd normally take.

Q: Then are coffee and tea good for me?
A: Depends on the hour.

Q: Can I drink too much coffee or tea?
A: Yes.

Q: Is caffeine addictive?
A: Undoubtedly. But it is not really an
addiction unless it causes you harm.

Q: Will cutting down help?
A: Only if your coffee disagrees with you or your wallet.

Q: Should I leave out the milk and sugar?
A: Only to suit your taste.

Most people begin their day with a cup of tea or coffee. Given our busy, demanding lives and pressing deadlines, there is no time to take it easy. We simply have to get going. Most of us would rather give up our smart phone than our morning cup of coffee!

Coffee and tea are many things for many people. But first and foremost they are drug mules, delivery vehicles for a chemical stimulant known as caffeine. Caffeine does nothing for the flavour or aroma of tea or coffee, but after we drink it, it quickly enters our brain and blocks the receptors that are responsible for dulling brain activity. So by blocking the dulling of our brain we feel a sense of invigoration, vigilance and subtle euphoria. This sensation is commonly known as the coffee buzz, but it is just as likely to happen after a cup of tea, which often contains as much caffeine as a cup of standard instant coffee.

Caffeine also puts the energy into energy drinks, rousing us from our slumber and providing the revitalizing energy to do the things that need to be done. It is sometimes said that no work would be possible without that cup first thing in the morning. So much so that caffeine has long been considered an inspirational muse, a bottomless source of creativity. Beethoven, Bach, Mahler, Balzac and Sartre were all famous caffeholics. Not that caffeine actually makes us more creative. Only less likely to be tired or hung-over, which may be just as valuable.

Instead of experiencing a buzz or a high, many people find their cup of tea or coffee a profoundly relaxing experience, giving them a sense of calm, comfort and focus, eliminating distraction in their mind, uplifting their mood and enhancing their feelings of optimism that everything is going to be all right. Ah!

In this respect caffeine intake is a lot like meditation, both quasi-ritualistic habit-forming practices, both achieving a focused state of attention and self-awareness. However, in this respect, they are both also profoundly uncreative. We make new discoveries by letting our mind freely roam about. How many good ideas have come to us while out walking or in the bath (eureka!)? How many are then quickly forgotten when we concentrate again? Caffeine, meditation and hard work for that matter (like fixing a hole where the rain comes in) all increase our focus on the tasks at hand, and stop our mind from wandering (where it will go). They may help us to be productive, but not truly creative.

The best analogy for caffeine is that it is probably the closest thing we have to a time machine. At least, it changes our perception of time. When we are sad, stressed or exhausted, our internal clock slows and time seems to drag. By contrast, caffeine stimulation speeds up our clock, so that time flies when we are having coffee, as much as it does when we are having fun.

The effects of caffeine on our brain begin soon after having our first cup. It takes about 15 to 20 minutes for the caffeine entering our stomach to reach our brain. Some people seem to experience their coffee buzz much earlier, sometimes within seconds of the first sip of their morning brew or just after smelling the pleasant aroma of coffee. This is not just the gratitude of reward or our sweet imagination. By simply tasting or smelling the bitter twang of caffeine our brain really becomes more alert. Equally, just swilling coffee in our mouth, even without swallowing, is sometimes enough for it to do its thang.

Caffeine is quintessentially a **performance-enhancing drug**. Many of us take caffeine literally to enhance our mental performance as required, in areas such as concentration, alertness and memory. For example, a small dose of caffeine before a lecture improves the chances of us remembering what was said, as well as staying awake through the whole thing. For the same reasons, low doses of caffeine can also improve our driving and road safety.

Caffeine can also have significant effects on our physical performance, increasing the strength of our heartbeat and delaying the time it takes for us to become exhausted. It's not a very big effect. But neither is the difference between winning or losing in many elite sports. This is why caffeine is one of the most widely used performance-enhancing drugs across many different sports.

The tragedy of the Cappuccino Kid

 Caffeine has been long recognized for its ability to enhance athletic performance. So much so, that from the 1960s, the International Olympic Committee considered the presence of elevated caffeine concentrations in the urine a deliberate attempt at doping. The allowable cut-off for caffeine was set at a level beyond that expected to occur with normal consumption of tea or coffee, meaning that anyone breaching it was probably deliberately taking concentrated supplements with a view to enhancing their performance.

In the 1988 Seoul Olympics, the furore surrounding all performance-enhancing drugs reached fever pitch, as sprinter Ben Johnson was disqualified and sent home in disgrace for using stanazol. However, he was not alone. Australian athlete Alex Watson, competing in the Modern Pentathalon, also ran afoul of Olympic officials in Korea. In his case, he was banned for having elevated caffeine concentrations in his urine. The media labelled him 'The Cappuccino Kid'.

Alex had drunk a cup a coffee approximately every hour over the course of the gruelling 12-hour fencing event. In theory this intake should not have been enough to exceed the limit. In fact, other competitors at the same event may have drunk as much or even more coffee, but did not exceed the threshold. The problem was that the urine test he had to take was not a reliable measure of his intake, and subject to considerable person-to-person variability. He was later cleared of wrongdoing and in 2004 the IOC completely lifted its restrictions on caffeine intake for athletes. Today, athletes can take as much as they need, recognizing that big doses are not actually required to enhance performance. A couple of cups is usually enough to do the trick. Any more and performance can actually go down.

The effects of caffeine on the brain are most pronounced in people who don't routinely drink coffee or tea. They can simply use it as a performance-enhancing drug as required. Most people drink at least a cup or two regularly every day. This triggers their bodies to make an adjustment and break down caffeine at a faster rate. So, for the same cup of coffee, regular drinkers will get half as much caffeine in their brain as occasional drinkers. The same goes for smokers, who get less caffeine per cup because cigarette smoke ramps up their caffeine metabolism. This may be one reason why caffeine and nicotine often seem to be bedfellows.

Caffeine's pick-me-up abilities also seem to work best when the dulling receptors are fully occupied in our brain, such as when we are feeling really tired or sleep deprived, during long and demanding tasks, or first thing in the morning as we are still waking up.

However, when we really want those same dulling receptors to do their job and appropriately dull our brain, for example when it's time to sleep at night, caffeine can interfere with the process. This is why caffeine is often used to ward off lethargy, and keep us alert and awake when we should be asleep (particularly when working or driving late at night). But this is also why some people find they can't get to sleep at night after they've drunk coffee in the afternoon (or especially in the evening). Even a few extra cups of coffee in the morning can be enough to cause insomnia in some people. However, most regular drinkers are almost immune to the effects of coffee and tea on their sleep, and can even take an espresso after dinner and not be kept awake.

Where can we get some?

The infinite variety of coffee beans and their processing into coffee means that there is also substantial variety in the amount of caffeine we get when we drink a cup. Overall, the caffeine content is broadly similar in a small serving of single espresso and a cup of percolated, latte or instant coffee. However, this can vary by a factor of two (up or down) depending on other factors, such as methods of roasting or grinding, formulation (strength) and brewing time and the type of coffee bean.

Lighter roasts generally have more caffeine than darker roasts because the caffeine is progressively destroyed by longer roasting times. Darker roasts are also therefore smoother and sweeter (or less bitter).

There are essentially two species of coffee used in commercial coffee enterprises. These are Arabica and Robusta. More than three-quarters of the coffee sold in the world today is Arabica, of which there are many varieties including Java, Mocha, Colombian, Blue Mountain and Bourbon. Almost all of the rest is Robusta. A tiny amount of coffee is Liberica. In the Philippines this is also known as 'Barako', the local word for male machismo or sheer audacity.

The Robusta coffee bean is lighter coloured and contains almost twice as much caffeine and modestly more antioxidants than the darker Arabica bean. Coffee that is 100 per cent Robusta is often described as earthier, more bitter or having a harsher burnt-coffee taste, while 100 per cent Arabica coffee is nuttier, smoother, richer, sweeter or much less bitter. Many coffees are a delicate blend of the two varieties.

The myth of the peaberry

 Coffee is made from the green seeds of the coffee plant. These are usually called coffee beans because they look somewhat bean-shaped. But they are not legumes and are completely unrelated to beans.

The bean shape comes about because there are normally two seeds in every coffee berry (or cherry, as it's also bright red). The twin seeds compete for space and butt up against one another, creating the characteristic flat surface on the adjoining side, while the free side stays rounded.

But growing twins is a tricky business, and sometimes one of the coffee seeds doesn't make it. This leaves room for the remaining seed to grow and fill the space, creating an unusual round seed. This is known as a peaberry.

On average about 5 per cent of all coffee seeds are peaberries. Some varieties can double this number, while others can halve it. A good crop generally has fewer peaberries, while a bad crop often has more, as the worse conditions make it more likely one seed will not survive. This is fortunate for the coffee farmers as inadvertently growing more of the higher priced peaberries can help sustain them through bad times.

Because of their rarity, and the challenges of harvesting these big babies, peaberries have achieved a mythical status amongst coffee aficionados. The experts claim they taste different. At the very least their extra size means they roast differently. Most of all they cost differently too. You can almost taste their exclusivity.

Green coffee beans can be decaffeinated before roasting, keeping many of the interesting flavoursome chemicals but removing 95 per cent of the caffeine, meaning a standard cup of decaf contains around 5 per cent of the caffeine contained in a standard cup of joe. This is still enough for non-drinkers to experience a lift in their mood.

Decaffeination is usually achieved by simply soaking green coffee beans in hot water. This is called the Swiss Water method, although it is essentially the same thing as throwing away the first steep of your green tea. Caffeine can also be removed by mixing beans with oils from spent coffee grounds, carbon dioxide or chemical solvents. This latter method is often erroneously called 'natural' decaffeination, as it uses ethylene acetate, a chemical solvent that is found naturally in apples. But there are no apples used in the process.

The caffeine content of a cup of tea is also highly variable and influenced by many different factors. On average, a typical cup of black tea contains about two-thirds the caffeine in an espresso. Unlike coffee, the darker the tea the higher its caffeine content. Caffeine is partly destroyed in tea processing so that minimally processed (green) tea will usually contain the same or greater amounts of caffeine than an espresso, depending on how long it has been steeped in water and whether the first infusion has been discarded, a common traditional practice to reduce the caffeine content and unpleasant bitterness associated with the first steep.

Milk and two sugars

 Some people add milk to their tea or coffee. Some people don't. There are no good reasons either way. It is just how we like it and the comforts of habit and tradition: 'We've always taken it this way.'

The reasons some people even started putting milk in their brew in the first place are as murky as the beverage itself. Adding cold milk certainly means the tea or coffee is not so scaldingly hot and is therefore drinkable sooner. Putting the milk in first also stops the porcelain cup from cracking from the boiling hot water.

Interestingly, milk fat also helps any brew stay warm for longer by reducing evaporative cooling. In this way the traditional workers' cup of joe could stay hot for the whole coffee break. This fatty insulation does not work as well with low-fat skim milk. But fortunately today, we get a polystyrene cup with a lid, so even hot water stays hot.

The strong, bitter taste of some tea and coffee can also be substantially softened by adding milk. Some tea blends (e.g. English Breakfast) are deliberately strong brews on the expectation that milk will be added. Milk does not interfere with the modest antioxidant potential of tea or coffee, so doesn't make it any more or less healthy.

Sugar is also often added to tea and coffee to allow those who don't really like the bitter taste a way to participate with their peers. But because our brain runs on glucose, especially under adverse conditions, sugar also provides the brain a pick-me-up. So mixing our beverage with a teaspoon of sugar or combining it with sugary food (e.g. a piece of toast, a muffin, a biscuit or cookie) really does provide a greater sense of energy than either alone.

For the health conscious, the idea of two teaspoons of white sugar per cup seems abhorrent. In reality, 15 calories per teaspoon is not very much compared to the 2000 calories we get elsewhere in out diet every day. So if we enjoy coffee with two sugars, it is really not something we have to give up for health reasons. The accompanying muffin that comes with hundreds of calories is probably far more dangerous than the spoonful of sugar that helps the medicinal coffee go down.

Other than coffee and tea, caffeine is also naturally found in the seeds, leaves and fruits of over fifty plants, including guarana and yerba mate. Extracts of these exotic plants are often added into energy drinks to increase the caffeine content, as well as enhance our belief in their exotic effects on our brain. Some soft drinks (sodas) and energy drinks are just fortified with caffeine. For example a can of Diet Coke has about the same amount of caffeine as a cup of black tea. A small can of energy drink is typically formulated to provide the same amount of caffeine as a typical cup of coffee.

The upside of coffee

Given the acute effects of caffeine on our brain, it is hardly a wonder that tea and coffee are widely viewed as vital tonics. But the long-term effects of caffeine also appear to be surprisingly positive for human health.

Most observational studies show that people who drink a cup of tea or coffee every day have on average a 10 per cent lower risk of dying during any set period than those who don't partake. This might not seem like a very big effect, yet the risk of dying is reduced by a similar amount when smokers give up smoking.

Some studies also suggest that people who drink tea and coffee have a slightly lower risk of diseases that might kill them, including the usual suspects like heart disease, stroke, diabetes, some cancers and dementia. Not by a lot, but still enough to add up.

How these positive associations come about is still anyone's guess. It is probably not even the caffeine. People who regularly drink decaffeinated coffee also seem to have similar health benefits per cup when compared to espresso drinkers.

Shampoo and conditioner

 If we weren't already believers In the many benefits of our daily caffeine fix, it turns out that it also prevents hair loss! And no, it's not because a shot of caffeine makes it less likely for you to pull your hair out with frustration or boredom. In fact, when you put caffeine directly onto your scalp it appears to block some of the effects of the male hormone testosterone, a common contributor to hair loss in both men and women. Consequently, caffeine is now found in many popular conditioners.

But while upending a cup of tea or coffee on your head every day could help prevent hair loss, it would be a terrible waste and would stain your hair more than it would save it from falling out. Better to buy the conditioner.

Unfortunately, you don't get the same head of hair from just drinking lots of coffee. Caffeine has to reach the hair follicles in order to have any effect. To get as much caffeine as in a caffeine hair conditioner you'd need to drink over fifty cups a day. Maybe this explains Beethoven's hair.

Coffee chemistry

Coffee is far more than just caffeine. As the coffee seeds/beans are fermented, roasted, brewed and filtered, over a thousand different chemicals can be liberated, including caffeine. Some of these chemicals could be theoretically beneficial for human health, including antioxidants, lignans, quinides and minerals (at least in the high doses used in experimental studies). However, none of these alone explains the association between coffee and tea and long-term good health.

Tea is also an equally complex mix of chemicals. The most widely drunk tea in Western countries is black tea, prepared from tea-leaves that have been fermented and oxidized. By contrast, oolong tea is only partially oxidized, and green tea is minimally processed before drying. This processing creates a range of different flavours, astringencies and caffeine content.

In each case the dried tea-leaf is steeped in hot or boiling water to release the complex mixture of polyphenols contained within, including the well-known flavanoid antioxidants (such as epigallocatechin gallate). Some of these antioxidants are lost or transformed during the prolonged drying and oxidization required to make tea black. But enough remain that for people who usually don't each much fruit, black tea is often their major source of dietary flavanols.

Minimally processed tea (such as green tea) generally has the highest concentration of antioxidants. This fact has led many health conscious individuals to flock to drinking green tea as a potential foundation of eternal youth. In support of this idea, it is well known that the habitually long-lived people from Okinawa, Japan (who have an average life expectancy that exceeds the average American by over ten years), prefer drinking green tea. However, this may have nothing to do with antioxidants. It may just be that drinking so much caffeine every day makes their lives seem not as long.

Herbal teas are infusions of herbs, flowers, seeds or fruit that contain no tea-leaves. They do not contain caffeine, but they still may be high in flavonoids and other antioxidants. Often herbal brews are used for the specific effects of their phytochemicals on our brain, such as stimulation or relaxation. The long-term effects of herbal teas on human health are uncertain and as variable as the brews themselves, although — given their long history and wide use — most can be considered safe, with some exceptions. For example, comfrey contains toxins that cause liver damage with chronic use. Chamomile can cause severe allergic reactions in those sensitive to ragweed (pollen).

The great escape

More than the caffeine, more than all the antioxidants and flavanols, our daily cup of tea or coffee has a real and predictable effect on how we feel. In so far as health comes from our mind, so it is with coffee and tea.

The purported health benefits of a regular cup of tea or coffee may have nothing to do with the drink at all. It might just be that stopping for a cup or two through the day is enough to make us feel happy, rewarded and relaxed, or at the very least less unfocused for a little while.

There is no doubt that happiness is an important means to good health. And knowing we can grab a coffee or sit down for a cup of tea means we know there is something in our day that will make us feel differently, that we have somewhere else we can go. Stop the world and let me off! Actually, depression and suicide are lower in those who find refuge in coffee or tea.

Coffee and tea are also often taken during breaks from work (e.g. morning tea or coffee break). As discussed elsewhere in this book, getting off our backside is good for our health in many ways. So one of the many useful things that coffee and tea do is to pry us away from our desk as well as our burdens.

Drinking coffee and tea is also often a social ritual, associated with convivial interaction with others, with the beverage as the lubricant. This is not a new phenomenon. For hundreds of years, coffee houses (shortened to 'café') and teahouses have been social hubs, and still are today. As Howard Schultz once remarked, it is amazing 'the power that savouring a simple cup of coffee can have to connect people and create community'. This social interaction helps our mood and alleviates our stress and, with it, improves our health. So it may be nothing to do with chemistry, but everything to do with the brew.

The dark side of caffeine

At the same time, caffeine is undoubtedly also a lethal poison. Fortunately, humans possess a remarkable tolerance to it. This is because each of us has enzymes in our liver that rapidly inactivate caffeine, breaking it down into harmless metabolites. In order to kill ourselves with coffee we'd need to eat half a kilogram of instant coffee or drink near to fifty double espressos in one sitting.

The protective enzymes are slightly less active in women, meaning that women generally get more caffeine from a cup of coffee or tea than men. This gender difference is even more marked during a woman's pregnancy, where a single cup of coffee achieves higher and more sustained levels of caffeine. By contrast, cats, dogs and birds have no protective enzymes at all. This means that very small amounts of caffeine can easily kill them.

Despite our own highly protective enzymes, it is still possible to kill ourselves with coffee. The most notorious reported case is the death of the French playwright Honoré de Balzac. Balzac was famous for his work habits, toiling through the night on his manuscripts, inspired by bottomless black coffee, allegedly sometimes up to fifty espressos a day and even eating coffee grounds. This kind of intake was not unusual. Bach, Beethoven and Voltaire were also said to be in his league.

Then, as today, it was widely viewed that coffee was an inspiration. Sir James Mackintosh attested that 'the powers of a man's mind are directly proportionate to the quantity of coffee he drinks'. But, as the ever-realistic Balzac was quick to also point out, 'as everybody knows, coffee only makes boring people even more boring'.

In the end, it is said that it was the coffee that did Balzac in. In his historical post-mortem, nothing is mentioned of his chronic lack of sleep, copious intake of French wine, poor nutrition or the lack of sanitary conditions in his writer's hovel. Even then, it was a better look to burn out than to fade away!

Some studies have observed that people who drink too much coffee or tea (e.g. more than five to eight cups a day) not only don't share the same benefits as those who partake in more modest amounts, but may also have higher rates of some diseases. The interpretation of such studies is always clouded by the reasons some people might drink so much more than others (like the extra stress they are under). But if there were small amounts of toxins in coffee and tea (actually there are: acryalmide and diterpene), then maybe drinking large amounts may eventually give you a big enough dose to start causing problems.

For people who don't take caffeine regularly, having a cup clearly also has a number of potentially unpleasant effects. Caffeine can make many unaccustomed drinkers feel tense, nervous and jittery. Drinking a cup of coffee will usually make them pee more. This is partly nervousness and partly because caffeine causes kidneys to make more urine. Caffeine also makes the bladder contract more vigorously when it is nearing fullness, increasing our urgency to go or go earlier than we otherwise would.

Again, this phenomenon is mostly in people who don't drink the beverage regularly. For most of the population who regularly take at least a cup or two every day, caffeine doesn't have much effect on their bladder beyond the volume of fluid they drink. Consequently, there is no particular need to consume a glass of water with our coffee to ward off dehydration. However, it is custom in Italy to have a glass of water with your coffee. But when in Rome, it is important to drink the water *before* rather than after the coffee, otherwise you would be implying their coffee was terrible and you were trying to wash away the taste!

Caffeine also modestly increases blood pressure levels. Again, this effect is most pronounced and probably confined to habitual non-drinkers and then only immediately after having an occasional cup. Importantly, a typical daily intake of coffee or tea (two to three cups a day) is not associated with an increased risk of high blood pressure in the long term.

The strength of our bones may also be influenced by the coffee and tea we drink. It is quite normal for our bones to become thinner with age. At some point, this age-related bone loss may become so significant as to compromise structural integrity, making it easier for our bones to break. This is called **osteoporosis**. During their lifetime, about half of all women aged fifty years or older will have a fracture through thin areas of bone.

Some studies have shown that people who habitually drink coffee or tea may have slightly thinner bones. This is often attributed to increased loss of calcium, our bones' main mineral and strength promoter, into the urine that we make more of when we drink caffeine. However, there is no clear evidence that coffee or tea leads to more fractures or more problems from them. There are many more important things to keep our bones strong than giving up our daily cup.

Coffee stains

 Coffee, tea and red wine all leave an indelible mark on our lives, and not just on our carpet, clothes and furniture. Have a look inside your favourite coffee mug and you will see a stain that simply doesn't wash off. The same thing happens with our teeth. They might look solid and smooth on the outside, but just like the porcelain of a teacup they are slightly porous, enough to let stains in and keep them there. Given that around half the population regularly drinks coffee, coffee is a major cause of teeth yellowing. However, it is often argued that, on a per cup basis, black tea has a greater staining effect because of its darker flavanoids.

There is no easy solution to coffee stains. Who has time to clean their teeth or rinse after every cup of tea or coffee? However, coffee stains any plaque on our teeth much more than the teeth themselves, so keeping our teeth free from plaque reduces the potential for them to become stained or need to be whitened.

Missing the fix

The other potential downside of our regular caffeine intake is how we feel when we aren't getting it, or at least in the amounts we are used to. Missing out on our chosen beverage can leave us with headaches (the most common symptom), fatigue, inattention, irritability and low mood. This is known as **withdrawal**.

Some level of caffeine withdrawal is probably experienced by about half of all regular tea or coffee drinkers if their regular drug supply is completely cut off. The more we drink and the more regularly we drink, the more likely we are to experience withdrawal symptoms if we ever go without. The feeling of relief we get from our morning 'fix' only serves to reinforce our addiction.

For regular coffee drinkers, withdrawal symptoms typically occur a day or two after removing all caffeine from the menu. Symptoms usually only last for a day or two but can sometimes last for up to week before subsiding. Caffeine withdrawal does not occur within a few hours of the last cup, despite the protestations of the habitual coffee drinker. What they are usually complaining about is coming down from the focused high experienced when caffeine levels were at their peak (a couple of hours after the previous cup).

The bottom line

Coffee and tea might seem some of life's luxuries, but that doesn't mean we have to give them up in the austere pursuit of good health and a long life. A regular intake is quite safe. Caffeine improves our mood and helps us to concentrate when our brain is dulled. It can also be a meditative escape to relax us and focus our mind in a distracting world or on those dull unproductive mornings when nothing seems to be working as we planned. At least we can stop and have a cup. Whether it is actually any good for us or only feels like it is unclear. At best, the effect on our health is not enough to warrant taking it up if we don't like it. But if we do, all the better to enjoy and share. I'll have a latte, please.

Do I really have to...

#4

Lose the waist?

Q: Is being overweight really a problem?
A: It is your biggest problem.

Q: How do some overweight people remain healthy?
A: Because they bank fat efficiently.

Q: Why will being overweight kill me?
A: Because fat accumulates in the wrong places.

Q: Why is it so hard to lose weight?
A: Our brain thinks we should stay big.

Q: Why do some men have man-boobs?
A: Fat creates hormones that make breasts.

Q: Will losing my waist really make a difference?
A: In the long term, yes.

The most important health challenge of our life will be keeping our waistline in check. How we (and our waistline) rise to this challenge will be the biggest determinant of what happens to our health and longevity.

Gaining more fat than is appropriate for our body shape and size is responsible for much of the excess chronic disease now affecting human beings. Each and every centimetre of extra fat around our waists can literally tip the scales progressively until our health is ultimately compromised. Those who accumulate body fat steadily to the point where they become obese will, on average, lose at least a decade of healthy life. Only being a smoker throughout our adult years would shorten our lives more.

Despite our best intentions and personal abhorrence of the notion of getting fatter, about a third to a half of us will ultimately become obese. At least half of all women put on one dress size (S to M, M to L, L to XL, XL to XXL = 5 centimetres or about 2 inches) every decade of their adult life, from their twenties to their sixties. A century ago this would have been unthinkable. Dresses could be handed onto children and their children too. Nowadays, well-fitting dresses hardly last more than a decade before we grow out of them.

The fat bank

In our body, energy is like money and fat is the perfect bank in which to store it.

Every day, we have costs. So we need to spend a little simply to get by, like paying the power bill to keep the lights on. But when we bring in more than we spend over the same time period, obviously our bank account expands.

This is a very useful cushion for those times when we want to spend a little bit more, like buying a car or a flat screen television or paying a large doctor's bill. It is also important for those lean periods when very little is coming in, sometimes even less than we need to live off. We always have a back-up squirreled away as an effective buffer against times of extra need or extra want.

For our bank account to grow, it doesn't really matter how the money comes in. A little bit extra every day or big lump sum deposits now and then are all happily tucked away. Each and every addition will work in the same way to make our balance steadily grow, as long as we don't spend more than we bring in. Where it comes from is immaterial. Even getting a little bit extra in non-money terms, like receiving a gift of a new handbag or a voucher for a birthday, is also a useful addition, as more of our money can be safely kept in our bank account for another day.

All energy in the human body ultimately comes from what we eat and drink. Food energy is measured in calories or kilojoules. Like money, energy is a vital commodity, so our body is intrinsically thrifty when it comes to the calories we eat. We want to hold onto whatever we can get our teeth into, whether it comes in small drips or large dollops. We can't afford to waste calories because of the historical possibility of lean times ahead, when food becomes scarce or crops fail; when it's all about survival of the fattest.

Our healthy fat stores kept us alive through the Stone Age. In the absence of shops and gardens, we couldn't rely on finding our next meal quickly. It was best to eat as much as we could during times of excess and bank the dividends. When it came to periods when there was less available, during famine, snowstorms and other calamities, we could just raid our piggy bank.

The piggy bank

 Why a pig (an animal known for gluttony) should be used as symbol for thrift and financial restraint is one of the world's great ironies.

People have long been saving up their spare cash in boxes, pots and jars. But unlike a pirate chest, the great innovation of the money jar was that it was completely sealed, save for the single slot cut in its side. You could insert coins any time you liked. But you couldn't change your mind (or steal from it). You couldn't just easily open it, take the money and then put the lid back on.

The only way to get your money out was to break the jar, which you were generally reluctant to do. So it was an ingenious way of encouraging saving — literally putting your money away.

Because they were eventually smashed open, the original money jars were made of cheap pottery clay called Pygg, and therefore the earthenware pots were sometimes known as Pygg jars. Hence, the term piggy (bank) may have had nothing to do with the actual animal.

However, in many countries, pigs are associated with good fortune. And these jars were literally filled with your fortune. Moreover, an earthy round jar that narrows to a short neck (like a snout), with a single straight slot (like an slanting eye) cut into the side, so resembles the cute face of a fortunate pig from side on that it's little wonder the name stuck.

Of course, if the three little pyggs were really three money boxes, then the moral of their different risk-averse investment strategies makes a lot more sense, with the Wolf of Wall Street gobbling up their savings (unless they were brick-solid investments).

~~~~~~

Those nutritionally impoverished days of hunting and gathering are long gone. The same thrifty traits we needed to ensure our survival in times past now make our modern life of excess an increasingly heavy burden.

Just like with our money, we naturally spend some calories in just getting by, as our continuous metabolism and intermittent physical activity need some energy to keep the lights on. But any calories that we don't spend end up as an energy deposit in our fat bank. Importantly, this means we always have plenty in reserve to cushion against any variability, such as if we miss a meal or two or if we need to be more physically active outrunning a hunting lion pack.

Our thrifty body banks any excess energy from everything we eat as fat, not just the extra fat in our diet. This is because fat is a very efficient way to store energy. Like bars of gold in a bank, fat can stack itself densely. It is also water repellent, so it takes up less space. If we stored all our energy as sugar, our back-up energy reserves would need to be over five times the size. Just to survive, we would all look like the Michelin tyre man.

Our fatty banks are usually very efficient at impounding fat and keeping it safe. We wouldn't be very happy with a bank that lost some of our hard-earned money from time to time! But a perfect bank account is also always accessible, listens to our instructions and can make automatic payments to the power company so that the lights remain on between pay cheques. In much the same way, our fat is also very efficient at releasing its stored energy in the right amounts and precisely when it is needed to satisfy the needs of the body between meal times.

Importantly, our body banks excess calories as fat. Regardless of its currency, whether it comes in as sugar, protein or fat, any and all energy in excess of our requirements is converted into fat. This happens either directly (i.e. the body makes fat or stores the fat we eat) or indirectly, by giving the body something else to eat, leaving our fat account to just happily sit there and steadily grow inch by inch. Pasta or pork, bread or butter, the end result on our energy balance is still the same.

A positive energy balance often happens through more or larger deposits. But just like a growing bank balance, we can also drift into the positive by keeping our spending down. If less goes out of the account there is more left behind (literally).

This is the usual mantra of governments that attempt to achieve a surplus by cutting costs without necessarily increasing revenue through new or extra taxes. So if our income can remain the same but our costs are reduced, then our balance will go into surplus. Good for governments, not so for waistlines.

In the human body the major variable cost is physical activity. So when we change our level of physical activity, even if we don't modify what we eat (i.e. same income), our fat balance also changes. For example, out weight stays much the same for a few years (i.e. we are in balance). But then we go through a busy period in our life when we are less physically active than usual. We don't eat any differently but now our energy budget goes into the black, and our coffers get fatter. Equally, if we find a way to get more active, even without changing our diet our energy balance will naturally shrink. If we go into the red, the net negative balance will cause our fat deposits to dwindle.

The challenge of balancing a budget can be readily appreciated when we tally up all the calories in our diet and how many we use up in our activities. For example, we need to go jogging for half an hour or do two hours of housework to burn off the amount of calories contained in one Snickers bar. A typical Western-style diet provides a deposit of well over 2000 calories every day. By contrast, our daily energy requirement is somewhere between 1400 and 1800 depending on our age, size, gender and level of physical activity. It is just a small mismatch: the equivalent of walking an extra 500 metres every day (a third of a mile, or maybe to the next bus stop) or not taking two bites of a meal. But after month after month, year after year of having continuously positive balances, our banked assets slowly but surely swell. And by the time we reach our middle age, our coffers are overflowing.

Overflowing coffers

When food energy is coming in in excess of our daily requirements, it is initially sequestered efficiently by our fat cells. These bankers live predominantly under our skin, in the buttocks, thighs and breasts. Eighty per cent of our fat is normally stored in these very obvious places.

We may not like its appearance. But this fat is not actually bad. In fact, it serves many important functions that keep us healthy. Most important of which is that it keeps our fat safe and out of the way when it is not needed, and then drip feeds it back when it is. In fact, people who are born with a reduced capacity to deposit fat in all the normal places have a real health disadvantage, even though they look thin.

If all the excess fat from under our skin, in our thighs, bottoms or breasts could be dissolved and sucked away (for example, using liposuction) we would not get any healthier, reduce our risks for poor health or live any longer. In fact, removal of thigh fat by liposuction mostly means any accumulating fat has to deposit itself somewhere else, like around our waist.

If energy comes in day after day without our needing to spend it, our healthy fat cells can get bigger, making extra room for the extra income. In some cases, fat cells can also multiply. But in every man and woman, there comes a **tipping point** when there is simply no more room in the vault. Then the problems begin.

What does our body do with extra energy when the place that it normally banks it is full to capacity? It's not like we can just throw it away. How many millionaires do we see deliberately throwing away excess money when they become rich?

The solution is pragmatic, but ultimately deadly. Faced with nowhere else to put excess energy, the body instead dumps fat outside where fat is normally stored. This is known as ectopic fat, from the Greek word *ektopos,* meaning 'out of place'. Most of these new dump sites are around our internal organs (also known as visceral fat) or inside them (known as steatosis). Ultimately, this 'out of place' fat means fat-stuffed organs can't do the job they are supposed to do and so we become unhealthy. This is why ectopic fat is sometimes called bad fat.

Although storage space eventually runs out in every body, some people just seem to have a greater propensity to accumulate fat in all the wrong places and get sick as a result, even when they don't appear to be overweight.

Equally, others can be very fat but have it partitioned safely off in all the right places, and as a result they are often quite healthy. It is thought that about a quarter of all people who get really fat have very little 'out of place' fat, despite appearing very large in size. It seems that they have more capacity in their bank or can expand it sufficiently instead of having to look elsewhere to dump their excess.

The capacity of the fat bank is very different in different people depending on their age, gender, body shape, race, genes and a host of other factors.

One idea is that early in our development and childhood the capacity of our piggy bank gets programmed. For example, periods of poor nutrition may have reduced fat banking capacity in babies born in Europe during or immediately following World War II. This may explain the higher rates of ectopic fat and its consequences now observed in these children. Equally, our modern environment may eventually foster adults with increased fat capacity and a greater buffer to the adverse effects of excess.

However, as we get older, our capacity to bank fat declines slightly, so that for the same calorie balance more of it ends up in the wrong places as we get older than when we were teenagers, when most excess was safely banked somewhere under our skin.

In particular, pre-menopausal women intrinsically have a greater fat storage capacity under their skin as well as greater expandability of this capacity. Both these factors are crucially important for the demands of pregnancy, breastfeeding and child-rearing. Women, it seems, are built for the long haul, with better banking and capacity to store extra fat to prop up the next generation. But this also means that, at least during the reproductive years, a woman generally has about 10 per cent more fat in her body than a man (mostly as bigger bum, thighs and breasts). The extra banking capacity means a woman can also put on more weight than the average man before reaching a tipping point at which she too starts to accumulate 'out of place' fat, and suffer its adverse consequences on her belly, as well as her health. This is potentially also one reason why women have a longer life expectancy than men and have a much greater chance of reaching one hundred.

Pears and apples

 A woman's figure changes through her life. This is mostly because of changes in how much excess fat she has banked and where she has banked it.

Under the influence of sex hormones like oestrogen (estrogen) following puberty, young women generally bank excess fat in their buttocks, thighs and hips, with more weight below their waist, creating a pear-shaped body if weight is gained. Their waist circumference is usually less than half their height.

But this is not true of all women. At least one-third deposit their excess fat around their waist, creating an apple-shaped figure, with a wide waist and belly, and more weight above the waist than below it. As in men, this distribution is associated with an increased risk of health problems and a shorter life expectancy.

After the menopause, when a woman's ovaries stop making oestrogen, her body shape changes again. Oestrogen helps keep the fat banking capacity high in women. But with its decline and the waning ability to efficiently store excess fat, older women become as prone as men to adding a spare tyre around their waist.

Because excess 'out of place' fat characteristically causes our waistlines to get bigger, an expanding waistline is often used as a surrogate marker for the presence and amount of ectopic fat. It's not a perfect marker by any means, but on a population level it gives a fairly good guide as to how many have reached their tipping point. In general, a woman with a white/European racial background probably has too much out of place fat when her waist circumference reaches 35 inches (88 cm) or above. For a man this is more like a waist of 40 inches (102 cm) or above.

By contrast, naturally lean people from Asia also generally have a lower storage capacity in their fat bank. This means that if they gain extra weight, they are more likely to reach their fat capacity sooner, allowing excess to spill over and become ectopic, or dumped 'out of place'. So in Asian women, a waistline above 32 inches (80 cm) and in Asian men above 36 inches (90 cm), means they are likely to have accumulated 'out of place' back-up fat, and it is beginning to affect their health.

Pis aller

Fat is supposed to be the perfect bank. The real problem with out of place fat is that it is not very good at its job. Moreover, it has selective hearing. It doesn't listen to some messages, and responds inappropriately to others when it does. It is really a makeshift solution, a last resort for a temporary imbalance. The French term for this is *pis aller* (*pis* meaning worse + *aller* meaning to go; literally 'the worst going'). And by not doing its job particularly well, many things can go wrong.

Ectopic fat is far less efficient at safekeeping its stores. It tries really hard to compensate. But it is just not very good at keeping itself contained. So instead of being efficiently stored away, excess triglycerides leach out into the bloodstream. This free fat is a free lunch for cells that normally only get drip fed slowly between meal times with the small amounts of fat they need to function. If fat is free, then it must be feeding time at the zoo. So our organs gobble up the free lunch, and so accumulate out of place ectopic fat in great globules that change their chemistry and the way they function.

For example, when fat overfills the pancreas, its ability to control the glucose levels in our blood can decline, and sugar levels rise dangerously. This is called **type 2 diabetes**. This is different from the diabetes that is caused when the immune system destroys the sugar-controlling part of the pancreas (known as type 1 diabetes), although both are the result of the pancreas not being able to do its job.

Type 2 diabetes now affects at least 460 million people worldwide and is a leading cause of premature death. It is not due to eating too much sugar. Rather, it is due to eating much too much of everything when compared to how little we really need to be eating. In short, type 2 diabetes is due to accumulating out of place fat. This explains why type 2 diabetes is more common in older people, in men more than women and people of an Asian background, because for the same food intake and size these people are more likely to have out of place fat.

When fat spills over into our liver, it also can't do its job properly. When more than 10 per cent of a liver is replaced by fat, it is called **fatty liver** (not surprisingly). The liver regulates many important things. For example, the liver normally responds to signals from the pancreas to control sugar levels. But a fatty liver also doesn't listen very well, pouring out an additional 60 grams of sugar (half an ounce or the equivalent of 15 teaspoons) back into the blood every day when it should be doing just the opposite. When excess fat is in the liver, the pancreas has to work doubly hard and, under the burden of its own fat load, not surprisingly gives out.

The other problem with 'out of place' fat is that *it knows* it's not very good at its job. It's a short-term solution to a temporary crisis of excess, not a long-term solution for a life of it. So once on the field, our ectopic fat soon puts its hand up and waves it about wildly, hoping to be replaced.

One of the messages it sends out communicates the stress that it is under. As discussed in Chapter 16, each and every stress we suffer contributes not only to our mood but also our overall health. This is partly because when we are under stress, we naturally stoke the fire of inflammation to make it burn stronger or longer to help defend ourselves better. But in the long term, this heightened inflammation results in collateral damage, which we experience as ageing and age-related disease.

In particular, there is a strong link between markers of 'out of place' fat (e.g. a big waist circumference, a fatty liver, or high amount of free fat in the blood) and heart attacks and strokes, together the leading killers of all human beings. For example, the greater your waist circumference, the greater your risk of heart problems. The heart is mostly muscle, and doesn't accumulate free fat to the same extent as the liver or the pancreas. But free fat is still damaging to it. Fat also accumulates around the blood vessels supplying the heart, hastening the narrowing and destabilizing process known as atherosclerosis (see Chapter 10).

At least a third of us will face cancer some time in our lives and almost all of us have some cancer cells somewhere. Having out of place fat probably makes this worse. All the major cancers that slowly kill humans (colon, breast, endometrial, kidney, oesophageal, liver and myeloma to name but a few) are all more common and more severe in people with too much fat. Overall, it is now thought at least one in every five cancers in the world is due to excess fat. Within a few decades, our excess fat will almost certainly unseat smoking as the major preventable cause of cancer in the world.

Whether cancers are really caused by being overweight or whether cancer cells simply enjoy the free lunch that excess fat offers is unclear. Some cancers are hurried along by changes in the hormones made by dysfunctional 'out of place' fat.

Fat hormones

Hormones are chemicals that specifically regulate many of our body's vital functions. Ectopic fat is especially good at breaking down the male hormone testosterone to make the female hormone oestrogen. As discussed earlier, oestrogen helps stimulate fat capacity, which is why women generally have more fat than men. So all the extra oestrogen made by ectopic fat is one way it tries to recruit new fat storage capacity, so that we won't need its replacement services any more.

However, all this extra oestrogen has other effects as well. After the menopause when a woman's ovaries stop making oestrogen, most of their oestrogen actually comes from ectopic fat, albeit in much smaller amounts than from their ovaries during their reproductive years. But this fat-derived oestrogen can be enough to keep the bones of larger women just a bit stronger as they age and may partly explain why they have a lower risk of bone fractures than habitually thin women.

But at the same time, the production of oestrogen after menopause and other chemical signals produced by excess fat can also promote the growth of hormone-sensitive cancers like breast cancer. Indeed, being overweight has emerged as the major preventable cause of breast cancer in older women.

Today, breast cancer is responsible for the death of around 5 per cent of all women in the world and one in eight women will develop breast cancer during their lifetime. Sadly these rates are still on the rise, particularly in Asian women, in whom breast cancer was historically uncommon. This is partly because in the past, Asian women were not very fat. But as this changes, so will the rates of cancer, diabetes and a host of other problems.

In overweight men, increased production of the female sex hormone, oestrogen, may also help them by increasing their fat storage capacity (mostly in oestrogen-sensitive areas like bums, thighs and hips). This can help keep fat in the right place instead of in and around the abdominal organs. However, the extra oestrogen made by ectopic fat can also sometimes lead to the development of small but significant breasts in men.

Man-boobs

 Men do not usually have breasts. Obviously!

The formation of breast tissue is triggered by the female sex hormone, oestrogen. Men normally make lots of the male sex hormone, testosterone, which stops breasts from forming. All men also make some oestrogen, although far less than women and not enough to overcome their testosterone. However, this balance can sometimes change.

For example, it is quite common for newborn baby boys to have obvious breast tissue when they are born. This is due to extra oestrogen transferred from their mothers. It is only temporary and usually resolves within a month or so.

During their early teens, breast tissue becomes more prominent in at least half of all adolescent boys. Although all sex hormones are rising rapidly at this age, oestrogen production can briefly get ahead of testosterone, promoting enlargement of the breast tissue. Again, this is only temporary and soon testosterone obviously gets the upper hand in all boys.

Sometimes medical conditions and some medications can also upset the balance of sex hormones and trigger breast enlargement in men, through either reducing male hormones or increasing female ones. For example, oestrogens can be used therapeutically to initiate breast development in male-to-female transgender transformations.

Many men who are overweight have prominent contours on their chest. This is usually due to excess fat deposited under the skin. These are not breasts. Breasts are special organs. Breasts are not prominent lumps of fat.

Real man-boobs can be easily distinguished from just excess fat because breasts fill in under the nipple while excess fat does not. And unlike fat, man-boobs don't melt away when men lose excess weight, especially if they have been there for more than a year or two.

Fasting

A good bank is more than just a cold store. It is also a regulator, chiefly through the messages it sends back about the account and how it's faring. For example, when we are thinking about buying a new car or a new house, having a baby or even checking out a new partner, it pays to have an eye on the bank balance (before doing anything hasty). In the same way our fat balance is not a lifeless lump of lard, but rather a dynamic regulator of many parts of our health, from our fertility and mood, to our appetite and even our rate of ageing. The messages our fat sends tell us what we can afford to do and what we can't.

Just like on our phone, during times when the energy is low, messages pop up saying it's time to switch to low power (energy conserving) mode. Accepting this, all workings become pared down and super efficient so that no energy is wasted while we are waiting for our next meal to charge us up.

This extra efficiency may be one explanation for why diets really low in calories may actually reduce some cancers, inflammation and other excesses that a streamlined body simply can't afford. In fact, limiting energy intake increases the lifespan of most animal species, from worms to primates (provided the subject doesn't become malnourished or die of hunger). The onset of many signs of ageing may also be slowed when running in lower power (energy conservation) mode. Whether this is really true for humans is still hotly debated. But it doesn't stop people from giving it a go.

The temperate life

 In 1605, Venetian nobleman and patron of the arts Luigi Cornaro was at death's door. He was only 40 but he had burnt the candle at both ends during his life and was now living to regret it. He suffered from chest pains, fevers, gout, ongoing thirst and disorders of the stomach. Despite consulting numerous doctors he was sinking fast.

His final solution was radical. He cut his diet back to '12 ounces of food divided among four meals per day' together with 14 ounces of wine (i.e. four small glasses with each meal). This adds up to no more than 800 kilocalories per day. Today we call this a very-low calorie diet.

Miraculously his health improved. He subsequently lived to the age of 102, almost unheard of in the 17th century.

His survivor story, *Discorsi Della Vita Sobria* (Discourses on the Temperate Life), went on to be a bestseller over the next three centuries. However, it is likely that many, many others died trying to survive on equally meagre rations. But, as the pirates say, 'dead men tell no tales', creating a bias that made Luigi's story look all the more credible.

Of course, if living on a bare minimum of calories prolongs life, today we live at the very opposite end of the spectrum. We spend much of our days eating or basking in its afterglow. By the time we add up breakfast, lunch and dinner, morning and afternoon tea, and the liquid calories we take in between, there are only a few hours through the night when our bodies need to switch into high-efficiency fasting mode.

One of the luxuries of living in a bonanza state of constant income and excess is that any loss of efficiency is less critical. A dollar lost here, a rebellious cell there, is unimportant to the bottom line, at least in the short term. But bonanzas are not supposed to last forever. Once charged we are supposed to use up our batteries before having them charged again. Continuous charging risks accumulated damage.

Recently it has been suggested that one opportunity for good health is to spend more time in a fasting state, i.e. being efficient rather than partying all the time without a care in the world. Many cultures undertake periods of fasting as part of their religious observance, such as during Navratras or Ramzan (Ramadan). Many people observe fasts on certain days every week. Fasting is not only important for their spiritual wellbeing, but is also an important part of their identity, culture and relationship with friends, family and community. Intermittent fasting has a number of benefits for health, including self-discipline and self-awareness, especially of our hunger and eating behaviours. Importantly, fasting can also contribute to waist loss and improved health.

One of the many current dieting methods involves intermittent fasting or time-dependent eating (i.e. eating only between certain hours of the day, giving the body at least twelve hours without energy coming in as food or drink). This actually works nicely for weight loss and is very easy to understand. Unlike many complicated diets where we have to eat different things, intermittent fasting just means cutting back one day and eating the same on another. This makes it a lot more portable than having to eat specific things all the time.

Whether such fasting strategies can also capture any of the benefits that long-term calorie restriction can provide is unclear. But what fasting changes the most is our mindset around food.

Mindset

While it is abundantly clear that being overweight is bad for our health and its long-term prospects, and most of us don't like being overweight and how it makes us feel, it is just not that easy to shift. We hang onto our fat just like we hang onto our hard-earned wealth.

We might go on a diet or do some exercise, spending away our excess fat on other pursuits. And these work, but only for a time, because we frequently slide back into our old ways and old behaviours. This is not just because old habits die hard. Another reason is because our brain wants us to. Our brain thinks like Goldilocks.

When Goldilocks ransacks the house of the three bears, she scopes things out first. A lot of things are not to her taste. She only feels really satisfied when things are 'just right'. After all, she is a little girl, and not a big bear.

Of course, if she were a big bear, her tastes would have been entirely different. She would have only felt comfortable sleeping in the big bed, sitting in a big chair and eating a big steaming bowl of porridge.

The Golden Mean

 Some things are just too much. Some things are just not enough. For the most part, the best course is right down the middle between the two extremes. This is just how Goldilocks chooses what is just right for her.

The middle road between two extremes has long been considered the best way forward. In Greek philosophy, virtue only existed between two vices, like courage exists somewhere between cowardice and bravado. Socrates taught that the way to happiness is to try to avoid the extremes on either side and know how to choose a golden mean that is just right for each individual. This Golden Mean is probably where Goldilocks (of the golden mane) got her moniker as well as her mental aptitude for choosing porridge

A central tenant of Buddhism is also the Middle Way, a path walked between the extremes of self-denial and abstinence (not enough) and self-indulgence and gluttony (too much). In the same way, instead of giving up chocolate or alcohol, or having too much of either, there is a golden middle way. Today, this is known as moderation, but it is simply channelling Goldilocks.

Our brain unconsciously weighs up these kinds of Goldilocks decisions hundreds of times every day, matching various choices against the kind of bear we are. Or rather, against the kind of bear it thinks we are.

For example, if our brain thinks we are really a big bear, then we will only feel 'just right' when we are eating from a big bowl. Equally, if our brain thinks we are little Goldilocks, we will only feel just right with the small breakfast bowl in front of us.

Most overweight individuals who are maintaining their excess body weight (instead of losing it) are eating a 'just right' amount for their body size, just as smaller individuals maintain their healthy weight by eating smaller amounts.

Our brain's keen desire to keep the status quo probably comes as an adaptation from past times of food shortage, when to accept weight loss was to accept defeat. Our brain thinks it knows what kind of bear we are based on the chemical signals it gets from our body, and especially our intestines and our fat. Over a period of time this information becomes hardwired and our mind becomes set on the answer.

And, of course, the problem with this mindset comes about when trying to change it. Goldilocks becomes as dissatisfied lying in the big bed or sitting in the big chair as Papa Bear would be eating only Baby Bear's insubstantial bowl of porridge.

The same thing often happens when we try to lose weight. Our brain defends the old (higher) mindset, even though there may be a billion extra calories still stored away in our fat tissue. It doesn't matter if we lose weight fast or gradually. If we get thinner, our brain makes us hungrier to get back to how it was before. It also delays when we feel full and reduces our enjoyment, so we have to eat more to feel 'just right'. It slows down our metabolism so that we burn fewer calories, allowing weight to be restored even though we still may be eating less. All of these factors drive us to unconsciously put the weight back on after we have tried so valiantly to consciously take it off. This cycle of weight goes down and then up again, like a yo-yo on a string.

It's not as though we want our diets to fail or we don't try hard enough. It's just that our fat-adapted biology works against us. Sadly, most diets that work in the short term fail in the long term. A couple of years later we often find ourselves back where we started, or sometimes worse. This has led some to argue that, at least in some people, repeated dieting makes us fatter.

Unfortunately the same systems that make us fight against weight loss don't get in the way of us gaining weight, possibly allowing us to make fat while the food is on the table or allowing Baby Bear to grow up and turn into Papa Bear (once the porridge-stealing Goldilocks is out of the way).

Some of the most successful long-term weight loss strategies work partly because they specifically resist these bounce-back mechanisms that try to put our weight back on every time we lose it. For example, by removing part of the stomach during weight-loss surgery, the appetite-stimulating effects that are triggered by weight loss are partly assuaged, leading to better and more sustained weight reduction than with conventional dieting. Some low-carbohydrate diets also work partly by generating ketones, fat-derived chemicals that also act to suppress our appetite even while we are losing weight.

But it is also possible to change our mind through psychology rather than physiology. This is because chemistry is not the only cue our brain uses to guide our consumption. It can also be entrained by other factors, like regular habits, smaller portions and even smaller plates. When presented with a big bowl most people generally just clean the plate. Regularly using a smaller plate with less food on it repeatedly signals to our brain that we are a wee bear after all.

Another important cue for eating is proximity. Sometimes the food is just there, sitting on the table waiting for someone to come by and eat it. So Goldilocks can't restrain herself. It is unlikely she would have ever gone into the bears' house without the fast food as a temptation. The idea she might have, as an intruder, gone to the pantry, got the ingredients, and turned on the stove to make the porridge herself is ridiculous. But because it was just there …

This is also how the human brain works (and how fast-food outlets make a killing). It responds to cues that help inform our behaviour. At the same time, changing our food environment can actually work to support our goal of waist management. We can make it harder to get to the calories and snacks (and easier to access the lower-calorie alternatives), so our Goldilocks brain stays out of the pantry.

Edging closer

Imagine that there is a crowd on top of a cliff. The crowd is getting larger. It slowly lurches forward. It has momentum. Disaster looms for those who are closest to the edge. Already some have fallen to their early death. How do we respond to this impending tragedy?

We could simply remove those at the front who are too close to tipping over. But they are hard to reach. Even if we could shift them, the empty spots would soon be taken by others pushing forward. We could ask the whole crowd to step back, but only those near the front would benefit. In fact, the majority would be inconvenienced for no gain whatsoever in the short term. Exactly the same dilemma exists for the public health management of obesity.

Some people are clearly very overweight and, as a result, their health sits close to the edge, with fat already beginning to tip over and get deposited out of place. The people at the edge really need to be helped back, or the consequences may be dire. So encouraging waist loss is a no-brainer.

Equally, for those who are a 'normal weight', just like they were when they were 25, there seems little reason to change what they are doing. Even though they might be creeping forward, they are nowhere near the edge.

But what about everyone else? In between these two extremes of big bears and little bears is where most of the world currently resides. Inside this zone some people are more efficient at storing fat in the right places, and get health advantages from safely banked fat. Others lay down fat in the wrong places even when they are not very overweight. In the middle zone, our weight or even our waist size does not fully answer the important question of whether we have the 'out of place' fat that is so bad for our health. How close are we to the tipping point?

If we were to average out the 'safe' bankers, those with overflowing coffers and everyone else in between, the net result of our weight on longevity would appear to be almost neutral. And this turns out to be the case. A number of recent studies have shown that those who are only modestly overweight do not actually die more frequently than people with a normal weight (at least in the short term).

This kind of data has led some people to rethink whether we really should be encouraging absolutely everyone to lose their excess weight. Maybe we should just accept our size and get on with the rest of our lives? If there is no net risk, maybe it's all just crisis hype to make us buy their product or feel like we are doing something worthwhile. Maybe only some people will benefit, while most of us will suffer the slings and arrows of outrageous diets? Why should we follow everyone else into disaster, like a lemming?

The lemming suicides

 In the Arctic tundra live small hairy rodents known as lemmings. They look a bit like hamsters, with long soft fur and short tails. They are famous for their population explosions followed by en masse migrations, like an army in search of greener pastures. These greener pastures are invariably downhill from their mountain burrows, so sometimes they fall over in their haste. Sometimes they drown crossing rivers. But they are not deliberately reckless.

Lemmings do not deliberately jump off cliffs or altruistically commit suicide to reduce population numbers for the common good. Nor do they automatically follow a leader if one accidentally falls off.

The myth of the crazed, suicidal lemming was brought to public attention by Walt Disney in the Oscar-winning *White Wilderness* nature documentary. Having heard of the single-minded migratory behaviour of Norwegian lemmings, Disney's film crew staged an event that captured the public imagination.

The filming took place on the outskirts of Calgary in Canada, far from the Arctic sea where the lemmings actually lived, let alone the true (Norwegian) lemmings that were famed for their mass migrations. So the crew imported as many lemmings as they could find. Disney paid locals '$1 a live lemming', mostly to Inuit children who kept them as pets.

The pet lemmings were all herded together to look like an army, and then coaxed to the edge of a cliff beside a river. None was crazy enough to jump, so some were thrown off. Others were collected in the back of a truck and simply tipped onto the rocks below. The whole thing was staged!

Although humans have been happily killing rodents around their homes for millennia, the seemingly self-destructive behaviour of the lemmings captured the imagination of people across the world. In 1958, when the film was released, the world was changing radically. Just as Disney had previously used a mouse to explore human traits, people could also see in this headstrong rush to disaster the same nihilism exemplified by the movie *Rebel Without a Cause*. In fact, James Dean had recklessly driven to his own death just over two years earlier. But humans are not lemmings, nor are lemmings human. Some are Mouseketeers. But not lemmings.

It is absolutely true that not everyone will fall over the edge. But that does not mean that putting up a sign saying 'Keep back from the edge' is not beneficial. In exactly the same way, health messages encouraging weight control are mostly a public control barrier applied universally in recognition of the dangers of tipping over.

The reason for the public health message calling for everyone to watch their weight is simply because if only those few who are really very overweight were told to lose weight, even if they could do it successfully, more people would still be becoming overweight all the time, because this targeted message is not addressing the surging forces that eventually tip people over.

So the rationale for telling everyone to get thinner (apart from the obvious sales in diet and exercise products) is not to make everyone healthy today. On average, they are not made much healthier by dieting. This is why, when we look at the data, the gains most people get from dieting in terms of improving cholesterol, blood pressure and other markers of health risk are modest at best. And the overall effects of weight loss on human health looks underwhelming. But this is a short-term view.

The more overweight we are today the more overweight we risk becoming tomorrow. The closer we stand to the tipping point at which we eventually deposit fat in the wrong places, the more likely it is that we will eventually tip over it. On average, our excess fat may not be that risky today or maybe even in the short term, but we should all still be stepping back from the edge.

The other reason to keep at it is that life is a slow-moving game, played over decades. It often takes a long time to realize the legacy of diet and lifestyle on our health. Moreover, once tissues are eventually damaged by excess fat, because of finite regenerative capacity, just like Humpty Dumpty, all the King's doctors cannot put him together again, no matter what diet they use. Hearts, brains, kidneys and the pancreas are just like eggs: once broken they can't be mended.

This means that in the very long term the latent benefits of waist control are much more substantial, even in those who are not hugely overweight. Having taken decades to accumulate our fat, it may take at least a decade to turn the same ship around. This is consistent with the few long-term studies that are following overweight people who are dieting and exercising and comparing their outcomes to those who are not, demonstrating that good things come eventually to those who do the good things. Moreover, their continuing legacy of better health, lower risks for disease and a lower probability of dying early can still be observed several decades later. And this is really why our efforts today to reduce our fat deposits, by spending them with physical activity or not adding to them by dieting, may not seem like we have made much difference in the short term, but will eventually be worth their weight in gold.

The bottom line

Most people have more fat than they need. This is not because they are gluttonous, self-destructive, undisciplined or indifferent to their plight. They are not crazy lemmings rushing headlong to their doom. They are simply the product of their environment, making hay while the sun shines.

Banking fat is not a sin. But it is deadly. Once it tips from the right places where it can be safely stored into the wrong places where it cannot, our health problems really begin. Staying away from this tipping point is the reason we all should aim to lose some weight and keep our waistline under control. It will not make us healthier in the short to medium term. It will feel like an unnecessary imposition and our body will fight to stay in position. But in the long term it will mean a longer, healthier and happier life on average.

This is all well and good. But how is it possible to achieve and sustain weight loss? Consuming fewer calories to add less to our stores and being more physically active to use more of them up is the simple answer. Most diets work only because they limit our choices, forcing us to follow a different menu (and eat less) instead of the diet that we are used to. We could also achieve the same thing by substituting lower calorie versions of the things we eat anyway, or by removing the calorie bonuses that really make our fat banks swell. What works best depends on the individual, where and when they get their calories. One diet will not fit everyone, no matter what the hype suggests. We all eat differently. So we have to find our own way like Goldilocks, taking a few wrong turns as we go, but finding in the end something that is just right.

Do I really have to ...

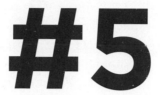

Get off the couch?

Q: What is wrong with a still life?
A: It only works for paintings.

Q: Can I make up for it by exercising?
A: Exercising helps, but sitting is still a problem.

Q: Should I get myself a better ergonomic chair?
A: So you can sit down for longer?

Q: How much more exercise do I need to do?
A: Go the extra mile.

Q: Do the fittest really survive?
A: The unfit certainly don't.

Q: What is the best kind of exercise?
A: The one that you'll do.

Most of us really aren't that active. This is not because we never go for a run, play sport or go the gym. It is simply because most of our lives are spent sitting at a desk, in a car, around the meal table or on the couch at home watching TV (or reading really interesting books). After hard days working like a dog, we're exhausted! But very likely this work involved sitting on our behind for the most part of 10 hours. Most of us haven't moved enough each day to burn as many calories as there are in a bowl of ice-cream. This is what's known as being **sedentary**, and is an all too common reality of modern lives.

In our distant past, we used to be 'hunters and gatherers'. We would walk or run on average somewhere around 16 kilometres (or 10 miles) every day, just hunting and gathering. This was the equivalent of taking the good part of 20,000 steps each day. For our well-adapted ancestors, being active was a matter of life and death. To survive the harsh and impoverished environment, we had to keep moving. This was our strength.

By comparison, today we hardly move at all. Modern adults take an average of 7500 steps each day (or just less than 6 kilometres or 4 miles). However, a typical modern office worker may only take 2000 steps a day. This is the equivalent of moving no more than 1.6 kilometres or walking a mile each and every a day.

Unlike our ancestors, we don't really have to move to survive. We won't be left behind. We can easily get by in our opulent world, taking public transport, driving in our car or just strolling along to the pantry, without going the (nine) extra miles.

But there's getting by, and then there's being healthy. The same adaptations that can keep us alive in one environment can become a killer in a completely different one.

For example, take the famous-but-true story of the spotty-coloured moth that liked to sit camouflaged on a spotty tree. The birds couldn't see him up there, and so he survived. His spots ensured his survival for millennia.

However, during the Industrial Revolution, pollution from coal fires darkened the bark of his tree and his mottled spots made him stand out in the gloom like a fast-food sign. So the same spots that once saved his life become his ruinous inheritance.

In much the same way, our evolutionary biology may be far better adapted to our own ancient environment (where we spent millions of years perfecting our survival skills) than to the few hundred years of post-Industrial prosperity, supermarkets and desk jobs that now make us show our spots. This is the obvious philosophy behind modern Palaeolithic diets. But we did a lot more during the Palaeolithic Age than just eat.

The big problem in today's environment is that not only do we eat very differently, but we are also over ten times less active. And this mismatch now affects our chances of survival. Our sedentary life increases our risk of developing many common health problems including obesity, heart disease, high blood pressure, diabetes, depression, weak bones and some cancers. For example, people who rarely undertake regular physical activity have, on average, twice the risk of heart attacks when compared to active individuals. A similar difference is observed if we compare an average smoker to the risks of a non-smoker.

It is thought that every year, about one in eight deaths in the world are now attributable to being sedentary, making it the fourth leading cause of death globally. This equates to more deaths caused by people being inactive than from smoking. If we truly want to survive, it means not only spending more time being active and getting fitter, but spending less time sitting still, being a couch potato.

Couch potatoes

We are not really 'couch potatoes'. This rather pejorative term was invented to describe the almost vegetative state some people fall into while glued to their television. Before the modern era of plasma and LCDs, all TVs were a giant glass tube. TVs in the sixties were sometimes called the 'boob tube', referring to the stupidity of the programs and their audience (as in the 'idiot box'), rather than any risqué adult content. Those who ecstatically loved and became co-dependent with their TV were called 'tubers' (the same name given to swollen root vegetables which, like the dedicated TV viewer, happily sit for long periods in the dark without moving). However, this clever term was far too esoteric and never stuck.

Potatoes are also tubers. Potatoes are also vegetables, drawing the unfortunate connotation of those in a persistent coma. So in the seventies the sofa-bound 'tuber' evolved into the common 'couch potato'.

Today, the computer screen and the smart phone has pride of place. Moreover, their tremendous adaptability (providing communication, entertainment, information and almost everything else), now means we spend more time in front of a screen today than even the most dedicated tuber of the 1960s.

This screen time may be an important source of daily productivity. You could even be writing a bestselling health book during your screen time. Yet the time we spend on our screen also makes a difference to our health and its future prospects. Generally, the greater our screen time, the more likely it is that we develop all sorts of health problems and have shorter lives as a result.

The reason is not just simply that couch potatoes are missing out on the health benefits of being active and the many other healthy things they could be doing if the TV/computer was turned off. In fact, the negative effects of sitting for prolonged periods are just as significant for those people who get plenty of exercise at other times. These people are sometimes called active couch potatoes or weekend warriors. They may go the gym, jog or go crazy on the weekends, but they still spend most of their day stuck on their chair. Even if we are at home all day we try to blitz all the housework so we can sit down and do some 'solid' work at the computer before the kids come home from school.

Conversely, people who sit for fewer than 4 hours per day but don't exercise at all can be at least as healthy as those who exercise at least 5 hours per week but spend most of their day sitting down. It is often argued that the health and slim figure of the fifties housewife had something to do with the long hours she spent on her feet doing the housework, walking to shops and around her neighbourhood. It is certainly true that modern life reduces housework and makes room for sitting screen time. However, the fact that we also eat far more than we did in the fifties and smoke much less might be a better explanation for our widening girth.

While it might feel comfortable on the couch, spending most of our waking hours not moving turns out to be directly damaging to our health in many different ways. This is particularly the case when we are sitting for long unbroken periods, sometimes for many hours at a time, and often cumulatively for 8 to 10 hours every day (at the computer, at the desk, in the car, on the train or in front of the television). However, every hour we continuously spend on our behind is associated with a shorter life expectancy.

On the buses

 The problem with sitting down all day was first conclusively demonstrated over 50 years ago in studies on the buses and trams of London, England.

The conductors moved up and down the bus, climbing over 500 steps per working day selling the tickets. On the other hand, the drivers spent over 90 per cent of their work time seated at the wheel. They both worked in the same environment on the same buses. But the physically inactive drivers developed 50 per cent more heart disease than the physically active conductors. In cases where both drivers and conductors developed heart disease, the drivers were more likely to die early from it than the conductors.

Bus drivers' uniforms were also found to be generally wider at the waist than their conductor colleagues. But even after adjusting for any obvious differences in physique, as well as other risk factors for dying young, the conductors still won out over the bus drivers.

The exact same phenomenon was also observed in postmen, where the ones who cycled or walked to deliver the mail had fewer heart attacks compared with the clerks who worked their day behind the counter. This phenomenon became known as the 'sitting disease'.

The negative effects of prolonged sitting are more apparent in women, in whom the normal protections against disease and the longer average life expectancy of women over men are both diminished by time spent sitting down. For example, women who are inactive and sitting for more than six hours a day have about twice the risk of dying in a given period as women who are active, and sit for less than 3 hours. This is even after adjusting for the kind of work they do and the different pay they receive for it.

Why is moving around so good for us? In order for a human body to move around, or even stand up, its muscles need to contract. This process requires energy, which is supplied by the sugar and fat absorbed and stored by our muscles while they are at rest. When we are sitting for prolonged periods our muscles don't move, so they expend little or no energy. Consequently our muscles have little need to take up any spare fuel. Inactive muscles also get progressively smaller (if we don't use them, we lose them), which further reduces their contribution to our energy-burning metabolism. Consequently, when we are sitting for long periods, more of the burden of calories we eat is placed elsewhere and ultimately ends up as fat. On average, the longer our siting time, the greater our waistlines become.

However, sitting down for long periods is not just an easy way to get fat (or fatter). In two women with exactly the same weight or waistline measurement, the one who spends most of her days in unbroken sitting has a higher rate of developing heart disease and a reduced rate of survival from it.

Bent out of shape

 Sitting down all day is also not good for our backs. In fact, it's awful for them. If there is one part of our spotty human body that now finds itself utterly exposed in our modern environment tied to our desk chair, it is our spine.

Prolonged sitting without back support alters the curve of the spine, especially the leaning-forward posture we employ when working at a desk and on a computer (in other words, most of the time!).

This bent posture puts extra pressure on the spinal discs of our lower back. Spinal discs are super shock-absorber cushions of cartilage that sit between each bony vertebrae, allowing our spine to bend. However, degeneration of the discs naturally occurs with age.

At the same time, the core muscles of our back and abdomen have little to do while sitting, so become weaker and reduce their ability to protect our back at other times. We also get heavier with our inactivity, putting even more shock onto our shock absorbers. Eventually, something's gotta give.

Initially we may just feel a bit stiff after being stuck at a desk all day. As we get older this progresses into intermittent back pain. Most people will experience back pain at some point in their life. In most cases it will be short-lived and self-limiting. But in some cases, back pain will become chronic and debilitating.

Good chairs and back supports can help our posture a bit. But even the best (expensive) ergonomically designed chair cannot solve the real problem — that we are sitting in it all day. For the sake of our back, we need to take a break (and preferably lots of them, frequently). So go take one now!

(Don't worry, this book's not going anywhere. It'll still be here when you get back.)

~~~~~~

It is not that breaking our day by getting up from our desk will help us get fit or lose weight. In fact, standing up frequently hardly burns any calories, let alone enough to lose weight (unless we also spend that standing time doing some kind of physical activity — like climbing stairs on a bus). So it's not simply working our backsides off by burning calories that makes getting off our backsides work for our health.

When our muscles are being active they send out signals to the body that make it run more efficiently. By contrast, inactive muscles are costly to our health, partly because they make the body believe that it is doing more than enough to get by and has no particular reason to do better. This is most likely the reason that sitting is harmful in the long term.

The potential solution is pretty obvious: we should break up long periods of sitting by getting up, at least once every hour. The more breaks we can take the better.

There are a number of different ways to conveniently break up our sitting time in our workplace (apart from changing professions). There are standing work-stations and touch-screen computer terminals. There is replacing the old office chair with a big, soft inflated ball (i.e. a fit ball) that requires constant muscle activity to prevent you falling off. There is just getting up and talking to our colleagues instead of sending them an email or text. There are untold opportunities to move everywhere we go.

None is a perfect solution. It's actually hard work standing all the time. It's easy to fall off the ball seat. Sometimes there are things that are better said in a carefully considered email than face to face. But for good health, we have to find a way out of our desk chair.

Television

More than any other part of our day, the relaxed time we spend in front of the TV is the least active. We just sit there, transfixed by our favourite shows, often with or after our evening meal.

Sure, we could get up now and then, but who can ever find the remote to press pause? And if we ever manage to get up, it's likely that we would just go to the kitchen and fix ourselves a snack. Furthermore, everywhere else in the house is dark and the kids are asleep, so what can we really do but sit quietly in the dark and grow older, like a potato tuber?

The association between screen time and dying young is more than just the effects of a lot of time spent sitting or not exercising. This is possibly because TV does more than simply transfix us. It also rewires our brain, subtly changing how we think in the real world. And no, it's not because of the electromagnetic waves. We needn't wear foil on our heads!

Just like all the things we see and hear in our lives, the content we watch on the screen influences our thought processes. For example, at least two-thirds of the food we choose to eat is in part influenced by information we get from our TV. Obviously, there are the food advertisements and the product placements. But there is also the behaviour and attitudes of our favourite characters whose fast-paced decisiveness we envy so much. If only we could say those cool words or do those things (impulsively) without thinking!

So we try. But the problem is that we live in the real world. Real-world choices don't need to work under the constraints of plot or program scheduling. And if we are impulsive like the characters we love on TV, a number of things can go wrong. One of these things can be eating too much.

Like a TV detective responding instinctively to clues, we get clues from our food-rich environment all the time. These draw us closer to the target. But instead of criminals, we are inexorably drawn to consume, because that is where the delicious clues are leading us.

Food porn

 Everyone loves cooking shows. There are more and more on our television screens, and even whole stations devoted to the subject.

These shows are sometimes derided as 'food porn'. This is because we imagine doing it while watching celebrities actually doing it. There is certainly all the same voyeuristic sensuality, temptation, excitement, adventure, doing things we'd never do at home. People vividly living their dreams with no consequences, no mess or dirty dishes in the morning. What's not to like? What's not to want?

Whether cooking shows are simply adult entertainment or actually influence our behaviour is debated. Some studies say they have an effect. Others suggest we know the difference between reality TV and real life. But when we see an exotic dish on special at the supermarket, aren't we just a bit more tempted than we would have been had we not watched the cooking show?

Finally, if we are eating when watching the TV, we are literally mindlessly eating. There is only so much attention we can spare, and TV shows are designed to grab it all (otherwise we'd be off channel surfing). So there's not much mind left to pay attention to our eating and stop when we are full. Often we wait for the end of the show to tell us that a meal is over.

Worse still is that the enjoyment of a meal in front of TV comes from the TV show that has our attention, rather than our meal. This makes a meal without TV (or eating a meal without any decent program to watch) seem unfulfilling, so we sometimes eat more to get the same pleasure we are used to getting. The solution is simple: don't eat meals in front of the TV. Food is food. TV is TV. (This also means less food falls down into the deep crevasses of the couch, down where the couch potatoes like to grow.)

Counter action

Sometimes, we try to make up for our mostly sedentary lives by dedicating some time for physical activity. This is **exercise**. It is probably the easiest way for most of us to get more physical activity in our days.

Regular exercise in significant amounts (we're talking at least an hour a day, every day) can partly counteract the time we spend inactive in our offices or in front of the TV. It does not fully eliminate its effects, but it can substantially reduce its impact.

The problem is that about one-third of adults do no exercise at all and most of the others only now and then in very small and short doses. Not only is this not enough to counter-balance our sedentary ways, it may also further compound them.

However, dedicated exercise is not the only way to live a more active life. We can also slot in more activity throughout our day by taking the stairs instead of the lift or walking the kids to school instead of driving. This sort of opportunistic activity can add up to make a real difference. Health outcomes are improved whether regular physical activity is performed as part of an exercise program or part of our daily life or part of our job. People who are habitually active (even if they don't exercise) live about five years longer on average than those who don't. But while opportunistic activity is important, unless we are doing a very physical job, it can be hard to get enough of it on a regular basis to make a very big difference to our health or fitness.

Freezing cold

 If we were ever to get really cold (and couldn't just put on a sweater, go inside or turn the heater on) our body would try to keep us warm. Cold causes our muscles to rapidly contract and relax in small movements, which we experience as shivering. This involuntary physical activity produces heat as a by-product to keep us warm. At the same time, special (brown) fat cells in our body also start burning fat to generate heat to keep us warm. Together these mechanisms help us not to catch our death.

This shivering and fat burning when we are cold is a bit like doing exercise. And like exercise, we don't get enough of it in this day and age. Better temperature control during our winters with modern heaters means that our bodies have no good reason to burn excess fuel to generate heat, so become less efficient at doing so. In fact, we are more prone to not make heat, in order to stay cool. We also now don't need to burn extra energy chopping logs or carrying coal for the fires.

So it has been argued, not unreasonably, that indoor heating has contributed to rising rates of obesity. But the problem with this catchy hypothesis is that those equatorial countries that experience very little change in temperature from month to month have also seen the same obesity epidemic as those who used to suffer a desperately cold winter. So we really can't blame global office warming for our woes.

If doing an active job, regularly getting cold or both (as they often go outside together) are not options, the easiest and most practical way to incorporate more activity into our lives is to exercise.

Since ancient times, it has been universally declared that exercise is the best medicine. Every great civilization contains some pithy adage that exercise both sustains good health and is a cure for all illness. Given the lack of effective alternative treatments in those days, it is hardly any wonder that exercise came out on top. Hippocrates may well have found exercise to be the best medicine simply because aspirin hadn't been invented yet. Yet today we have a very different environment. What protected us in ancient times may not do the same now. And besides, now we have drugs and surgery, as well as an endless array of medical supports.

Exercise also carries the expectation of success. This is partly because sick people find it hard to exercise. So we only see the really healthy ones out on the cycle paths or in the gym, which biases our perception of how good exercise really must be for us.

Most people think that exercise works by just burning calories that would otherwise be deposited around our waistlines as fat. It does burn energy but not as much as most people think. For example, the total fuel burnt walking for an hour is contained in a single Snickers bar or a single can of soft drink. So even if we set aside a whole hour every day for walking, this won't offset the excess calories we consume in our modern diets. To create the negative energy balance we need to lose weight requires us to exercise quite a lot more or, more practically, eat fewer calories as well as exercise.

Importantly, the value of doing regular exercise in promoting human longevity is apparent not just for those who are overweight, but equally for those with a healthy waistline already. It is also good for our health regardless of whether or not we lose weight while doing it. This means that exercise can't just be calorie burning. It must also be something else.

When we exercise, our muscles send signals back to the body that improve and maintain the way it functions. Some of these signals are sent via the nerves while some are chemical signals released into the bloodstream (known as **exer-kines**). The identification of these chemicals makes it theoretically possible that one day we will be able to mimic the beneficial effects of exercise with a pill. However, today we must rely on our own signals to trigger the benefits we crave. It doesn't seem to take much to reap these positive effects. Even as little as 5 minutes a day appears to better than nothing at all.

High on exercise

Anyone who has ever gone to the gym or for a run will know that afterwards it is not just our body that feels different but our mind as well. And if we feel better, we do better and we are better. In so far as our health is determined by our emotional and psychological wellbeing, one of the most important reasons why exercise keeps us alive is because it affects our mind.

The runner's high

 Almost everyone who exercises regularly sometimes experiences a sudden feeling of profound exhilaration and relaxation. This is known as the 'runner's high' but it can also occur after other kinds of physical activity.

It is popularly thought that this sensation occurs as our brain naturally releases chemicals that have similarities to mind-altering drugs like opium, cannabis and amphetamines. In this paradigm, exercise is like a drug, and gym-junkies are its addicts. However, endogenous drug levels after exercise are nothing like those taking hard drugs, and though exercise is habit forming, it is not usually addictive.

Another hypothesis suggests that the same pathways that give us the sense of satisfaction after a meal also work during our exercise high. This may be another reason why regular exercise helps curb overeating. By augmenting the reward circuitry of our brains, it helps us to reach our pleasure zone without having to overeat.

Ever had a great idea pop into your head when doing exercise? Exercise not only makes us feel better but also makes us think better. This is not just when we are doing it. In the long term, regular exercise also directly enhances our capacity for learning and memory function and slows the decline of both as we get older. This is because we learn and remember things by changing and remodelling the connections in our brains. This is known as plasticity.

Exercise enhances plasticity and stimulates the growth and development of brain cells, increasing our capacity for attention, thinking, processing, remembering and coping with challenges on the run. This is probably why exercise also has protective benefits for several diseases of the brain, including dementia and Parkinson's disease.

Survival of the fittest

What does not kill us makes us stronger. Precisely because vigorous physical activity is taxing, the stresses and strains it places on our body cause it to adapt. Cumulatively, these adaptations are what we call 'getting fitter' or 'getting into shape'.

These changes are far more than just bigger, stronger muscles, or acquiring the contoured body shape of athletes and body builders. These adaptations also lead to complex changes in many other areas, including our heart, circulation, brain, nerves and hormonal functions. Cumulatively, these changes also add up to a substantially improved health outlook and longer survival time for the fittest.

The many 'getting fit' adaptations that occur after regular exercise essentially come about to improve our capacity for future physical activity and its associated stresses and strains. However, these adaptations also have important spin-off benefits on other processes, many of which are relevant to our health and resilience. This explains why being fit is good for our health beyond the fact that fit people are getting the benefits of doing exercise or spending time not being a couch potato.

Being 'unfit' essentially means that our body is not physically adapted to do the job it is asked to do. So it doesn't have the capacity to do what we ask of it. We experience this as exhaustion, which comes more easily to unfit people than fit ones.

For example, muscles that are regularly used will adapt to become bigger and stronger, meaning they are more capable of getting the job done next time with less effort and less fatigue at the end of it. Of course this makes it easier and safer doing things ourselves, like carrying the groceries or the kids. But at the same time, exercise changes the metabolic capacity of our muscles and our body overall. For example, bigger muscles are also more efficient at taking up and burning fuel. This is a bonus response and helpful for keeping fat under control and reducing its consequences on our health.

The six pack

 For men, nothing defines physical health better than six-pack abs. The sexy appearance of six bulges (in two rows of three bulges, one row on either side of the tummy button) is said to resemble the profile of six drink cans arranged on their side.

This appealing definition can only happen in those who are lean enough for the muscles to be seen through the layer of fat that normally covers the abdomen. Consequently, six packs are an endangered species. Extra tummy exercises (such as crunches) can make the abdominal muscles (abs) a bit larger. But it's getting rid of the fat that really reveals what lies underneath.

Most people have six packs hidden away. But some people only have a four pack (most famously Arnold Schwarzenegger). Others have eight or even ten. This has nothing to with athleticism, specific exercises or techniques. It's just anatomy and the way strands of connective tissue bind around the abs, like knots in a string of sausages. Still, the fewer the knots, the bigger the sausage.

The original six pack of drinks was invented by Coca-Cola to improve sales and ease mass transport for the average consumer. For the same reasons, this strategy was also subsequently adopted by beer companies. The irony is that soft drinks and the beer belly are the arch nemesis of six-pack abs. So perhaps calling your toned tummy a six pack is strangely appropriate — a way you can forgive your enemies but never forget their name.

Regular exercise can also get our heart into shape. Following regular exercise our heart gets a little bigger, allowing it to pump out more blood. And by pumping more strongly, the heart needs to beat less often to maintain the same output, the same way a bigger engine needs fewer revs to get up a hill. So our heart rate and blood pressure at rest will fall with training.

Important adaptations also occur in our bones. When we exercise, especially during weight-bearing and impact exercise, the density of our bones increases to compensate, even if our bones are already thin. This is especially useful as we get older, where typically there is a decline in bone strength that increases the risks of fracture. Exercise also strengthens muscles to reduce the risk and number of falls, meaning that the risk of fractures is doubly lowered by regular physical exercise.

The greatest improvements in health outcomes with physical activity are seen in those who can achieve and sustain improvements in their physical fitness. In fact, more than just doing lots of exercise or getting off our backside more often, people who are physically fit are about a third less likely to die in any given period.

Curiously, some people are intrinsically fit, even without doing much exercise. It doesn't seem fair. But at school, as in life, there is always some kid who could beat the pants off everyone else without raising a sweat. This is probably because they are born with or develop at a young age adaptations that make exercise easier. Most people need to work for their adaptations.

Physical fitness can be improved in most people by regularly undertaking some kind of activity that is taxing. Some people find this easier and make greater fitness gains than others when they exercise. This is not because they are already intrinsically fit. In fact, there is no correlation between a baseline, intrinsic fitness level and its response to regular exercise. Even the most inactive people can get fitter when they undertake regular exercise. It's just that some people seem to get a head start. Others catch up faster, and some just seem to be left behind no matter what.

Importantly, adaptations that occur with getting fit are reversible. For example, gains in muscle mass will go away after stopping going to the gym. Loss of muscle bulk and strength is also often observed in people who are inactive as a result of illness, and the elderly due to frailty. Equally, a small decline in heart size can be seen three weeks after stopping exercise. For this and many other reasons it is important to make a lifetime habit of exercise, and not see it as a temporary fad or just a health kick. And this means doing something we are willing to do season after season. Obviously, this is the best selling point of sport.

What should we do?

There are many different kinds of exercise we can do. Each has its own benefits and limitations. The best exercise is the one we are able to do regularly and enjoy, rather than as an optional 'add on' that we sometimes do 'when we have the time' (in other words, almost never). We don't keep doing something from which we derive no pleasure. That is called a punishment.

Some kinds of exercise are aerobic. This means physical activity that burns fuel using oxygen as the catalyst. It easy to recognize aerobic exercise because we have to breathe harder to get the oxygen we need. Most continuous activities of more than 3 minutes are aerobic, like walking, jogging, cycling, swimming, rowing, dancing, hiking, and sports such as football, soccer, squash and tennis.

It is generally recommended that all adults should undertake regular aerobic exercise in sessions of 30 minutes or more three to five days a week. Ideally we should get some aerobic exercise on most days. The aim is to get us to a point where we are breathing harder for extended periods of time. At the same time our heart will be beating faster to deliver the oxygen to our muscles. This combination allows aerobic training to increase the healthy capacity of our heart, lungs and circulation.

Another kind of activity is anaerobic exercise. This means undertaking short bursts of intense exertion at nearly 100 per cent effort, like sprinting or resistance training. Because the energy required for this kind of activity is at or above the maximal ability to supply oxygen to fuel the muscles, anaerobic exercise must rely on fuel already stored within the muscles themselves. This energy store is limited and maximal exertion cannot be sustained for more than 2 to 3 minutes before exhaustion sets in. By specifically burning up our muscle stores, anaerobic exercises set in motion adaptations that build strength, endurance and the size of our muscles. Exhausted muscles are also hungry and need to replenish their stores, which helps to keep our stored fat levels down. This is why some people believe that weight loss is better with anaerobic exercise than aerobic sports. But it probably matters more that we do it regularly than what we actually do.

Aerobic and anaerobic exercises are often combined (and probably best combined) when short bursts of high intensity (all-out) exertion are mixed with intervals of lower-level aerobic activity.

One obvious example is sport: sudden maximal exertion mixed with aerobic movement while being competitive or having fun. Another more formal way to get both aerobic and aneorobic training is known as 'high-intensity interval training (HIIT)'. For example, deliberately incorporating short periods of jogging as part of a walking program, progressing to sprints with alternate periods of walking or jogging. Interval training is more effective in burning fat and getting fit than sustained moderate intensity activity for the same or longer period. It is also time efficient, making the most of limited time to exercise. It can also be quite gruelling. But that's actually the point.

The bottom line

If we truly want to survive for the longest period of time that we can, we need to spend more time being active and getting fitter, and less time being a couch potato.

This is harder than it sounds. Add in 5 minutes every hour of the day dedicated to moving instead of sitting. Then add a dedicated exercise time on top, to make up for what we lose by sitting. And do all this regularly enough to get fitter than we were before. All this takes time. But of all the things we can do for our health, the dividends from any investment in physical activity may be more meaningful than anything else we can buy into.

Do I really have to ...

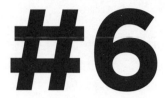

Eat less fat?

Q: Is fat really a problem?
A: Look at your waistline and decide.

Q: How much fat should I be having?
A: Less.

Q: Why is burning fat a bad idea?
A: Ever heard of tear gas?

Q: What about taking fish-oil supplements?
A: Fish oil only works in fresh fish (otherwise it smells fishy).

Q: Should I care about trans-fats?
A: You mean the poison disguised as fat?

Q: Is margarine better than butter?
A: They are both over 80 per cent fat.

We like to think that all the important choices are black and white; that some things are obviously good for us and others are clearly undesirable or harmful. Lots of stuff sits in the grey zone, so we can safely ignore them or do them without thinking too hard. But we like to separate the rights from the wrongs. The things we think are good for our health we should really go for. And the things that we think are bad for us, we make them outlaws or villains; we cut them out without remorse and leave them behind on the plate or in the shop.

The fat in our food has a bad name. And for good reason. More than any other component of our diet, fat is regarded as the archenemy of our waistlines and, consequently, our health. So much so that, at least until relatively recently, cutting out fat and the 'low-fat' label were synonymous with the (good) healthy alternative.

Fat has a number of characteristics that make it appear especially villainous. Pound for pound, the fat in a meal provides twice as many calories as the same amount of sugar or protein — which leaves a lot more to go straight to our hips. Consequently, many low-fat diets are also low-calorie diets, which helps us to lose weight, or at least not gain it as easily.

But we aren't simply what we eat. Just because we eat fatty food doesn't mean we are fat or going to get fat. Equally, eating a low-fat diet does not mean we will always lose weight. Any extra calories from any source ultimately leads to more fat in our body, no matter if it started out as fat, sugar or protein. Overeating anything and everything with calories will still make us fatter, even if it is branded as the healthy low-fat choice. It's just that we need to eat more of the low-fat diet than our standard fare to pack on the same number of pounds.

Regardless of what we eat, if we eat more than we need our body generates its own fat for energy storage. This is useful, like having a pantry or fridge to store food in our house. What we don't need to use today, we pop into storage so that when we come home hungry on another day, we can just open the door and take something out. The problem is that if we find somewhere else to eat — like when go out for dinner or stop for fast food/takeaway — there is no need to raid the stores at home and they just remain there.

In the same way, when we dine out on anything that contains calories, whether savoury, fatty or sweet, we leave the previously deposited fat stored in the pantry around our waistlines largely undisturbed. Often, we eat more than we need, so we add any leftovers to our store, stockpiling even more fat that we never seem to be able to use up.

Unlike our fridge or pantry, we can't just throw out anything we don't want anymore. It won't go off. We have to eat our way out.

Fortunately, the human metabolism means we are always burning fat. So getting rid of our excess fat is simply a matter of using the fat in our pantry to feed our metabolism, rather than going out and having another meal. This is also why just reducing the fat we eat (or changing the kind of fat we eat) is not enough to lose weight and reduce our waistline. We simply have to eat fewer calories to empty out our pantry.

Stocking up for the winter

 Bears are able to pile on the fat when the living is easy during summertime. This extra fat not only insulates them during the cold winter months, but also feeds them for almost a hundred days.

Migratory birds also stock up their fat store before their extraordinary long-distance flights to warmer climes, knowing that they will need all of it to get where they need to go without stopping for a snack along the way. Many double their weight in fat before take-off.

Humans can double their weight in fat too. But we don't hibernate, and every long-distance flight we take is usually accompanied by very little exertion and a meal trolley to boot.

Some animals (e.g. squirrels) and insects hoard their food in underground caches. Aesop recounts the story of the 'good' ant that works hard to store up food for winter, while the 'bad' cicada (or grasshopper) spends the whole summer singing. Of course when summer ends, the cicada is starving and asks for a meal. But the ant is reproachful and tells the cicada to buzz off.

The cicada's song is the loudest of any insect, as loud as any rock band. Anyone who has been kept awake by the racket made by cicadas outside their window understands why a frustrated ant might feel uncharitable.

Although the moral of the story is obvious, the adult cicada is dying anyway. After emerging from many years underground, the job of an adult male cicada is actually to sing as loud as it can, mate frequently and then starve to death, all in a matter of a month or two. Its singing is not frivolous in the least.

Ants divide their labour across their society. A queen does what a queen does. The other ants are assigned to different tasks, from caring for the young, cleaning or defending the nest. The grumpy old males are sent out to forage. They are sterile and expendable, so have no reason to sing themselves or even appreciate a love song.

Most things in nature have a purpose. This is known as dharma: the spots on a moth, the fat on a bear, the song of a cicada. The ant is wrong to think a cicada should toil like an ant. The cicada is wrong to think he should eat and survive the winter as the ant does. The true moral is that everyone should follow their own dharma which, even when performed badly, is far better than following someone else's.

Straight up

Some people think that it's not how much fat we are eating that is the problem, but rather the kinds of fat and their unnatural proportions. To understand how the fats in our diet potentially work for or against us, it is necessary to talk about their chemistry. Fortunately, it's really not that complicated.

Just imagine three long chains all linked to a single short backbone, something like a cricket wicket or the letter 'E'. Each stump is called a fatty acid. The three long stumps are linked to one another by a special sugar (called glycerol), which looks like the bails on the top of the wicket. The whole complex is called a **triglyceride**.

Triglycerides are the main energy store in all animals. Plants also store triglycerides inside their seeds, nuts, corn and other grains. Some plants also add triglycerides in the fleshy pulp around their seeds (e.g. olives, avocado and palm seeds). Altogether, over 95 per cent of the fat we eat is in the form of triglycerides.

All the triglycerides we eat can be used as fuel in our body. But they are not all the same. The length of their fatty acid stump/chains, as well as the presence of double links between adjacent carbons in the chain, changes their physical properties. When double bonds are present in a fatty acid chain, these are called **unsaturated fats**. Fatty acids without double bonds are said to be **saturated**. All natural products have a balance of saturated and unsaturated fats.

The reason a double bond or two makes a real difference is because it introduces a slight kink into the structure. This is like a pack of cards when some of the cards have been folded or bent – they just don't stack neatly together the way they did when they were all crisp and flat. In much the same way, without any kinks in their structure, straight saturated fat makes a great way to pack lots of fat into a small space.

This is one reason dieticians go on so much about how much saturated fat we include in our diets. For the same volume, denser saturated fat brings in more calories. For example, spreading our toast with butter, which is rich in saturated fat, adds more calories than the same volume of polyunsaturated margarine, even though both are over 80 per cent fat.

About 40 per cent of the triglycerides languishing in our body fat are saturated fat. This is also true for most animals. So when we eat animal fat in beef, pork, chicken, a burger or a sausage, about 40 per cent of the fat we are eating is going to be saturated fat.

Dairy products like cheese, milk and ice-cream have even more fat and about 60 per cent of it is saturated fat. Low-fat milk has half as much fat as full-cream milk, but 60 per cent of what it has is still saturated fat. Skim milk (made when all the cream is removed) has about ten times less fat than low-fat milk. Consequently, cream has ten times more fat than low-fat milk.

Adding together all the meat and all the dairy we eat constitutes about half of all the saturated fat we normally eat. Lacto-vegetarians cut all of these out and so usually eat half as much saturated fat as everyone else. But they still eat saturated fat. This is because saturated fat is also contained in many of our staple foods made from cereal grains (e.g. bread, pasta, cake, breakfast cereals, etc.), as well as vegetable oils and spreads. Although these products contain much lower proportions of saturated fats than unsaturated fats, given our high intake of them it all adds up in our diet.

The dense packing of saturated fats is also how fatty things like butter, lard, tallow and cocoa butter can stay solid at room temperature. Even coconut oil will start so solidify if the temperature drops below 24°C (76°F). When heated, saturated fats are still able to melt. This is very useful on toast. But it is also widely used in cooking to give us that pleasing melt-in-the-mouth sensation, as in chocolate or pastry.

Bread and butter

 Butter happens. When milk/cream is churned, the fat coalesces eventually into large enough globs that can be collected. This is butter.

We have had butter almost as long as we have been collecting milk. It only takes 30 seconds of sloshing before we have what the Irish poet Seamus Heaney called 'coagulated sunlight', which is not far off the mark.

Why we would put butter on bread is still a mystery. Is it the silky smooth melt-in-the-mouth taste? Is it waterproof lubrication for the jam or honey that would otherwise sink into the bread? Is it glue to stick the topping on top?

Sandwiches were said to have been invented by the Earl of Sandwich in the 18th century. Tired of all his toppings falling off his bread while trying to snack and play cards at the same time, he conceived of the notion of adding another slice on top, keeping both his hands and the card table clean.

Of course wraps have been around since bread was invented. But sandwiches would never have worked without the butter to bind the whole. And the dry bread just acts as a wick to watery cucumbers and quickly becomes soggy without a thick waterproof coat of fatty butter.

Kinky

All the kinks in unsaturated fats mean that when they are purified they are generally liquid (an oil) at room temperature, like most vegetable, corn and seed oils.

Some fats have many double bonds in their chains. These are called **polyunsaturated fatty acids**. Some have only one kink in their chain. These are called **monounsaturated fatty acids.**

Having only one kink makes monounsaturated fats more flexible than solid straight saturated fats. Consequently, monounsaturated fats are found in all animals and plants where they provide extra flexibility to membranes while being oily enough to keep the water out. Around 55 per cent of the fat stored as triglycerides in our body is monounsaturated (chiefly oleic acid). Similarly, the major fat in the beef, pork, chicken breast and egg yolk we eat is also monounsaturated fat. About one-third of the fat in dairy products is also monounsaturated. Consequently, all the things that provide saturated fat to our diet are also the major sources of monounsaturated fat too.

The one kink of monounsaturated fats also confers the useful culinary property of being liquid at room temperature but still having the capacity to become solid when refrigerated. This means that oils naturally rich in monounsaturated fat, like peanut, avocado and canola oils, don't take kindly to the freezing cold.

The polyunsaturated fats have so many double-bond kinks in their structure that we usually call them oils rather than fat. Polyunsaturated oils with their multiple kinks such as corn, soybean, cottonseed, linseed (flaxseed) and safflower oils, can stay oily well below the freezing temperature of water. This is one of the reasons they are found in such high amounts in krill and cold-water oily fish (but more on fish oil later in this chapter).

Today about 20 per cent of the fat we consume is polyunsaturated, over half of which comes from seed and vegetable oils used in cooking and another quarter from the wheat and other cereal grains in our diet. Interestingly, less than 3 per cent of our body fat is made of the kinky polyunsaturated variety. This is not because we don't use it. As detailed below, there are actually many things we use it for. It's just that the extra kinks in polyunsaturated oils do not lend themselves to efficient mass-storage in humans.

By contrast, plants usually store triglycerides in a polyunsaturated form. Some have a larger component of monounsaturated fat (e.g. olives, peanuts and rapeseed). Occasionally, special plants (e.g. coconut, cacao) use saturated fat for storage. This is why different vegetable oils can have very different properties, both in the pan and in the pantry.

The Emperor's new butter

 Although margarine is often thought of as a polyunsaturated spread, this is mostly advertising. Standard margarine still contains about 20 per cent saturated fat. By contrast, around about half of the fat in butter is saturated fat. Both butter and margarine are still at least 80 per cent fat.

Margarine has always been an imitation of butter, rather than a culinary stalwart in its own right. The original margarine was said to have been conceived in response to a challenge laid down by the French Emperor. In 1869 strikes swept across France. The workers were revolting. The army was hungry and about to go to war. There was not enough butter to spread around. But rather than tell them that instead of buttered croissants they should all just go and eat brioche (you actually also need butter to make brioche), the Emperor hatched a scientific competition to find a cheap alternative to butter.

Supposedly there was only one entry, which naturally won. It was simply to mix beef fat (tallow — mostly saturated fat) and leftover skim milk (milk after the cream has been taken out). It wasn't yellow but it effectively put the creamy fat back. It was only subsequently, when tallow was replaced with vegetable oil and the whole concoction was dyed yellow, that the margarine alternative became the new butter.

Spoilers

The same double bonds that make unsaturated fats oily are also their Achilles heel, because they make them uniquely vulnerable to attack by oxygen, especially when they are heated. In other words, those double bonds mean that unsaturated fats like vegetable oil can go off (or spoil). This is the main reason that humans have historically preferred using saturated fats from butter, lard and tallow (i.e. fat from animals). Saturated fats do not have double bonds and don't go off as easily, so can be stored for long periods or left in the pantry at room temperature without smelling out the place. Of course, copious preservatives are added today to polyunsaturated fats to achieve a longer shelf life. So going off is not an issue for modern polyunsaturated oils and spreads made from them, like margarine. But preserving unsaturated fat is tricky or impossible for whole foods, like fish. For example, a fish can get pretty smelly if it is left out of the water for a prolonged period of time. This is mostly because of the spoiling of the polyunsaturated fats in fish oils. And this is also why fish must be stored carefully on ice or in the fridge and used as soon as possible. Even then, fish starts to smell bad long before it is actually rotten.

Splatter

 Have you ever heated a frypan of oil to the point it sizzles and spits burning oil all over the kitchen? It's not because you have the cook top on too high or you're not doing it like the celebrity chefs on TV. It's just chemistry.

Actually, pure oil doesn't spit and explode at all when heated. But water does. We all know the riotous bubble of boiling water on a stove.

Oil doesn't dissolve in water and water does not dissolve in oil. They separate into their own layers. The water sinks to the bottom while the oil floats on the top, like an oil slick on the ocean.

In an ocean there is more water than oil. But in our frypan there is usually more oil than water. So any water that gets accidentally mixed in with the oil while we are cooking gets trapped underneath the oil slick. As we heat up the pan, this trapped water gets hotter and hotter until it suddenly flashes into a bubble of steam, which rises and explodes from the surface of the oil, showering little globs of oil everywhere.

One way to stop this from happening is to heat the pan first, before you add the oil (thus evaporating any water from the pan). Another trick is to store the pan with a paper towel or give it a dry wipe before use, thus eliminating any stray water from the frying pan.

Another time we often get spitting oil is the moment we drop our food into a hot frying pan. We hear it crackle in the pan (and feel splashes of the hot oil burning our bare arms). This only happens because free water on the surface of the food immediately sinks below the oil, gets really hot, becomes steam and then explodes, creating the sizzling effect that characterizes cooking with oil.

Patting down our food with a dry towel first will reduce spattering. Leaving the food out for a while before frying it (e.g. in the fridge without the wrapping on) will also allow its surface to dry. Coating the food in batter or flour will also soak up any moisture, as will parboiling (blanching) before drying and then frying.

And if nothing else works you can always wear an apron and quickly put the lid on.

Having only one double bond makes oils rich in monounsaturated fats (e.g. olive oil) more resistant to going off in the pantry or needing as many preservatives in the bottle compared to polyunsaturated oils. This makes cooking with monounsaturated fats historically very popular in the kitchen, especially in Mediterranean cuisine.

Double bonds also make a difference to the toxic fumes that rise from the pan when we cook with them. The best known are aldehydes, which form as fatty acids and are blown apart under heat. The hotter it gets the more they form, so toxic fumes are greatest while deep-frying or pan-frying, although we can still get some while stir-frying. Cooking oils with lots of double bonds generally produce more aldehydes and other toxic species than those with few or no double bonds. But regardless of what we use, if we heat it enough, some smoke will get in our eyes.

Smoke point blank

When oil is heated hotter and hotter, at some point (known as the smoke point) it will vaporize, releasing a bluish smoke as it rises. This urgent smoke signal means that the oil is far too hot for cooking. You need to immediately take it off the burner (as if this wasn't completely obvious) otherwise your kitchen and your house will fill with toxic smoke particles and the pungent smell of burnt fat.

That (all-too-familiar) fast-food restaurant smell comes from burning of glycerol (the bails on top of the three fatty acid stumps in the triglyceride cricket-wicket analogy, remember?). Consequently, toxic smoke can rise from any cooking oil whether it is predominantly saturated, monounsaturated or polyunsaturated.

However, saturated fat burns a little faster in the pan (i.e. smokes at a lower temperature) than polyunsaturated oils. This is because, without double bonds, the heat (energy) has nowhere to go. Consequently, we generally have to use more saturated fats (e.g. lard, coconut oil) when cooking over high heat than polyunsaturated oils, or the frying pan dries out.

Other things mixed in with the oil can also lower the smoke point. For example, the less-processed, extra-virgin olive oil has a smoke point 100 degrees lower than light (highly refined) olive oil which has had the colour, flavanols and other elements that can easily catch fire removed. This is also why clarified butter (known as ghee) works and is so popular in cooking, as it has had its milk proteins (which readily go up in smoke) removed, thus raising the smoke point by 50 degrees.

Being pure and saturated are not the only things that make oil smoke. Re-using the same cooking oil again and again progressively lowers the smoke point by freeing up the fatty acids and glycerol from the triglyceride-complex, and so aiding their escape. This is partly why those old chip shops (well known for re-using their oil) were so smelly.

Tear gas

 When heated excessively, the glycerol in triglycerides breaks down into a chemical called acrolein. Acrolein is nasty stuff and highly irritant. In fact, it was used in World War I (under the codename of 'Papite') as a kind of tear gas.

However, it didn't work that well as a weapon of mass destruction. This was because, when exposed to air, acrolein undergoes a spontaneous reaction that effectively neutralizes its toxic effects (although it stays smelly).

The problem was ultimately solved by two chemists working in the French Department of Chemical Warfare. In their experiments they discovered that other chemicals could be added in minute amounts to block the neutralizing reaction. Importantly, they also realized the broader potential for such chemicals in preserving other things from going off, like food, rubber and a whole range of other products that decayed in air. They called the compounds 'anti-oxygenic'. Today, we know and love them as antioxidants. But it all came from finding a better way to gas the Germans.

Big fat Greek

Whether it is saturated, mono- or polyunsaturated, fat provides energy for our metabolism. All fat will make us fatter if we eat too much of it relative to our level of physical activity. So whether one kind of fat or another is a dietary hero or villain ultimately comes down to whether it has any other effects beyond its impact on calorie balance.

One of the reasons we have been told for so many years that it's not how much fat we eat but the kind of fat we are eating that's the problem is the so-called 'Mediterranean paradox'.

The story goes that in the 1950s, when things were going so wrong in the United States in terms of heart disease and diabetes, Mediterranean countries like Greece and Italy were experiencing record low rates. This made no sense, because their diet contained large amounts of fat, and fat was supposed to be bad for you. Ignoring the fact that the Mediterranean had been decimated by war a decade earlier (so people were not so well off and were living off the land rather than mass-production), the idea emerged that perhaps there was something special about the Mediterranean diet that conveyed a protective effect. But the critical ingredient(s) behind this rough magic remained to be established.

A classic Mediterranean diet is a pattern of eating lots of unprocessed cereals, vegetables, legumes, fruits, nuts, fish and olive oil with reduced amounts of meat, milk and milk products and sugar. Wine, as a rule, is taken with meals and in moderation. Essentially this all adds up to a high ratio of calories from (whole) plants compared to calories from animal products or highly processed foods.

But of all the many different ingredients in the Mediterranean diet, the finger was pointed at the large amounts of monounsaturated fat they ate compared to the supposedly heart-stopping saturated fat that dominated in other countries. While Americans used butter, lard and shortening, Mediterranean cooking had olive oil at its very heart.

Extra Virgin

 As you press and squeeze the flesh of an olive, an oily yellow juice emerges — this is extra virgin olive oil.

The virgin part simply means the oil was produced only by squishing olives, without any refining, heat, additives or chemical treatment. To get the rest of the oil out of the pulp you need these things. This is usually called pure olive oil.

Because of its key role in Mediterranean cuisine, many studies have looked at the potential health benefits of olive oil in its own right. For example, in one study investigators gave a few spoonfuls of extra virgin olive oil to subjects every day, and found the risk of having a heart attack or even dying young was significantly reduced.

All olive oil is almost 100 per cent fat, mostly of the monounsaturated variety (55–85 per cent) with a smaller component of saturated fat (8–25 per cent) and polyunsaturated fat (5–20 per cent). If it was only the special combination of fats that made olive oil so good for you, then extra virgin would have no advantage over pure olive oil. It is certainly true that eating nuts, which are also rich in monounsaturated fat (but are otherwise very different), shares many of the same health benefits.

However, extra virgin olive oil also contains all sorts of other things that come from olive flesh and give it its unique taste, aroma and colour. Today, the focus has switched from healthy fat to the possible benefits of some of these other things (e.g. the polyphenols), so refinement makes little sense to the health conscious.

In Mediterranean cuisine, extra virgin olive oil is generally used unheated or at low temperature. However, in most Western countries we use oils in high-temperature cooking, when frying, broiling and baking. So while we may buy the expensive olive oil for our health, the disadvantage of all the other things contained in extra virgin olive oil is that they don't take the high heat of a frypan so well. Any benefits may therefore be more easily lost in smoke.

Cholesterol

The logical explanation given for the Mediterranean paradox was that while saturated fat was driving up cholesterol levels in America, the Greeks' preference for olive oil and only a moderate intake of animal fat meant that they had much lower cholesterol levels and therefore fewer heart problems.

It is perfectly true that diets rich in saturated fat have a greater effect on our blood cholesterol levels than unsaturated fat (see Chapter 7 for more details). And if there are any benefits from cutting out foods that are high in saturated fat (e.g. butter) or switching to foods that are lower in saturated fat (e.g. margarine, olive oil), they are almost entirely due to lowering the levels of bad cholesterol in our blood.

Because of the link between cholesterol and saturated fat, and the link between cholesterol and heart attacks, saturated fat has been unequivocally vilified in the latter half of the 20th century. So effective has this campaign been, with even doctors advising their patients to eat margarine, that modern generations now eat less than half the saturated fat of fifty years ago.

The greasy counterfeit

 In 1972, New Zealand was an isolated agricultural island nation. Its dairy industry had lobbied long and hard to prevent margarine from ever being sold in the country. In fact, it was actually illegal to buy margarine without a doctor's prescription, and you had to go to your pharmacy to get it.

However, the tide was changing. Data from many countries started linking saturated fats, like those in butter, with blood cholesterol levels and rising rates of heart disease. Already in America, the margarine message was making inroads and for the first time margarine consumption began exceeding that of more highly priced butter. Although New Zealand-made butter had a cost advantage (being comparatively cheap in New Zealand) there were serious concerns of a quiet invasion of a counterfeit butter intended to deceive consumers. Like in the movie *Invasion of the Body Snatchers*, one day Kiwis would wake up and find their new world was filled with alien butter duplicates.

You can't hold back the tide, however. And the Margarine Act of 1908 was amended in 1972 to finally allow margarine to flow. In a last-ditched attempt to retain market share, the New Zealand dairy lobby hatched a grand scheme to mandate that all margarine be dyed blue, so consumers would immediately be able to spot the difference between local butter and alien margarine. It failed.

It wasn't the first time that such a suggestion was made. Vermont, South Dakota and New Hampshire state legislatures had all passed laws requiring margarine to be dyed pink at the beginning of the 20th century, only for these unconstitutional laws to be struck down by the Supreme Court.

But while cutting out saturated fat was the only way to lower bad cholesterol in the seventies, its effect was only modest at best. Today we have many much better ways to achieve this (see Chapter 10). Moreover, the ultimate cost to our health of eating more unsaturated fat may not have been worth it.

Imbalance

During the latter half of the 20th century, the amount of fat in the average diet changed radically. We were not eating much less fat as a proportion of our diet. Rather, based on the Mediterranean paradox and the supposed explanation for it, people started to replace saturated fat with polyunsaturated substitutes (e.g. replacing butter and lard with margarine and vegetable oil). Today, only a third of the fat in our diet is saturated. The great majority of the remainder is monounsaturated fat with some polyunsaturated fat on the side making up 8 to 10 per cent of the total fat we eat.

The problem with this shift is that the fat in our diet is far more than just a danger to our cholesterol levels or our waistlines. It also has a range of vital functions in the human body, from maintaining our immune system and brain function, to regulating blood flow and protecting against injury.

Some polyunsaturated fats are positively essential for our health. In fact, they were once known as vitamin F and must be obtained from the food we eat, just like all the other vitamins. This is because, while our body is able to generate and store all other kinds of fat, we can't make the useful ones that have reactive double bonds, specially placed exactly three or six links from the end of a fatty acid chain. Omega is the 24th and last letter of the Greek alphabet, so the end of a fatty acid chain is called the omega. These essential fats are usually called the omega–3 (-3) and omega–6 (-6) fatty acids. Their unique chemistry makes these fats very useful for creating other things, including essential regulatory and signalling chemicals.

Although humans can't make these special fats, plants have no trouble at all. Similarly fish and animal fat can also contain useful amounts of these essential fats (because they eat mostly or entirely plants).

But the fact that we can't get by without them doesn't mean that they are essentially good for us in the very large doses and the unnatural ratios we often take them.

Omega–3 fats and omega–6 fats look pretty similar to each other (they just have one double bond in a different place), so they compete for many of the same chemical reaction pathways in our body. However, the products of the reactions that occur when using omega–3 fats are very different, chemically and functionally, than those that occur when using omega–6. So the net result of what happens when we eat polyunsaturated fat also depends partly on how much omega–3 is present versus omega–6.

It is thought that a one-to-one ratio of omega–3 to omega–6 (or as close as possible) is optimal for good health. But in a typical modern diet, for each omega–3 fat we consume there are at least a dozen omega–6 fats, and very often much more than this. Undoubtedly, this imbalance can alter the balance of signalling chemicals being made, and potentially have consequences on our health, including depression, heart attacks, stroke, arthritis, osteoporosis, inflammation and some forms of cancer.

To address this imbalance, it is now widely recommended for our health that we increase our intake of omega–3 fats. The most common sources of omega–3 fats in our diet are the plants we eat, as well as any fat from the animals that eat them. Egg yolks are mostly saturated fat, but the amount of omega–3 they contain can be enhanced by feeding chickens with omega–3-rich plants (e.g. linseed/flaxseed, santolina) or sometimes fish-oil. This is because omega–3 polyunsaturated fats are especially high in cold-water oily fish and in the oil that is extracted from them. This why most guidelines recommend that we should eat them more often than we do and many people take fish-oil supplements in their stead. And, of course, there are the Eskimos.

A fishy story

 It is appealing to think that reverting to 'natural' dietary habits will allow us to avoid the ills of a modern Western diet.

Long before the Paleo diet was popular, it was believed that the Inuit population of Arctic Greenland had paradoxically low rates of heart disease despite eating vast amounts of saturated fat (in seal and whale blubber), which at the time was thought to be a potent cause of heart disease. They also ate no fruit and vegetables, which was another dietary no-no.

Maybe they had developed a secret genetic immunity? Maybe something extra in their diet gave them special powers to defeat the fatty villain that was poisoning America? Maybe if we could have a little of what they were having we would be saved too?

Inuits did have higher levels of omega–3 fats in their diet (from eating oily fish and other things that also ate oily fish). So maybe it was the fish-oil? Great idea. This is why one of the most popular health supplements found in every pharmacy is fish-oil.

The problem is that Inuits aren't actually protected from heart disease. In fact, they generally have a higher rate of strokes and a shortened life expectancy compared to everyday Europeans. Moreover, recent trials of fish-oil supplements have failed to confirm any clear benefits in reducing heart problems. So the whole story smells a little fishy.

The same reactive properties that make omega–3 useful for health also make it hard to store at room temperature for long periods without spoiling. And once spoilt, these rancid fish fats not only don't work, but they are smelly and may actually be bad for our health. At least in Greenland there is no shortage of ice.

~~~~~~

As well as raising our intake of omega–3 through fish-oil and the like, another recommended way to bring the omegas back into healthy balance is to lower our intake of omega–6 fats. This is one of the key aims of the Paleo diet, which reduces the intake of grains, seeds and their oils (i.e. most of the polyunsaturated omega–6 in our normal diet), replacing them with monounsaturated fat-dominant oils (like olive oil) and saturated fats like butter. Used in this way (and in modest amounts) the reformed villain — saturated fat — is made to work for us instead of against us.

Maleficent

In the seventies and eighties, avoiding saturated (animal) fat at all costs was the central tenet of a healthy diet. Out went butter, lard, tallow, palm and coconut oils. This created an opening for a new kind of fat to enter our bodies called trans-fat. Although hailed as the saviour, in the end it turned out to easily be the most maleficent fat of all.

Trans-fats are typically created when unsaturated fats (usually from vegetable oils) are overheated. This may be deliberate, for example, to make solid shortening (e.g. Crisco) or ghee from liquid vegetable oil. For example, some Vanaspati (vegetable ghee) products sold in India may be over 20 per cent trans-fat.

Sometimes trans-fats are created accidentally, for example, when products that come out of the frypan carry the stain of trans-fats generated in the overheated, reused vegetable oil in which they have been fried.

The discovery of how to make trans-fats was so revolutionary that its inventors received the Nobel Prize in 1912.

Trans-fats are a deceptively clever piece of work. Instead of double bonds creating a nice kink in its structure like other unsaturated fats, trans-fat gets twisted around, which paradoxically results in a super straightening and stiffening of its carbon backbone.

This upright chemical structure means trans-fat looks and behaves like a saturated fat when it comes to cooking. It could pack in tightly and be semi-solid at room temperature, just like butter. It could equally have melt-in-the-mouth texture on heating and provide a palatable alternative to other fats in making baked goods. In fact, head to head, trans-fat more reliably produces uniformly fluffy pastries than butter.

Being tricky, trans-fat also has a longer shelf life, and is less prone to going off (spoiling) than polyunsaturated fat found in conventional vegetable oils. Trans-fat also doesn't burn as easily as saturated fat, so there is less fire and smoke at fast-food outlets. It is also cheaper to mass-produce than butter.

All this culinary chemistry without the price tag. With trans-fats on board, products could now be considered healthy (and became popular) because they did not contain the nutritional devil, saturated fat, and its deleterious effects on our cholesterol levels. No wonder we all switched our butter to margarine and vegetable oils in the seventies.

The fall of margarine

 There was once a time that margarine was king. It was cheap and almost indistinguishable from butter. Doctors extolled its virtues and recommended all their patients switch to margarine as it was low in saturated fat and free of cholesterol, both important causes of heart disease.

However, a study following 120,000 nurses over eight years in the late seventies and early eighties clearly showed that those with the highest intake of trans-fats also had the highest risk of heart disease and death from it. Subsequently diabetes, sudden death and other problems became associated with eating trans-fats. And in 1980, margarine was the major source of trans-fat.

It looked good on paper and in the kitchen. But the doctors were wrong, and they had struck a bargain with the devil. And we all know how that turns out. Trans-fat looked like a panacea, but was really a poison. People died and margarine sales went straight to hell.

It turns out there really was a (hidden) catch. The same super-resistant chemistry that made trans-fat a culinary wonder also made it deadly for our health. In fact, pound for pound trans-fats increase the risk of dying prematurely more than any other component of our diet. There appears to be no safe limit for trans-fats. Even a small intake may be sufficient to begin increasing the risks for death and disease.

Recognizing this, most of the previously common sources of trans-fats, like margarine and vegetable shortening, have had their shot at redemption. Today most of them contain less than 0.2 per cent trans-fat. However, some processed foods and spreads still contain trans-fats. The chief offenders include microwave popcorn, certain biscuits, cakes, potato crisps and savoury pastries. Sometimes the trans-fats are listed on their nutritional labels. If they aren't listed then it's a fair bet the producers don't really care about your health. It is likely that mandatory testing and listing of trans-fat content will soon be required in many countries.

All the reputable mega-chain takeaway and fast-food restaurants have also switched their oils to canola oil free of trans-fats. While this makes them less unhealthy it still does not make them healthy. Deep-fried foods from unscrupulous operators still run the risk of generating trans-fats, especially those reusing vegetable oils to reduce costs. Again, it is likely that regulations will eventually catch up with them, as there have been calls for banning all trans-fats from restaurants and fast-food outlets. In some places they are already outlawed. However, in many developing counties, trans-fats remain a major concern, especially in India and South Asia, where vegetable ghee and deep-frying are culinary icons and staples for cooking at home.

Finally, some trans-fats do occur naturally in meat (fat) and in dairy products like cheese and butter. But these are not the synthetic ones that caused so many problems for margarine and are chemically different again, containing both trans-fat and unsaturated fat elements. These natural trans-fats are not thought to be a major problem to human health.

The bottom line

It's a topsy-turvey world. Saturated fat was bad and now it's not. Trans-fat and polyunsaturated fat were the solution, but now they are the problem. Fish oil saved the Eskimo, but now it just smells fishy. Reducing our dependence on a low-fat diet was essential, but now we are eating too many sugars/carbs.

Paul Newman once said from the inside of his racing car that it was useless to put on the brakes when the world was upside down. This is exactly how many people feel about their diet. If you're crashing anyway and nothing makes sense, why slow down? And what good would putting on brakes do, anyway?

But we are not there yet. We still have plenty of time to turn the wheel and slow down. And targeting the fat we are eating can make a big difference.

The fat we eat is not intrinsically bad or good, only made so by how we use it. Obviously, eating too much fat readily adds to our calorie count and ultimately to the pantry around our waist. So cutting out unnecessary fat is one simple way to cut calories as well.

Most of the saturated fat in our diet comes from meat and dairy. So if we can only make a habit of eating the lean meat or substituting an amount of something else that doesn't have the fat (like legumes for mince) we lose nothing except for calories.

Most of the unsaturated fat in our diet (as well as a quarter of the saturated fat) comes from oils and spreads, which together contribute as many calories to our waistlines as all the saturated fat we currently eat. It is possible to cook without oil or at the very least with less oil. Today we have non-stick cookware, a zillion herbs and spices, steamers, slow-cookers, an abundance of whole unprocessed foods and a host of other opportunities to ditch the oil. This means fewer calories, not less food. It also means less tear gas.

Do I really have to ...

#7

Eat less added sugar?

Q: How much added sugar is really in a soft drink (soda)?
**A: On average there are about eight
teaspoons of sugar in every can.**

Q: And how much added sugar should I be having?
**A: It is recommended we aim for six teaspoons added
sugar a day (across everything we eat and drink).**

Q: Isn't that impossible?
**A: Difficult but not impossible. If it is not processed
(i.e. whole food), sugar can't be added.**

Q: Should I only worry about fructose?
A: Half of table sugar is fructose.

Q: What about my sweet tooth?
A: It's not to blame.

Q: Are artificial sweeteners dangerous?
A: Not more than added sugar is.

Almost every organism on the planet burns some sugar to generate the energy it needs to function. But the human brain only burns sugar. Having sugars in our blood is as essential to our brain as the air we breathe. Without it for more than a few minutes, our brains would shut off. Just like being starved of oxygen, we would lose consciousness and die.

Because of the importance of sugar to all forms of life, and the fact we eat other animals and plants that also rely on it, almost all of the food we eat contains some sugars. We call all the sugars in our diet **carbohydrates** (or carbs for short). About half of the energy (calories) we get from our food usually comes from the carbs that we eat.

Carbs can be divided into essentially two types. Firstly, there are the complex carbs. We usually call these starch and fibre. These are discussed in the next chapters. Then there are the **simple sugars.** We usually just call these 'sugar' for simplicity.

Simply sugar

The simple sugars are the ones that our tastebuds can recognize as sweet, including ones like sucrose (the white 'table sugar' used in cooking and added to our tea and coffee), lactose (in milk) and fructose (in fruit and honey). Inside our blood circulates another simple sugar called glucose (or dextrose when used in food). This is why fresh blood has a sweet but salty taste, if you've ever licked a cut on your finger.

Simple sugars are naturally abundant in all naturally sweet foods, like fruit, milk, corn and honey. But when people talk about the bad effects of sugar on their health, they are usually only talking about the sugar/syrup that has been added in food processing and to a lesser extent by consumers (e.g. into our tea or coffee). This is why the more descriptive terms '**added sugar**', 'sweeteners' or 'sweetened' products are also often used when talking about sugar and health.

About half of the all the sugar in our diet comes from naturally occurring sugars in fruit, vegetables and milk. The other half comes from added sugars. Any sugar is still sugar. But the big difference is that fruit/vegetable/milk bring other useful nutrients into our diet other than sugar. Added sugar only brings sugar. This is why calories from products high in added sugar are often called 'empty calories'.

A lot of people are worried about all the extra added sugar in our diet. So much so that from mid-2018, all nutritional labels in the US will specifically list both the amount of 'added sugars' in a product and how much this relates to the recommended daily intake. For good health, it is recommended that we should all try to eat and drink less than 25 grams of added sugar every day (or six teaspoons' worth), with an absolute limit of no more than 50 grams a day. A single can of regular soda usually contains over 35 grams of sugar or the equivalent of about eight teaspoons of added sugar. So the new nutritional label will say that this single soda can contains 70 per cent of your daily sugar limit. Drinking a standard 600-millilitre (20-ounce) bottle will be shown to represent 130 per cent of your daily limit. In other words, you've blown it!

Obviously this new label will graphically bring the issue of added sugar squarely home to the consumer, and encourage them to choose something less sugary. It also may force manufacturers to find something else to put in their products, or face a consumer backlash. The same strategy has recently worked for trans-fats (see Chapter 6).

Although some conscientious manufacturers are already listing their content of added sugar, in most countries only the total amount of sugars is required to be listed on the nutritional label, usually under the carbohydrate heading. Total sugars includes all added sugars as well as any sugars naturally present in ingredients like fruit, vegetables or milk. This stops products claiming to have 'no added sugar' while at the same time adding large amounts of natural sugars (e.g. from fruit concentrates). However, no daily limit is usually provided for total sugars, so we have to make sense of the numbers ourselves.

Across the population, the major single source of added sugar is found in what we drink. Soft drinks (also known as sugar-sweetened beverages), energy drinks, sports drinks, fruit drinks and the like account for at least a third of all the added sugar in the average diet. In the US this figure is closer to one half. To put this into context, this is about the same amount of sugar we'd get each day from all the fruit and vegetables we eat.

Apart from drinks, the other big source of added sugar is baking. Cakes, cookies, donuts, pies, crisps, cobblers and muesli (granola) bars together add another two teaspoons of sugar every day to out diet. More added sugar in our diet is hidden in plain sight in everyday products, from breakfast cereal and bread to yoghurt and sauces. These products don't always taste sweet. But sugar is subtly added to improve the taste or offset other tastes that we would find less agreeable on their own. For example, one tablespoon of tomato sauce contains about one teaspoon of added sugar. A typical bowl of breakfast cereal contains five teaspoons of added sugar. A typical slice of white bread contains one to two teaspoons of added sugar. None of these tastes the same without added sugar.

Looking at how many, many things in our diet have added sugar in them, it's very easy to understand how few thoroughly modern people stay anywhere close to the target of less than six teaspoons a day, let alone the ceiling of twelve teaspoons. One bottle of soft drink (soda) and we have already blown it!

In general, most of us will eat and drink more like twenty teaspoons of added sugar a day. So a teaspoon of sugar in our tea or coffee is just a drop in the bucket. At least one in eight adults regularly eat and drink over thirty teaspoons of added sugars (125 grams) every day without ever troubling the sugar bowl.

On top of everything else we eat, the added sugar we consume mostly adds calories that we don't really need. Consequently, simply ditching those things with lots of added sugar or replacing them with less calorific alternatives is one practical way that most people can control their waistlines. Just halving the amount of added sugar that we eat each day with a few simple product choices can improve our calorie balance to almost the same extent as running for half an hour every day. For example, there's drinking water and having a piece of fruit instead of just drinking juice. We could also swap our flavoured yoghurt for unsweetened yoghurt with some berries to halve the added sugars.

Together alone

Added sugar in processed food comes in many different chemical forms. The most popular is **sucrose** (also called **table sugar**). Sucrose/table sugar is itself made up of two other sugars, glucose and fructose, which are naturally bonded together to form a chemical pair. This bond is only broken during our digestion. Consequently, sucrose is just a convenient delivery vehicle for glucose and fructose into our blood.

Brown sugar

 The white sugar we use on our table (sucrose) is manufactured from sugar cane or sugar beets, which are then juiced, dried and processed to become raw sugar. The raw sugar is further refined to produce clean white sugar crystals, leaving behind dark molasses.

Commercial brown sugar is essentially white sugar with some dark molasses mixed back in.

Raw sugar is essentially white sugar before all the molasses has been removed.

This makes raw and brown sugar stickier as well as more complex in their flavour. They are not any healthier just because they are raw, naturally brown or less processed.

In fact, because raw/brown sugar crystals are much smaller and pack in far tighter than standard white table sugar, there are more calories (and less air) in each teaspoon of dense brown sugar than one of balancing white sugar crystals.

Instead of adding table sugar (sucrose) to processed food and drink, it is possible for manufacturers to cut out the middleman and simply add a mixture of glucose and fructose to their product. This makes it just as sweet as adding table sugar.

On its own, pure glucose is not actually that sweet. By contrast, pure fructose is very much sweeter. Some people find it too sweet. Eating pure fructose can also cause diarrhoea in some people. For the sake of tolerability as well as taste, products containing fructose are always mixed with some glucose, either in a one-to-one ratio (just as in table sugar) or 55 per cent fructose to 45 per cent glucose (just as in honey). This mixture provides roughly the same sweetness and syrupy fullness as table sugar. As it is digested, sucrose is broken into fructose and glucose anyway. So both strategies essentially create the same result inside our body.

Fructose is found in nature in things like fruit, honey and some vegetables. Sweet corn doesn't naturally have fructose. It does, however, have lots of glucose and starch, which can be converted to fructose by industrial processing. Mixing back the natural glucose from corn with the fructose created by its enzymatic processing creates an artificial product, known as **high fructose corn syrup**. In many countries, this cheap alternative to sugar cane (sucrose) is the major form of added sugar.

Bonanza

Everybody knows that eating too much sweet stuff can make us fatter, and in doing so can lead to the diseases associated with being overweight like diabetes, heart disease and some cancers. These issues are discussed in Chapter 4 of this book. Whether any of these problems is a unique feature of eating too much added sugar, or will happen if we eat too much of anything, is still hotly debated. Much of the danger probably lies in the fact that added sugar is just about the yummiest source of excess calories we don't need.

But beyond the fact that sweet things contain calories, and that these calories are agreeably delicious, there is some argument that the added sugars in our food and drink have special effects on our body that cause them to add more to our waistlines than any other part of our diet.

In particular, it is thought that the human body treats the **fructose** component of added sugar differently to the glucose part. Glucose is naturally present in our body all the time. Our brain depends on it. And so it is carefully regulated and never used up unnecessarily. The availability of fructose (as naturally found in fruit and honey), on the other hand, naturally changes with the seasons.

The Garden of Eden

 In Palaeolithic times, there was no added sugar. In fact, it wasn't until the 19th century that it became widely available. The only significant fructose our ancestors gratefully received was obtained from fruit and berries. These became ripe, sweet and wonderfully abundant for only very brief periods, each in its particular season.

To make best use of the fleeting bonanza, our thrifty human body has made a special place for fructose, specifically in our liver. Here any fructose that we eat is very efficiently converted into fat. Unlike glucose metabolism, the metamorphosis of fructose into fat is not tightly regulated. The only thing controlling it is how much fructose we have eaten.

This sugar-to-fat conversion shunt was obviously critically important for our long-term survival as a species. The next fruiting season may have been some time or distance away.

Fat in the liver is more than just a useful energy store for lean times ahead. Fat in our liver, at least in the short term, also triggers other adaptations. For example, with extra fat in the liver, the hormonal signals that call for sugar to be taken up and used by the body for energy are blunted. This leaves more sugar available for the growth and processing power of our brain. Those sweet (fructose-rich) ripe apples we gorged ourselves on in the Garden of Eden may really have been the wellspring of all human knowledge.

As making the most of fruit when it's in season is so important for all animals, including ancient human beings, some people also argue this is why sugar may be less filling (or satiating) than other kinds of nutrients. In other words, we are perhaps supposed to end up eating much more sugar before we feel full enough to stop than with other nutrients. And this also makes eating too much sugar far easier than other nutrients. But this makes perfect sense only if we were an animal dependent on seasonal fruit to survive. Eat fruit while it's ripe, make fat while the sun shines (winter is coming, and all that). But how true this is for modern human beings is unclear.

Of course, gorging on ripe fructose in season was not really a problem when we were very active and lean. The problem today is that the ubiquity of fructose in our modern diet (either as added sugar or corn syrup in almost everything) makes it seem to our Palaeolithic physiology that fruit is ripe and in season every single day. And this means that our liver is habitually making extra fat we really don't need. This is why some (but not all) people think that it's the excess of added sugar in our modern diet that is our biggest health problem, and the main cause of our fatter societies.

An alternative view is that fructose itself is not really toxic, evil or poisonous. After all, when in its primary natural form (i.e. whole fruit) fructose is not actually associated with any major health issues. If anything, the human body uses up more energy to deal with fructose (turning it into fat) than with glucose. This view has sugar as just a yummy source of calories; no better or worse than other energy sources in our diet. Except of course for the fact we like its taste lots and we usually eat far too much of it! The bigger problem may be eating sugar out of its natural context, without the fibre and other healthy plant nutrients it's supposed to come with.

Sweet pleasures

It's universal to the human condition to like something sweet. Even in previously uncharted parts of the world that had never had any access to added sugar, every time that the sweets have been handed around they have been met with unanimous delight.

In many languages, the word sweet has come to mean not just something that tickles our tastebuds but also something that is inherently pleasurable or appealing: sweetheart, sweet-talk, sweet dreams, sweety, sweet as, *la dolce vita* (the sweet life).

Enjoying sugar is not just hedonism. There is obviously an evolutionary advantage to seek out a rich energy source in the form of sugars. For our ancestors, sweet meant ripe, and ripe meant more energy and a better food safety profile. In fact, having a preference for sweet foods is generally associated with greater fruit consumption. So the next time our kids ask us for sweets, we can console ourselves by thinking how well adapted they are (to life in the jungle).

Sweet tooth

 A penchant for sweet things is often called a 'sweet tooth'. But it actually has nothing to do with our teeth.

The expression 'sweet tooth' is used in the same way as we might use phrases such as 'a head for heights', 'an ear for music, 'a nose for trouble' or 'an eye for a bargain' to denote a particular talent or a proclivity towards it. In more recent times, this latter meaning of sweet tooth has dominated. Having a sweet tooth has become synonymous with a tendency for overindulging in sugary things rather than any talent in our tastebuds.

In animals, the ability to taste sweet and the preference for eating sweet things are closely linked. For example, cats have no sweet receptors at all (as they are carnivores), and would rather chew cardboard or grass than something sticky and sweet. By contrast, bears possess sweet sensors and, as a result, have a well-known fondness for honey.

However, this relationship doesn't seem to hold for humans. How well we are able to taste sweetness doesn't have anything to do with how much we like it or whether we will eat lots of sweet things. So the sweet tooth is neither super-sensitive nor overcompensating because of lack of sensitivity.

Nonetheless, it's still widely assumed that most overweight people have a sweet tooth and the over-consumption of sugary delights got them there in the first place. However, the perception or the liking for sweet things doesn't actually affect our body weight. Obesity is much more complicated. We can't just blame it on our (sweet) tooth.

Our sugar preference (or sweet toothiness) is influenced by a range of different factors, including our age. Children have more of a sweet tooth than either of their parents. In fact, sweetness also turns out to be the most important feature determining what our well-adapted children are willing to eat. The little bears! However, their liking for concentrated sweetness fades rapidly during adolescence, as their tastes change both literally and figuratively.

Some people suggest that women have more of a sweet tooth than men, who are more often salivating over the savouries. This is also the basis of the old wives' tale that if a pregnant woman craves sweet things she is having a girl: 'Sugar and spice and all things nice. That's what little girls are made of.' Having salty, savoury cravings on the other hand means you are having a boy. And, of course, experiencing both may mean you are having twins. Fortunately, it doesn't actually work this way in reality.

All of us like a little sweetness. But only up to a point. From then on we can be loosely divided into two types. In some people, increasing levels of sugar beyond this point leads to further enjoyment or, at the very least, no reduction in enjoyment of sweet treats. For these people (with their sweet tooth), there is no such thing as too sweet. However, other people reach a point when things get far too sweet for them and how much they like what they are eating falls off dramatically. Yuk, too sweet!

Taste is more than just biology. There is also an important link with our past experiences and future expectations. Sugar is our first drug experience. And the more enjoyable, rewarding or relaxing we remember that experience, the more likely we'll reach for it again.

As we grew up, sweet usually meant something special. So the sweet placebo takes us back there in our mind every time.

Sugar rush

Many people eat a sweet snack to give them a much-needed emotional lift, often at times of the day when their energy is sagging or they are under stress. Part of this boost comes from the simple pleasure of eating something sweet. The same boost can happen if we get a compliment, or something goes our way. While we can't buy a compliment or a dose of good luck, chocolate or muffins are always for sale.

When simple sugars hit our tastebuds they send a chemical message to our brain. This not only tells our brain we have just eaten something sweet, but it also triggers the release of chemicals normally associated with feelings of reward and pleasure. The most well-known of these is dopamine, but there are many other chemical changes that in total add up to the pleasing sensation we get after eating sweet things.

This sensation is not unique to sugar. Our brains can get the same happy (dopamine) jolt from other good things. In fact, to a greater or lesser extent, all the food we eat can stimulate the release of reward chemicals in our brain. The more calories we eat, the greater the reward to our brains. This is why banquets and feasting are such an important and enduring part of human culture. Just think of Christmas dinners past or Thanksgiving, and we are already salivating.

But more than simply the reward of taste and calories, the sweet things in life are special. Most of us have been conditioned from our childhood that sweet things are literally a reward, treat or a gift for special occasions. Do this and we will get (sweet) dessert or a treat. Later, in adulthood, it's little wonder we turn to the sweet stimulus to recreate that feeling of accomplishment.

Our brain learns in proportion to the amount of reward chemicals that are made. In other words, the bigger the prize, the stronger the memory. This programming is probably designed so that we better remember (and are less likely to forget) to do good things again and again, as well as desire to do them when they are not around.

Eventually our brains learn to expect this. The bigger the rewards become, and the more frequent, the stronger these feelings can become. Even when there are other ways to make ourselves feel better, our brain has trained itself to do the one action it is used to doing and knows will be satisfying. Even if it is bad for us, habit is stronger than logic.

High on candy

 Many parents believe that sugar makes their kids bounce off the walls. Sugar has an uplifting effect on adults when they eat dessert. So why not our kids as well?

It sounds logical. However, the association between sugar and hyperactivity is mostly due to context and connotation, rather than sugar itself. It's a party for goodness sake. It's Halloween. They should be excited.

We can reward kids in many ways to make them hyperactive. They are over-excited at Christmas, even before the first bon-bon is torn apart. They are uncontrollable at birthday parties even before the cake has been cut.

But if we believe it to be true, then it is. We can see little candy monsters everywhere we look. One study found that when children were all given a diet soft drink (soda) to drink, those mothers who were told their children had received a regular soft drink rated their kids as more hyperactive than the mothers who were told their children really had received the diet drink. Sugar is all in our mind.

One of the reasons that cocaine is so addictive is that it causes a build-up of the reward chemical dopamine in the brain. This makes everything seem more intensely pleasurable than it actually is. Caffeine has similar effects, although to a far lesser extent. But for the same reasons, when the reward chemicals go away, everything seems less rewarding and our brain misses that intoxicated state of mind.

Whether sugar is really addictive or not is still debated. At least in mice, sugar is just as addictive as heroin. In humans, however, it is mostly the pleasure and comfort that comes from sweet sugar pushing up our dopamine and driving our behaviour. Once something works, it can be habit forming, especially if we enjoy it. It can even become compulsive (i.e. doing something repetitively without necessarily leading to pleasure and enjoyment). But there's not really any sugar addiction we suffer from.

A sweet alternative

Given the significant and largely unnecessary energy contained in added sugar-rich processed food and sweetened beverages, a popular way to reduce their impact on our waistline (without having to give up sweet things entirely) has been to swap out any added sugar with other chemicals that still activate our sweet tastebud receptors but don't contain the calories. These chemicals are knowns as **sweeteners** or sugar substitutes, because that is what they aim to do. This is the principle behind the many diet drinks and low-energy products now on the market.

The most commonly used ones are artificial or synthetic sweeteners, like saccharin, aspartame and acesulfame K. All these different chemicals have a very intense sweet taste, much more potent than table sugar. This means they can be used in very small amounts to produce a roughly similar sweetness to sugar. Moreover, because of the very small amount of sweeteners we'd need to use, the calories contained in diet products are also far fewer (compared to regular sugar-sweet versions).

Sweet accidents

 Constantin Fahlberg was a sugar chemist hired by the H.W. Perot Import Firm in 1877 to make sure its sugar shipments were pure. They found him space at Johns Hopkins Hospital to do his work, and after he was done he stayed on in the laboratory to focus on purifying chemicals found in coal tar.

One night, having picked up a bread roll for dinner, he found that it tasted remarkably sweet. But so did his hands that, in his haste, he had forgotten to wash. Back in his lab, he rediscovered the sweet tasting chemical that had got onto his hands and then onto his food. This became known as saccharin.

Fifty years later, a second artificial sweetener (known as cyclamate) was discovered in similar fashion when graduate student Michael Sveda, who was working on an anti-fever medication, put down his cigarette on a lab bench. But when he put it back in his mouth, the taste was now sweet.

The sweetener aspartame was also accidentally discovered by scientist James Schlatter in 1965 when he licked his (contaminated) finger to lift up a piece of paper. The same thing happened in the discovery of acesulfame K in 1974, when Karl Claus accidentally licked his finger to turn a page during an experiment.

You may notice a pattern here, but please don't randomly lick your fingers. For every success there are probably another ten thousand poisoned scientists wishing they hadn't.

~~~~~~

However sweet, the taste of artificial sweeteners is not quite the same as sugar. Get the dose wrong and saccharine can taste metallic. Sugar also contributes to the 'thickness' or 'syrupiness' of a product, particularly in a drink, so products using artificial sweeteners can feel 'thinner' or 'watery' in the mouth when compared to the usual sugar-laden products.

To solve these dual problems, many diet products are usually complex mixtures of both artificial sweeteners and bulking agents (e.g. soluble fibre) to approximate a syrupy sugar-like sensation. However, even when perfectly formulated, so that we swear we can't taste the difference, our unconscious mind can still work out which one is the diet drink.

Another group of chemicals used as sugar substitutes is the so-called '**natural sweeteners**' including sucralose (also known as Splenda), stevia and monk fruit (*luo han guo*). Sucralose is just ordinary sugar (sucrose) that has been chlorinated. This makes it over five hundred times as sweet as sugar, so we need five hundred times less to achieve the same sweetness as sugar. In addition, only 15 per cent of it is absorbed into our body (as compared to nearly 100 per cent of regular sugar), so its footprint on our calorie count is very small.

Extracts of *Stevia rebaudiana*, a herb originating in Paraguay, are also used as natural sweeteners and are gaining popularity. Again these chemicals are much sweeter than table sugar, meaning we need to use very little to get a sweet fix. Moreover, in every teaspoon of stevia (not that we ever need a teaspoon) there are seventeen times fewer calories than in a teaspoon of sugar.

When used in recommended amounts, both artificial and natural sweeteners have no obvious adverse effects on human health, at least in the short term. The problem is that we often don't use recommended amounts and if we see something labelled as a diet drink or product we often feel liberated from guilt and guzzle much more than we otherwise would. It's only a diet drink! However, excessive use of sweeteners can definitely lead to stomach upsets in some people. The potential for more serious effects is unclear.

Although it sounds like a perfect solution for cutting down the calories, people who regularly use low-cal sweetener alternatives aren't radically thinner or healthier than those using the regular (added sugar) products. Remember, on average only 20 per cent of the added sugar we get comes from soft drinks (sodas). So while cutting down on soft drinks can be helpful in some people, on its own it will not eliminate most of the added sugar we eat at other times.

Another reason for this finding is that those people who routinely use diet drinks may feel free to eat other things. Equally, those who are justifiably worried about becoming overweight are more likely to use diet products. Another argument is that super-sweet chemicals can change the response to real sugars in our diet, and this might lead to us wanting more of the super-sweet life instead of less of it.

The bottom line

If you listen to the media, sugar seems like the new pariah of modern diets: pure, white and deadly. The mere act of adding two teaspoons of sugar to a cup of coffee nowadays is almost as heretical as lighting up a cigarette or ordering a soft drink with our meal. And just like with cigarettes and soft drinks, there are calls for taxes to dissuade consumers corrupted by their addictive pleasures.

But the same 'toxic' sugars found in a can of soft drink are also naturally found in fruit. One large banana or one apple contains as much sugar as two cans of soft drink. No one complains about apples or tries to ban them from schools. They might even keep the doctor away. So it can't just be the added sugar that's causing all the problems. It certainly adds to our woes, but we are getting fatter not because we eat too much added sugar, but because we just eat too much.

The biggest problem with added sugar is not so much what it adds, but what it doesn't. Sugar on its own behaves differently when it is part of an apple than when it is found in a soda can — not because the sugar is different, but because the apple also has fibre, resistant starch and other phytonutrients. The soft drink is just empty calories. When over 10 per cent of all the calories in a diet come from added sugar you're never going to be getting enough of the important things. The average intake of added sugars in the American diet is more like 15 per cent of all calories. So you know there must be something missing.

Just taking away all the added sugar is not the solution, however. It makes a diet less flavoursome and less rewarding. Regularly eating a fresh, flavoursome diet makes added sugar superfluous. Sugar then need only be added for special occasions, when it can be happily enjoyed without guilt.

Do I really have to ...

#8

Cut out the starch?

Q: Did our ancestors eat any starch?
A: Not until they started cooking.

Q: Will going low-carb help my waistline?
A: Eating fewer calories is what will help your waistline.

Q: What about low-GI food?
A: Eating less sugar and foods with sugar that take longer to metabolize both have advantages to improve health. Better with both.

Q: Do I need to eat more fibre?
A: Almost certainly. But avoid the cardboard.

Q: Why does bread make me feel bloated?
A: Because some starch is resistant to our digestion, so feeds our gut bacteria, releasing gas.

Q: Will eating my crusts make my hair curl?
A: Hairdressers work better.

The majority of sugars in our diet do not taste sweet. Instead of being simple and free to tickle our tastebuds, most sugars we eat are tied up in complex structures, containing hundreds or even thousands of individual sugar molecules all bonded together, like links in a very long chain. These are all known as **complex carbohydrates.**

The kind of links between the sugars in complex carbohydrates determines what happens in our bodies when we eat them. Sometimes, the links align the sugars in a tight coil, like a slinky spring. This slinky linking allows the chain of sugars to be packed tightly into semi-crystalline granules. This is known as **starch.**

Starch is how most green plants store the energy they get from sunlight during the day, so they will have the fuel to help them spring through the night. This means that most plants and plant-based foods are rich in starch. These include many of our favourite staples: bread, cereal, corn, potatoes, legumes, pasta, noodles and rice (and beer, of course).

The clever cook

Raw starch is normally so tightly coiled and packed that our comparatively short intestines can't digest it very well. Other animals that live off eating raw vegetables, such as gorillas, make do because of their much larger intestines and prolonged time spent chewing before swallowing. Even our ancient ancestor, *Homo habilis,* had a far bigger gut than that found in modern man. If we tried to eat starchy plants raw (like chomping into an uncooked corn cob), the starches would only be digested very slowly and incompletely by our intestines. This is why raw starch is often called resistant starch, because, in effect, by being supercoiled and granular it is physically resistant to the enzymes in our intestines that want to break it down into its constituent sugars.

Brainpower

 Roughly 20 per cent of the energy we consume every day is used up by the workings of our brain. Sometimes even more when we are stressed. By contrast, primates like gorillas, chimpanzees and orangutans are able to devote only 10 per cent of their energy to their brain, at best.

This is simply because, for our body size, our brain is over twice the size of that found in apes. It also contains about 86 billion brain cells (called neurons), which is about three times as many as in a gorilla.

But the price of having this super-computer in our head is the high power bill. To keep it running, a human brain needs sugar. Apart from honey and the occasional ripe seasonal fruit and berries, there was little natural sugar in our ancient raw diet. Certainly not enough to go around for the big demands of big populations and big brains. Just eating roots, shoots and leaves does not provide enough energy to keep a human brain running.

It's okay for a gorilla. But even so, they have to spend most of their day eating to sufficiently fuel their smaller brains. There are simply not enough calories or enough hours in the day to expand it any further. And so gorillas and chimps have stayed pretty much gorillas and chimps.

On the other hand, around 1.8 million years ago, humans discovered a clever way to circumvent the problem of resistant starch and extract enough sugar from starchy roots and tubers for our brain to double in size and expand in power. The solution was simply to cook them first.

In the presence of a little heat and water, the slinky-coiled structure of raw starch opens up. This is known as gelatinization and turns firm starch into something soft and wobbly, like cooked spaghetti. This creates access for our digestive enzymes, which can then chop otherwise resistant and unusable starch into large amounts of usable glucose (the chief fuel for the human brain). For example, we get much more glucose from eating a cooked potato than from swallowing the same one raw. So unlike gorillas, we don't need to spend six hours every day just chewing before we swallow. The development of cooking not only gave us bigger brains, but also afforded us more free time to use them.

Glucose from starch also gave us the carb loading our muscles need to run for long periods (and in particular run down our prey). Glucose is also the main source of energy for the efficient growth of a baby in the womb. Consequently, many consider that the discovery of cooking and the novel access to sugar it provided, is the key transformational event in human evolution.

If, as in the movie *Space Odyssey*, aliens came to the earth two million years ago to help us along, it would not have been weapons they gave us. It would have been cooking lessons. Today, we literally can't survive without cooking.

Eliminating the resistance

Human evolution did not end with the discovery of cooking over fire. To make the most of the stored energy inside any grains we had gathered, we also needed to add some preparation. In particular, we needed to remove the coating from the grains because it forms a physical barrier that is partially resistant to both cooking and our digestive juices.

Soaking is generally not enough to soften up grains for our digestion. It is also time consuming. However, if we crush the grains first (e.g. spreading the grain on a slab and beating it with a stone), some of the barriers are broken down, allowing us to make more use of the starch within. Generally, the more processing that is undertaken (i.e. the more refining) the more barriers to digestion are removed. For example, wholegrain wheat has over five times the amount of resistant starch as highly processed (fine and white) wheat flour. By contrast, the same amount of highly processed (fine white) wheat flour can provide over twice the glucose of an equal amount of wholegrain wheat.

Through human history, our diet has progressively become more and more processed (or rather, less raw), especially in modern times. In other words, our food has become easier to digest and more able to supply the needs of our brain without needing to eat very much at all. This was essential for sustaining large populations, where literally earning a crust or stealing a loaf of bread was critical for our very survival.

The bread riots

 Times were tough in the 1780s in France. The average worker spent over half his daily wages just on bread. He was literally the bread-winner.

But then things got even worse. Crops failed and the price of bread increased even further. Not surprisingly, something had to give and the masses rebelled, blaming the ruling classes for their condition. On 14 July 1789, a gathering that started as a bread riot ended with the fall of the Bastille and eventually the end of the French monarchy.

The French queen at the time, Marie Antoinette, never uttered the now famous words 'Paysans n'avaient pas de pain. Qu'ils mangent de la brioche', which translates as 'The peasants have no bread … let them eat brioche'. Only fifty years later, as her reputation became tarnished on partisan retelling of the French Revolution, was it claimed she had.

The word 'brioche' is often mistranslated as cake (as in 'let them eat cake'). However, brioche is not cake. It's really just a kind of luxury bread made from flour, butter and eggs.

Anyone thinking that you could simply eat something else if the toast had run out, as you might at a breakfast buffet, just proved they had no idea really about anything, including the plight of the peasants, the shortage of ingredients or indeed how you needed flour to make both bread and brioche.

Of course, today is a different story. The masses may be revolting but they are not starving. It is quite apparent that we eat far too many calories rather than too few. Although more access to accessible starch was the solution in 1789, it has become part of the problem 200 years later. The starch we consume so readily adds to our calorie imbalance, and now potentially threatens our very survival.

By contrast, resistant starch — which was the bane of early man and the starving masses and has been so thoroughly removed from modern foods — is now considered to be a potential solution. A number of diets specifically use resistant starch, from raw potatoes, uncooked oats and even green bananas, as the magic ingredient to lose weight. Certainly, it has fewer available calories yet still makes us feel full.

Low-carb diets

For most people, starchy foods are their major single source of sugar (carbohydrate) and therefore their major single source of calories. For this reason (and others discussed later in this chapter) starchy foods are widely vilified. When most people think about going on a diet, after cutting out the fat and the sweet things, starchy foods are usually next on the hit list. Sometimes even higher.

In recent years, low-starch (i.e. **low-carb**) diets have become very popular. Low-carb diets are those in which the carbohydrate components typically make up less than 20 per cent of the total energy intake. This compares to a standard diet where carbs (mostly starch) typically make up about 50 per cent of all calories we eat.

To reduce the carbs in our diet by this much almost always means cutting out the starchy foods and replacing them with other foods containing proportionally more protein or fat (e.g. meat, poultry, fish, shellfish, eggs, cheese, nuts, seeds and peanuts) or eating plant-based foods that are naturally low in carbohydrates (e.g. non-starchy vegetables, green leaves and tomatoes).

The Banting diet

 William Banting was a funeral director in the 19th century. In fact, he was a funeral director in London, taking care of the Royal family no less, including presiding over the funeral of Prince Albert, consort of Queen Victoria.

He was also sixty and overweight. He could read the writing on the wall. He wrote, 'I could not stoop to tie my shoe ... nor attend to the little offices humanity requires without considerable pain and difficulty, which only the corpulent [grossly overweight] can understand; I have been compelled to go down stairs slowly backwards, to save the jar of increased weight upon the ankle and knee joints, and been obliged to puff and blow with every slight exertion, particularly that of going up stairs.'

He tried every diet available: fasting, vigorous exercise, Turkish baths, sea air and even horse riding. He spared no expense. Nothing worked. But after consulting the best doctors in Harley Street, he finally discovered the trick for him was to give up bread, milk, sugar, beer and potatoes (i.e. sugar and starch).

He lost 20 kilos (46 pounds) in one year and his health was restored. He was so taken with the diet's relative success, in 1863 he published, at his own expense, a booklet describing his personal affliction and ultimate redemption 'which might almost be termed miraculous had it not been accomplished by the most simple common-sense means'.

Not surprisingly his *Letter on Corpulence* became an international bestseller, and the forerunner of every other celebrity diet book that now fills our shelves. The message is straightforward. Because it worked for me, it will work for you too.

Perhaps the best-known examples of modern low-carb diets are the Atkins and Paleolithic (Paleo) diets. However, there is a huge range of other diets that share roughly the same principles with respect to carbs, although they vary in regards to other macronutrients (e.g. fat or protein). For example, the Atkins diet does not restrict the amount of fat you eat, while other low-carb diets reduce both fat and carbohydrate, so the relative proportion of energy from protein goes up (which is why these diets are also sometimes called **high-protein** diets instead of low-carb).

The attraction of low-carb diets is that they are very easy to understand and it's simple to work out what not to eat: the sweet stuff and the starchy foods. However, because many of our staple foods are rich in carbs, generally food choice is reduced when going low carb. This is probably the most significant reason why low-carb diets work well in the beginning. We eat much less because we've much less to choose from. Additionally, eating more protein and fat helps our stomach to fill fuller with a meal and can reduce our appetite. Cutting down the carbs can also work rapidly to produce weight loss. This can give us early positive feedback when we are wavering about our diet and whether to stick with it or not

The big problem is that, in the long term, removing carbohydrate-rich foods from our diet means we don't eat widely across all the food groups and miss out on many of our favourite or most interesting and enjoyable meals. This can lead to us becoming bored with our new restricted menu and reverting to old habits. So the weight rapidly goes back on again when we fall off the wagon. In the long term, low-carb diets are only as good as any other diet we are prepared to stick to.

Cutting out the carbs sometimes also means we eat too much fat instead, which has its own problems (see Chapter 6). If we are not careful, taking away the starch in any low-carb diet can also sometimes mean not getting enough of the other things that starchy foods provide for us, including fibre and resistant starch, minerals, and vitamins like folate.

Fibre

Some of the sugars in our food are not coiled as starch but instead are linked solidly together in long, straight rods, like the long, firm cables that bring the phone and internet into many homes. They are both called **fibre**.

Meat has chewy bits too, which are often indigestible. But this is not fibre. Fibre is only found in plants. Some parts of plants are particularly rich in fibre, like the seeds, grains, nuts, beans, berries, vegetable and fruits (especially their skins).

Cardboard

 Fibre on its own tastes terrible. Have you ever tried eating a bowl of unprocessed bran? It tastes like cardboard. In fact, cardboard is actually made by pressing together bits of fibre derived from wood pulp.

Although we all say, 'Oh, it tastes like cardboard', no one actually eats cardboard. Rabbits and guinea pigs are able to eat wood, so eating cardboard isn't much of a change for them. Cats love to chew and shred cardboard, but they don't usually eat it. However, it's important to remember most of the material in cardboard is recycled, so cardboard often also contains unwanted chemicals that you'd not want to feed your pet, let alone taste yourself.

Whole plants solve the cardboard-taste problem by packing the fibrous parts they'd like you to eat with naturally tasty flavours and many appealing colours. This is yet another reason why eating whole fruits and vegetables is one of the best ways to get the fibre we need for our digestive health.

Unlike slinky starch, the long cables of sugar in fibre are tough and can't uncoil easily. This means that fibre generally can't be digested, even if we cook or boil it. So fibre doesn't add as much to our calorie intake or our waistline.

But this does mean that fibre is not wasted in regards to our health. When fibre is mixed with water, it is able to soak some of it up. This naturally thickens the fluid and makes it feel viscous or gelatinous in our mouth if we ever drink it (like in a fibre supplement). Not all fibre is fully soluble either, so sometimes it can feel a little gritty. Overall, it's a bit like drinking slightly grainy jelly. Jelly, by the way, is made from gelatine, a fibrous protein that comes from the skin and bones of pigs and cows (jelly anyone?).

The same sort of gritty, thickening reaction also happens when the plant fibre we eat is mixed with other foods and the digestive juices inside our intestines. This reaction is important because human digestion is a bit like a washing machine (or cleaning a small child). It takes more than just water and soap to make the process work. It also needs some agitation.

Watery liquids are easy to whip up, like with a teaspoon, and can quickly dissolve things, like sugar into our coffee. On the other hand thick, sticky mixtures like cake batter take a lot more beating and it's a sure bet you are going to need a bigger spoon to get the sugar fully mixed and dissolved.

This is where adding soluble fibre (e.g. beans or green leaves) to a meal transforms the contents of our stomach into a sticky batter. It takes much longer for the digestive enzymes to mix the batter through. This actually slows down our digestion process so that any meal releases all its nutrients more gradually, and not just those contained in the beans or leaves.

When fibre is mixed with water it also causes it to swell. This provides bulk, which helps make us feel full much sooner than if we ate an identical food devoid of its fibre (like wholegrain bread versus a slice of white bread). It is then less likely we'll feel hungry later and the urge to snack between meals is reduced.

If we digested and used everything we ate, we would have no need to poo. Much of the indigestible fibre in a meal remains undigested and holds water, which serves to keep things from drying out too much, while the bulk makes things easier to shift along the digestion tract. For example, there is a good reason why fibre-rich foods like prunes and rhubarb are known for their laxative effect!

On average, we consume less than half the amount of fibre required for optimal digestive health. One reason is that most of the grain products we eat in our diet today are heavily processed and refined, meaning that most of the fibre-rich bits have been removed and only the inner starchy part of the grain left behind (like white rice and white bread). These are just ready and waiting to hit our digestion and settle comfortably on our waistline.

By contrast, wholegrain foods retain the fibre-rich coating called **bran**. For example, flour made from whole grains (which keeps the bran intact) contains over ten times the fibre of standard white flour used to make standard white bread. Similarly, white rice has less than a tenth the fibre content of brown rice. Just by replacing all refined products with wholegrain equivalents, we are able to more than double our intake of fibre without ever really changing our diet.

Sugar diabetes

Most people mistakenly believe that diabetes is caused from eating too much sugar. And as starch is usually the major source of sugar it is commonly believed to be the main cause of sugar diabetes. For sure, there is too much (glucose) sugar in the blood of people with diabetes. But as discussed in Chapter 4, the reason it gets there in the first place is more about having too much 'out of place' fat through eating too much of everything, than it is about being overindulgent specifically on the sweet or starchy stuff.

Yet, when people realize that starchy foods like bread and potatoes carry a hidden sugar load (or indeed represent our greatest daily source of carbohydrate/sugar), they try to avoid starchy foods specifically in order to reduce their risk of diabetes.

It seems rational enough. As we have discussed, although starch does not taste sweet, its locked-up sugars are readily released from their chains when milled and digested, meaning the (amount and speed of) sugars delivered when eating starchy white bread or a mid-morning muffin, for example, are broadly similar to those delivered from eating a bar of sweet milk chocolate. In fact, the risk of developing type 2 diabetes from regularly consuming white rice (i.e. mostly starch) is about the same as if you regularly consumed soft drinks. So cutting out the white rice (starch) makes as much sense as cutting out soft drinks (which makes a lot of sense).

Insulin

 When any sugar is digested, whether simple and sweet or complex and starchy, it triggers the release of hormones that coordinate our body's response. The most important of these hormones is insulin, which controls the efficient delivery of sugars into storage sites for later use in between meals.

The amount of insulin that is needed for efficient metabolic functioning depends on:
- how much sugar we have just eaten (i.e. the carb count)
- how quickly the sugars from that bit of food are digested and absorbed (i.e. the glycaemic index or GI of food)
- how well the insulin is able to do its job (i.e. how insulin sensitive or resistant our metabolism is).

If an appropriate amount of insulin cannot be made in a timely fashion, blood glucose levels will rise uncontrollably. This is type 2 **diabetes**. It is not caused by the sugars or starches we eat, but rather our failure to respond to them appropriately.

Certainly, one of the ways to manage diabetes is to eat a lower-carb diet. Eating fewer carbs may help the pancreas to make sufficient insulin to deal with them or allow the condition to be more easily controlled with medication.

Another way to manage diabetes is to change the kind of carbs to ones that only release their sugars slowly. Like a low-carb diet, these **slow carbs** are slow to release their sugars and can reduce the amount of insulin the pancreas has to make to deal with them.

The rate at which a sugar is absorbed can be estimated by the **glycaemic index** or GI of a food, which ranks different foods on how quickly and how much they raise glucose levels after eating a fixed portion of food, relative to eating the same amount of glucose itself.

A low GI score of less than 55 on the index generally means foods deliver their sugar load more slowly than ordinary or table sugar. The slow delivery of sugars means less insulin needs to be made less quickly. It also means we are less likely to want to eat again soon and tend to eat less overall, which helps for weight control. Many (but not all) low-GI foods are also high in fibre, which may partly explain some of their benefits.

By contrast, high-GI foods (those with a score of 70 and higher) release their sugars quickly following their digestion. This causes a rapid surge of glucose into the bloodstream and the requirement for a rapid surge in insulin in response to prevent glucose control from getting out of hand. Many of the major sources of starch in our diet (flour-based products, such as bread and other baked products, and potato products) can have a high GI, sometimes even higher than eating straight honey or table sugar itself. High-GI foods also don't make us feel as full, or if they do, it quickly wears off and we're left feeling hungry again.

The problem with this diet strategy is that it can be challenging to spot a low-GI alternative. Some packaging will show a GI value, but many staples will not. Moreover, the value on the packet is just a rough guide, and can vary quite a lot between people and between different kinds of meals, the way they are mixed with other meal components and even how they are prepared.

For example, having some protein and fat at dinner can lower the GI of dessert by slowing its passage through the stomach and subsequent digestion. So sweet is not so bad if it comes after savoury. But sweet on its own, like in a soft drink, fruit juice, a piece of white toast, a cake or a muffin with nothing else to slow it down is a sure-fire recipe for sugar load. Drinking alcohol with meals can also lower the GI of both the meal and the alcohol.

Al dente

 It is often recommended that pasta, vegetables, rice and beans are ideally served al dente, meaning still firm when we bite into them with our teeth ('dente' — as in 'dent-ist').

Crunchy (raw) pasta is not bad for us. In fact, it is high in resistant starch, which can be good. However, like green bananas, raw pasta may generate a bit of gas in high doses. It also tastes a bit too starchy for most of us!

On the other hand, no one likes soggy spaghetti! We can't get it to twirl around our fork without it breaking. Overcooked macaroni simply dissolves into a cheese sauce as we stir it in.

The other advantage of al dente pasta is that it has a lower GI and contains a bit more resistant starch than pasta that is cooked to become soggy. This means a slower delivery of starch so we become full sooner and stay that way for longer.

Another culinary trick is to undercook the pasta and then leave it to cool before finishing the job later. This technique (known as al forno) allows the starch to reform into bigger, more stable crystals that are more resistant to our digestive enzymes. Providing the second cooking is at less than 120°C (or about 250°F) this resistant starch is retained, thus providing slower sugar and fewer calories to our count. Of course, if we eat the pasta cold after cooking (e.g. in a salad) the same benefits can be achieved.

The same principle also applies to reheating (or just eating cold) cooked potatoes, other starchy vegetables and grains like rice. It also explains why sushi, cold pasta or even potato salads can give some people gas.

It is important to remember that only foods that contain carbohydrates are ranked on their GI and the GI only ranks carbohydrates on their effect on our glucose levels. It doesn't rank how healthy they are. For example, ice-cream's low GI doesn't make it a healthy product — it's the fat that slows down the delivery of sugar but adds to our waistline that is more the issue.

Beyond weight control, there is also data to suggest that diets naturally rich in fibre (including lots of wholegrains, legumes, nuts, fruits and vegetables, etc.) are associated with a reduced risk of developing diabetes. Consequently, entirely cutting out all the wholegrain bread, legumes and starchy vegetables may remove some of the very things that are keeping diabetes away, like the fibre, resistant starch and other nutrients.

A more sensible solution to preventing diabetes is not to give up starches entirely, but substitute the key offenders like white rice, overcooked pasta and products made of refined wheat flour (which, like soft drinks, are mostly just sugar) with more nutritious alternatives (e.g. wholegrain foods, green leafy vegetables).

Regular with a chance of wind

For every cell in the human body, there are about ten times as many bacteria that share the ride with us. In fact, inside every person there are numerically more microbes than there have ever been humans walking on the face of the earth — about a hundred trillion in total and weighing up to 2 kilos, or about 4.5 pounds.

These bacteria are not just along for a free ride. They pay their way by performing a number of important chores, including removing toxins and producing chemicals that keep us and our insides healthy. However, our bacterial passengers can also sometimes contribute to poor health. In fact, many common conditions (including obesity, diabetes, heart disease, bowel problems and some cancers) have all been linked to changes in the composition of gut microbes or the chemical products that they make.

The make-up of the bacteria that line our intestines is significantly modified by what we eat, and particularly what we don't digest and leave for them to chew on. These bacteria love fibre, resistant starch and other indigestible sugars. These sugars are collectively known as **FODMAPs** (standing for Fermentable Oligosaccharides Disaccharides

Monosaccharides And Polyols). Because we don't digest and absorb them ourselves, FODMAPs are the major nutrients that reach down in our colon to feed our resident bacterial hoards.

By regularly eating food rich in FODMAPs, we are able to support or even enhance our gut bacteria. This is why adding fibre, raw vegetables, unprocessed starch or indigestible sugars to meals is sometimes called **prebiotic** (as opposed to antibiotic strategies, which kill bacteria).

The downside is that FODMAPS that feed the bacteria in our large intestine also result in the release of **gases** as they are fermented. For example, beans increase gas production because of their rich content of poorly digestible sugars, fibre and resistant starch.

Breaking wind

 Most people are contentedly flatulent. On an average day, we quietly release somewhere between 2 and 3 litres (4 to 6 pints) of gas, mostly hydrogen, carbon dioxide and methane. This is about the same volume of gas as that inside a blown-up party balloon.

However, some people are really troubled by all this gas. The stretching and distension of their intestines can create an uncomfortable sense of fullness, bloating, cramps, burping, gas and sometimes diarrhoea.

In fact, the most common reason that many people (and particularly women) prefer to avoid starchy foods is to avoid the 'heavy' sensation that often follows eating them. In severe cases, it is sometimes called **irritable bowel syndrome** (or IBS), which is usually caused by too much gas or increased sensitivity to it.

The more FODMAPs we eat (e.g. whole cans of baked beans), the more gas we make. Any time we increase the amount of FODMAPs in our diet we will also increase gas production, especially if it's done suddenly. For example, if we are used to having white toast for breakfast and then one day decide to go on a health kick and have a bowl of raw oats, the next day we'll probably be more flatulent than usual.

The most commonly eaten foods that contain FODMAPs are those that also have lots of starch, such as breads and cereals, pasta and bananas (especially when they are not fully ripe). Many vegetables also contain FODMAP sugars that we can't digest (but our bacteria can), including beans, mushrooms, broccoli, cauliflower, Brussels sprouts and other members of the cabbage family, onions, garlic and other members of the onion family. Equally, apples, pears, avocados, plums, prunes, watermelon and stone fruit can also give some of us wind.

Some people also have a reduced capacity to digest certain natural sugars like fructose or lactose. This means that should they have too much of them (e.g. lactose in milk, or fructose in sweets) more of these sugars will pass through to their gut bacteria than would occur in most people. Their bacteria will then gorge on the extra sugar and produce as much gas as if they had eaten an excess of FODMAPs, like a can of baked beans. This sometimes creates unpleasant symptoms known as intolerance (e.g. lactose intolerance or fructose intolerance). Most people can eat dairy products and have their fill of sweet desserts without these problems, because they absorb these sugars pretty much fully, so none of them reaches the bacteria in the large intestine to be fermented into gas.

For a significant number of people, cutting down the foods naturally high in gut-fermentable FODMAPs can substantially improve how their tummy feels after a meal. This can be achieved in a number of different ways, depending on where the FODMAPs in our diet are coming from to begin with. However, for many people their major source of FODMAPs is cereal grain in bread, baking, breakfast cereal and a host of other foods. So to get rid of the grains, they go gluten-free.

The gluten blues

Products made from wheat contain more than just starch and fibre. They also contain many different proteins that are naturally present in wheat grains, the most abundant of which is **gluten**. As the name suggests, gluten is a sticky glue-like substance. Gluten is essential for holding a loaf together as the bread dough rises in an oven. Without gluten, bread is either flat or dense and unpleasantly crumbly.

Gluten is only found in the grains of wheat and related species like rye and barley, as well as wheat-hybrids like spelt, kamut and triticale. This means that any product containing these grains also contains some gluten. There are the obvious gluten-containing wheat products such as bread, cakes, biscuits, pastries, cereal, pasta and the like. But then there are also many not so obvious sources of gluten, like sausages, beer, ice-cream, sauces, stocks and mayonnaise.

Over the last few decades, gluten has assumed a bit of a pariah status, and is often viewed in the same way as other dietary evils like cholesterol and saturated fat. This is mostly because a small number of people (maybe 1 to 2 per cent of the population) are allergic to wheat or react to gluten specifically. The latter is known as coeliac (or celiac) disease.

Coeliac disease

 Coeliac disease affects between 1 to 2 per cent of all adults. Coeliac disease is caused by the immune system attacking and damaging the intestines whenever any gluten is eaten.

To stay healthy it is essential for people with coeliac disease to avoid all gluten, which means avoiding all wheat products and other products that contain wheat in their diet for the rest of their life. Even tiny amounts of gluten are enough to set off a reaction. There is no other cure and it can only be treated this way.

Oats do not contain gluten (and in some countries can be labelled as gluten free). But oats have something similar and so can cause the same reaction as wheat in some people with coeliac disease. Oats are also often contaminated with small amounts of wheat, which is also unsafe for some people with coeliac disease.

Although symptoms vary from person to person, if someone with coeliac disease should eat food containing any gluten it can cause intestinal problems like chronic diarrhoea, distention/bloating, abdominal pain and gas. Consequently, many people with coeliac disease don't realize they have it, just thinking it is their grumbly tummy or irritable bowels. However, once diagnosed and treated, the cause of their symptoms is usually obvious.

Outside of providing special gluten-free products for people with coeliac disease, gluten-free is mostly a marketing ploy. For the 99 per cent of the population that doesn't have coeliac disease, there is no evidence that gluten itself is in any way harmful or causes intestinal problems. Nonetheless, the fact that going gluten free is the only treatment for coeliac disease is enough for the majority of people to misinterpret the grain-free, gluten-free option as the obvious intrinsically healthy one. Just because some people need some treatment for their disease, does not mean that everyone else should also take the treatment themselves.

There are, however, some positives from going gluten free that have nothing to do with gluten. For example, the resistant sugars present in wheat products can generate gases and upset the bowels of some people. So they may feel less bloated and uncomfortable when going gluten free. But this is actually due to avoiding FODMAPs, not due to avoiding gluten (unlike coeliac disease). And wheat is not the only source of FODMAPs in our diet.

But there are downsides too for gluten-free products. Special gluten-free processing and substitution of other grains that are fully gluten free (like chia, quinoa, amaranth, rice, potato, etc.) adds to the cost of gluten-free products, compared to the mass-produced and therefore cheaper wheat-based products.

Getting rid of all the wheat in our diet also means getting rid of a major dietary source of fibre, minerals and vitamins like folate, a vitamin essential for the health and development of babies while in their mother's womb. If women are not taking supplements while planning for their pregnancy or eating the green foliage of leafy vegetables (hence the term folate), then folate-fortified bread is their biggest source of folate. It makes little sense to give it up.

And when we are replacing all the wheat, what are we replacing it with? Often if a product is gluten free, it contains more fat and sometimes more sugar to make it just as palatable as the regular dough. Bitter pills only seem reasonable to swallow if they are worth the price of health.

Eat the crusts

Children never eat their crusts. No matter how much we ask. No matter how much we complain. They are treated with the same disdain as a banana peel or the rind of an orange.

It is hard to understand why. It's all bread after all. It all starts from the same dough made from exactly the same ingredients. However, evaporation of water from the outside creates a dry, firm brown **crust** that contrasts with the soft, porous inside (known as the crumb).

The rate at which water is lost from the surface of baking bread can be adjusted by changing the oven temperature, humidity or flow of air. This allows bakers to accurately control the thickness and hardness of any crust and create the same perfect culinary results over and over again.

In the same way, it is very possible to make effectively 'crustless' bread by baking at low heat, high humidity or heating from inside rather than the outside (e.g. by microwave or electricity). But somehow this concept has never caught on, despite our children's obvious dislike of eating their crusts, and our dislike of their apparent wastefulness.

Curly locks

 A famous old wives' tale suggests that eating bread crusts makes hair curl(ier). Kids certainly have less curly hair than adults. But this is not because they don't eat their crusts. Young hair is just finer, shorter and less susceptible to curl. Natural curls are largely a matter of genetics rather than diet.

Having curly hair was once considered an important sign of affluence. What medieval woman had so much time on her hands that she could ornately curl her hair? One who didn't have to work hard making a crust?

And what would you do with the leftover crusts if you had them? They would be fed to the pigs, whose tails are intrinsically curly.

The nursery rhyme goes:

Curly locks! Curly locks! Wilt thou be mine?
Thou shall't not wash dishes, nor yet feed the swine
But sit on a cushion and sew a fine seam
 And feed upon strawberries, sugar, and cream.
Just like the upper crust would.

In preservative-free, olden days, the crust of bread had an important effect on its shelf life. But by being on the outside, the crust is also in contact with the external environment, and all the fingers, flies and other contaminants that touch it on its way to our mouth. In avoiding the crusts, maybe our kids are just being hygienic? (Like when did that ever happen?)

The same chemistry that makes crusts brown (appropriately known as the **browning reaction**) also leads to the generation of more complex and more intense flavours than are found in the rest of the loaf. Most adults prefer these tasty chewy bits over the bland interior of white bread. But our children do not.

Children generally prefer sweet and dislike bitter tastes. The highest concentration of bitter chemicals in bread is found in the crust. The same taste preferences also see children happily consuming their starchy potatoes but avoiding their green vegetables, rich as they are in flavour and nutrients. They drink milk while we love our bitter roasted coffee.

This taste preference may be a very important survival mechanism, an instinct to spit out any bitter poisons before we know any better, while avidly consuming things which are sweet and energy rich, as and when they become available.

The same (browning) chemistry that gives crusts their flavour also creates other chemicals that have the potential to impact our health. Some of these (in pure form) have been shown to have anti-cancer effects. Some also have the opposite effect. So the net health result of eating our crusts is unclear.

The bread crust is probably no healthier than the rest. This is mostly a myth concocted by exasperated parents. The crusts don't contain more fibre or antioxidants, because they start out from the same dough as the inner part does. Just because the crumb inside has air pockets and the crust hasn't, that does not mean it's a radically different kind of bread. It's only denser, and there is less of it.

However, for the most part, bread is not consumed on its own. It is generally an edible platform for the delivery of butter, jam, honey, cheese or a number of condiments. (And if it doesn't spread over the edges, what is the point of eating any further?) The same argument goes for the dry pizza crust, which seems unappetisingly bland when compared to the sumptuous topping inside it.

Some companies have attempted to solve this problem by coating a pizza crust with additional ingredients, sweetening or salting it to mask the bitter products of browning. But it still doesn't work. It's only a spoon, a Popsicle stick, a cheap utensil with which to shovel pizza topping into our mouths. It's just the crust.

The bottom line

Starchy foods like bread, cereals, rice or potatoes are more than just the sum of their sugars or their calories. Make no mistake, sugars and calories count in regards to our waistline and our health. And while abandoning these foods by going low carb or low GI can have an immediate and obvious effect, in the long term they are no better than other methods for weight control. They might work fantastically for some people, like William Banting, but work less well for others for whom taking away their bread or other grains is a great hardship that inevitably leads to rebellion.

At the same time, if we are not eating enough vegetables (which, let's face it, we are not — see next chapter) our major source of resistant starch and fibre is the starchy grains we are planning to give up. In so far as gut bacteria are a key determinant of our health, feeding them even less makes little sense, unless they are causing issues like pain, bloating or excess wind.

The obvious solution is to compromise and have a foot in both camps. Eat a little bread but maximize its fibre. Eat rice and pasta but maximize their resistant starch. Eat more beans, nuts and wholegrain cereals. And importantly, when changing our diet, we should do it gradually, so the wind doesn't stop us.

Do I really have to ...

#9

Eat more fruit and vegetables?

Q: Does it really matter?
A: Yes.

Q: Do vegetarians live longer lives?
A: Not because they eat their vegetables.

Q: Will vegetables make me stronger?
A: Beetroot, maybe.

Q: Will vegetables help me see in the dark?
A: No.

Q: Does an apple a day keep the doctor away?
A: Yes ... or a banana.

Q: What about all those superfoods?
A: Mostly marketing hype.

Q: How do I get the kids to eat their vegetables?
A: Focus on the joy.

From the time we first sat at the dining table, we have been told to eat our vegetables. Our parents didn't mind so much about other parts of the meal. We could even skip dessert (not that we would!). But the one thing they insisted on was that the vegetables were not optional. But why? Because they are really good for you. (Please, eat your carrots!)

Vegetarian

The notion that eating lots of fruit and vegetables is good for us comes partly from what we think happens to those people who regularly eat lots of fruit and vegetables. One obvious group of people who do are vegetarians.

In most Western countries, 3 to 5 per cent of people consider themselves vegetarian, with women much more likely to be vegetarian than men. However, in some countries, like India, the percentage of vegetarians is at least ten times higher.

Vegetarian heresy

 Most people are not vegetarians. Those who are have long been ostracised for being divergent. Vegetarians were considered to be heretics by the Roman Inquisition. Even today, many people still perceive the vegetarian minority as liberal, alternative, high-minded, fanatical or even feminist.

In 1999, a high school student in South Jordon, Utah, was suspended for wearing a sweatshirt with the word 'vegan' on the back. The suspension was later upheld by the Federal court, ruling that the school had the right to suspend those wearing 'gang attire'. Some gangs in the area were thought to have taken up veganism and understandably 'gang attire had become particularly troubling since two students wore trench coats in the Colorado School shooting'.

Vegetarians aren't the only people who eat plenty of vegetables. And being vegetarian has many challenges, too, to ensure the diet is complete with all the vital nutrients. But if there was really something about eating vegetables, vegetarians would likely have it in spades. And interestingly, vegetarians do seem to have slightly lower rates than everyone else of some major diseases like heart attacks, strokes, obesity, diabetes and some forms of cancer. Whether this is in any way due to the fruit and vegetables they prefer to eat is unclear.

Obviously, one reason that vegetarians might appear to be a bit healthier is partly because the kind of people who chose to eat only or mostly vegetables are also often the kind of educated people who do all the other healthy things too, like pick out their diet more carefully, exercise more, not smoke, moderate their alcohol and control their waistline better. In essence, they are more likely to follow all the health messages. They also probably listened to their parents when they were asked to eat their broccoli! Many people are vegetarian for reasons other than their health (e.g. religion, animal welfare, environmental impact, etc.), but health is usually part of the reason.

Importantly, after adjusting for all the other healthy things that vegetarians do, the chance of dying over a 5- to 10-year window is about the same in vegetarians and non-vegetarians.

This does not mean eating our vegetables does nothing for our health. On the contrary, a lack of fruit and vegetables in the diet is a leading cause of illness and premature death in the world. It's just that there comes a point when probably enough is enough.

We get most of the benefit we are going to get out of maybe three serves of vegetables and three of fruit every day. If most people are doing this anyway, as in the above study, going vegetarian and eating many more serves of vegetables each day doesn't seem to add much more to the average prospects for long-term survival. On the other hand, if most people almost never touch their vegetables (e.g. in the US the average vegetable intake is far less than two serves a day) vegetarianism looks like a panacea by comparison. It's all a matter of perspective.

One more apple a day

Calorie for calorie there is something special in fruit and vegetables that we just can't get anywhere else. One the most important is probably **fibre**. As discussed in the previous chapter, fibre is that indigestible part of plants that we use to feed our gut's bacteria, which in turn look after our health in many different ways, including reducing the risk of heart disease, diabetes and some cancers.

Fibre is only found in plants. But the grains from plants we eat are usually so processed and refined that most of the fibre is gone from them. That leaves fruit and vegetables as our major sources of fibre, and because we seldom eat our vegetables (and even then mostly as starchy potatoes and, to a lesser extent, corn, pumpkins/squash and carrots) the greatest source of fibre in most diets is generally the fresh fruit that we occasionally remember to consume.

There is an enormous variety of fruit now available. Yet we eat mostly apples and bananas, which are everyone's favourite and available all year round. On average, we're over five times more likely to eat apples and bananas than berries, oranges, stone fruit and melon combined.

An apple a day

 Everybody knows that old saying: an apple a day keeps the doctor away. Apples have been reported to have effects on human health since Adam was a boy. However, this phrase seems to have first cropped up only in the 19th century in the far south-west of Wales.

Apples thrived in the cool damp conditions of South Wales. The most famous of all was the Gwell Na Mil (better than a million) which was well known for its medicinal as well as culinary qualities. In England and America, this apple was also known as Seek-no-Further (for obvious reasons).

In the 19th century, constipation was considered the 'root of all ills' and 'the shortest road to old age, wrinkles and decay'. People's health was being corrupted by their own excrement (known as autointoxication). To treat constipation (usually caused by eating mostly meat, as Welsh farmers were wont to do) they'd have to call for the doctor. Therefore, eating an apple a day (and the fibre laxative therein) was an obvious solution for keeping the doctor away.

Much of the fibre of an apple is found in the skin, so peeling it reduces its overall fibre content by about half. We also throw away one-third of its vitamin A and two-thirds of its vitamin K. The peel also contains some interesting and potentially beneficial antioxidants (e.g. quercetin, ursolic acid and other triterpenoids) and helps to protect the white inside of an apple from going brown when exposed to the air. Still, eating a peeled apple is better than not eating an apple at all, and is a good place to start with the young ones before they get the teeth for chomping into the real deal. Apple juice is no substitute, as it has no fibre (unless it is a juice smoothie made from whole apples).

A peeled banana contains as much fibre as a peeled apple. But unlike the apple peels that we usually eat, we always throw away the banana peel (or leave it to become brown and disgusting until someone else finds it in the bottom of the school bag and throws it away).

The peel or banana skin as it is often called, is actually edible, though somewhat fibrous, waxy and slightly bitter (becoming less so as it ripens). Still, it can be happily thrown into a banana smoothie with no ill effects (but do remember to take off the sticker and wash it first).

When bananas are green and unripe, they do not taste very sweet as most of the sugars are locked up as resistant starch. As a banana ripens and turns yellow, more of these starches are broken down, freeing the sugar and sweetening the taste. This is the same for most ripening fruit, but the taste transition in bananas is the most dramatic.

The potential advantage of eating green bananas is that the large amounts of resistant starch can boost the health of our intestinal bacteria. Consequently, green bananas have become a popular diet element, partly by avoiding the sugar rush of a ripe banana but also via the tummy-filling sensation that only happy microbes and their gases can give us. Apart from the taste, the only other disadvantage is flatulence and bloating, as our gut microbes go bananas.

How to peel a banana

 Bananas are perfectly packaged. Getting into them without squishing their contents takes skill. Give a banana to an infant and you will see how challenging it can be!

Most people dive into a banana by partly cutting or snapping the stem on one side. We then pull the stem downward, dragging the attached peel away from the naked flesh underneath. This opens a rift so that adjacent peel can also be pulled down from the top in two or three different sections until the inner banana is fully revealed.

This is not the only way to skin a banana. Monkeys start from the other (non-stem) end that has that little crunchy brown tail, which is the residue of the banana flower. If you carefully pinch it at this point, the peel splits, coming off in two clean sections. You can then hold onto the stem and use it as a kind of lollipop-stick while you eat the banana right down to its end.

Or you could just cut it in half with a knife and share some with your little monkey.

It is widely recommended that we eat at least two servings of fresh fruit (e.g. two apples or one apple and one banana) every day. Pretty simple, yes? It doesn't seem like much. But less than half of adults routinely meet this mark. Women more than men, children more than adults, but only just. Despite all their fruity abundance, the majority of people still don't regularly eat enough fresh fruit every day. As a result we seldom get enough fibre in our diet to keep us healthy.

If we all ate just one more serving of fruit every day (e.g. just one more apple a day) over 80 per cent of people would reach this (at least two fruit a day) target. This is significant because large studies in China have demonstrated that increasing fruit consumption (from a low baseline) by as little as one extra serving a day could reduce the chance of dying by 6 per cent across the population. This would be mostly due to a lower risk of dying of a heart attack or stroke. In the same study it was noted that people who ate three or more serves a day did not survive much better than those who just had the regular recommended two servings a day. As with vegetables, at some point enough is enough. But for everyone else, and in particular those many people who ate almost no fruit at all on a regular basis, their chances of an early grave were significantly decreased by adding an apple a day.

Seeing in the dark

One of the reasons we often rationalize that eating vegetables might be good for us is that we think they are good for our eyesight and, in particular, may help us to see in the dark.

It's not that easy to see in the dark. We need the very special cells (called rod cells) that line the back of our eyes to be activated by the tiny amounts of light that still exist in the dark places we'd wish to see. Each eye contains about 100 million of these rod cells, whose only job is to work in low light. These cells are very sensitive to light. This means that they are fully switched on by bright daylight, so don't provide much help to our vision during the daylight hours. But at night or in dim light, these cells come into their own and are vitally important in determining whether we can see or not.

Rod cells can't make out colour, which is why things look pretty much like shades of grey in the dark. However, in this modern world of streetlights and LEDs, it is uncommon to have so little light that no colour is visible.

Bright eyes

 Many animals have much better night vision than humans. This is obviously the case for nocturnal animals that have to see in the dark. But even dogs and cats have far superior vision to their masters in low light.

This is partly because these animals possess a special layer of crystals at the very back of their eyes that reflects incoming light forward. This reflected light can then bounce back into their eyes again, essentially to amplify the signal and allow them to see in what would appear pitch black to us.

This is also why when we see animals at night their eyes seem to have a strange colourful glow (known as **eyeshine**). This can be anything from green or blue to reds and oranges. The colour reflected usually depends on the species, allowing clever spotters to identify an animal by just the shine of its eyes. For example, in the forest of the night, a tiger's eyes would be burning bright green. Bright eyes on a rabbit glow blood red.

Humans also naturally reflect light from their eyes but, without this special crystal layer, to a far lesser extent. Consequently, we can only see the reflected light from our own eyes when we are accidentally caught straight-on by a flash photographer. This causes the unphotogenic red-eye effect in some of our worst photos.

The rod cells we use for night vision possess a special chemical to detect incoming light. This is made from vitamin A, most of which comes from our eating fruit and vegetables. In plants, vitamin A is present in yellow, orange and red chemicals (known as **carotenoids**), which are converted into vitamin A when we eat them. This is why orange and red vegetables and fruits are often recommended as a good source of vitamin A. Some examples include carrots, sweet potato, pumpkin (winter squash), capsicum (bell pepper), tomatoes, strawberries, mango, apricots, rockmelon (cantaloupe) and watermelon. But even the rich green ones like spinach, kale, broccoli and lettuce contain just as much. In all cases, fresh and whole is best, as vitamin A can be depleted during preparation, cooking or storage. Those wilted spinach leaves in the bottom of our fridge contain only a fraction of the nutritional boost (as well as flavour) as freshly picked leaves sourced from our own garden.

We can also get vitamin A from some animal sources. For example, astaxanthin is a pink carotenoid found in high concentrations in salmon and shrimp. Pure vitamin A is only found in products from animals that have eaten plants and stored it in their tissues, especially in liver, eggs and milk.

Consuming too little vitamin A in our diet can lead to **night blindness,** as the rod cells don't have the vitamin A they need to make the key chemicals required to see in low light. This is a big problem in many developing countries. It can be fixed by eating more coloured vegetables, like carrots. So, in a way, our parents were partly right. Eating our vegetables can help us see in the dark — but only if we were likely to be very short on vitamin A. Outside of really extreme diets, this almost never happens in the developed world (even if we don't eat all our vegetables).

There is no point in taking much more vitamin A than we need. Eating all our vegetables all the time or munching on a couple of carrots every day will still not make us see as well in the dark as our cats can. But at least we can turn on the light if we need to see.

Vegetables make us strong

On its own the human body cannot manufacture all the essential elements it needs to function properly. Any elements we can't make ourselves have to be obtained by eating the things that can make them. The vital elements we obtain from our diet are known as **vitamins**.

Vitamins do more than help us see in the dark. Almost all of our body's complex chemistry relies on vitamins to keep functioning, and stay healthy and strong. And in the days before multivitamins and fortified food, the best place to get vitamins was fresh fruit and vegetables. Vegetables made us not weak. Which was as good as inferring that they made us strong.

Oranges and lemons

 Perhaps the best example of how eating fruit and vegetables once actually made us strong is the historical plight of long-distance sailors.

Far from land for many weeks at a time, with no access to fresh food, the crew developed vitamin C deficiency (also known as scurvy). They slowly lost their strength and eventually their lives. It was not unusual for fewer than half of those setting out on a sea voyage never to return.

Eventually, an antidote was found. All they needed to do was eat fresh vegetables or fruit to obtain the vital element (vitamin C) contained therein. The most reliable and stable source were citrus fruits like oranges and lemons. This is probably the basis of the famous nursery rhyme, 'Oranges and lemons, sang the bells of St Clements'.

St Clements was in the market area down by the docks where you could buy produce for your next sea voyage or on your return. At least when you could afford it, after you'd grown rich. If you couldn't pay five farthings (the cost of maybe a few lemons) you might well have been sent to the debtor's prison via the Old Bailey courts.

The last lines have a different metre and were probably added later as an afterthought. The final vivid image of 'here comes the chopper to chop off your head' is an inappropriate punishment for a debtor let alone a citrus thief. However, in a disease-infested debtor's prison you may well have met the Grim Reaper and his chopper.

Ever since the 18th century every sailor has known that fruit and vegetables keep them strong and provide an essential substrate through which the vigorous manual work while at sea allows them to actually become stronger.

The most famous reworking of this lore is the briny cartoon superhero Popeye the sailor man, who achieved his superhuman strength simply by consuming a can of spinach. Why it was that canned spinach (rather than baked beans or something else) made his muscles bulge and helped him rescue his fickle Mediterranean babe, Olive Oyl, is now the stuff of folklore.

It is often suggested that early scientific studies had erroneously determined that the iron content of spinach was ten times higher than it actually was, making it look like a superfood. And of course iron is the stuff that steel is made of. It was also well known that iron deficiency led to profound weakness and lethargy, and in the context of an iron-deficient seafarer with little access to fresh meat, the iron contained in spinach would have definitely made him a little stronger, though not superhuman like Popeye.

Along with citrus, fresh greens were well known to transform scurvy sailors into sturdy seamen, literally overnight. In his voyages around the world, Captain Cook had collected green vegetables at every opportunity for their anti-scurvy properties. It is little wonder that people believed that vegetables made them stronger. Because sometimes they really did!

By the early 20th century it was understood that vitamins were the real reason. Spinach, of course, was well known to be extremely high in vitamins, including vitamins A, B1, B2, B6, C and K. Spinach was the closest thing to a multivitamin pill. Of course many other vegetables are also high in vitamins, such as carrots. However, carrots, being taken by a rascally rabbit and only known for helping you see in the dark, left spinach as the next one picked.

The fact that spinach could be canned was also probably an important factor for Popeye. Canned food is ever-ready, portable and has a long shelf-life. On the other hand fresh vegetables are seasonal and hard to keep longer than a few days. It would not have worked if Popeye had to go searching in a vegetable garden every time Olive Oyl got kidnapped. Canned food was literally fast food. It is still used in many households today, with cans of beans or spaghetti on hand to feed those in urgent need of an energy boost.

Beetroot

 In retrospect, Popeye probably should have been eating canned beetroot (often known simply as beets). Beets are surprisingly rich in nitrates, chemicals that provide an easy substrate for our body to make nitric oxide. And nitric oxide is perhaps the most potent natural chemical for relaxing human blood vessels, allowing them to dilate and facilitate the flow of blood to where it needs to go.

This improvement in blood flow is thought to be why taking beetroot is able to improve endurance in sport. More blood flow means less oxygen is needed to do the same task, and more tasks can be done with the same oxygen cost.

The effect is not huge. But neither is the difference between winning gold and silver. This is why many athletes, as well as occasional competitors, now take beets for a boost.

Eating whole beets is probably better than taking beet supplements or nitrate salts, as whole beets provide other beneficial things like sugar and fibre. Concentrated beetroot juice, as found in some supplements, can also cause gastrointestinal upset in some people.

The only issue with eating beets is that its red colour (that comes from the chemical betanin) is not broken down by the human body. Instead it is excreted intact. This can temporarily cause the urine to take on a pink–purple hue. Consequently, the popularity of beets in recent years has seen drug testing at the Olympics take on a completely different colour.

Popeye was not the first to be transformed by fruit and vegetables. In Christian religious history, Adam received knowledge from eating the forbidden fruit. In Chinese legend, the Eight Immortals achieve their immortality through eating a peach. More recently, Banana-man gets his super strength from eating a banana. Sadly, there is absolutely nothing in spinach, beetroot, peaches, apples or bananas that conveys superhuman prowess. But that does not mean they can't be super for our health.

Superfoods

It is also widely believed that many plants also contain some super-special chemicals that are super for our health. These are often called **phytochemicals** or phytonutrients (simply meaning these chemicals/nutrients are found in plants).

It is absolutely true that some plants really contain unique chemicals that have dose-dependent actions on the biological functions of the human body. Many are poisons. But some can work as medicines. Aspirin was originally identified in the bark of the yew tree, and is still widely used for treating fevers and headaches. Quinine (again from the bark of a tree) is still used to treat malaria. Another super-chemical is folate.

Fortification

 Folate (or folic acid) is a vitamin. It is super essential for human health as well as fertility. Folate is especially important during early pregnancy. During the first month, even before a woman may know she is pregnant, the folate she eats is critical for the developing baby in her womb.

Folate is highest in the foliage of leafy vegetables, which is where its name comes from. So the leaves we normally eat like lettuce, spinach, chard and Brussels sprouts are a major natural source of folate in our diet. Folate is also naturally found in significant amounts in legumes (peas, beans, lentils, peanuts, etc.), broccoli, asparagus, avocado, rice, and wholegrain cereals and seeds. Apart from plants, folate is also present in high concentrations in liver and products made from it.

The problem is that we don't always eat as much foliage and legumes as we should. And we almost never eat liver anymore.

To prevent the serious complications that could result from inadequate folate in early pregnancy, flour, cereals and orange juice are now all fortified with folate. This has approximately doubled average folate levels in adults and reduced the numbers with really low folate levels from 24 per cent of all adults to now less than 1 per cent. This super intervention has significantly reduced the number of babies born with serious birth defects. In addition many women take additional folate supplements while planning for a pregnancy, as well as during pregnancy and breastfeeding to facilitate their babies' development.

The effect of folate supplements on adult health is still debated. Clinical trials of giving people folate supplements or folate-fortified food have not replicated the clear benefits of eating a diet naturally high in folate. This may just be because these diets must also be high in beneficial fruit and vegetables. It may have nothing to do with the folate. It may also be that following fortification, folate is no longer a limiting factor. So supplements don't give the kick they used to, while fruit and vegetables remain just as super and can never be replaced by a pill.

Some plants and particularly some parts of plants (e.g. berries) are especially rich in phytonutrients. Many people believe that a cure for cancer or heart disease exists right now in some plant, if only we had Sean Connery to find it for us deep in the Amazonian jungle.

Today, many of the nutritional marvels of the plant world are widely promoted as superfoods. Sadly, this is mostly a marketing ploy. There is no magic berry that provides super health.

But they are super in one respect: what they have is almost always in a slightly more concentrated form than we can find elsewhere. They offer more bang for our berry.

Obviously, during times past when people were malnourished with not a lot to eat, those superfoods that supplied, in a concentrated form, the vitamins and other essential elements we needed to survive, would have been an enormous boon. Especially when we'd have to track down and eat much more of the other ordinary foods that were far lower in these same elements to get us out of our jam. This is how most of these super plants got their mythical status. They really did once save people's lives!

The problem today is that we almost always have too much food rather than too little. In a balanced modern diet there is very little chance for any significant life-threatening nutritional deficiency to occur. Many foods are fortified and many people often take multivitamins over and above this. Only when it is not possible to eat a good variety of healthy foods (e.g. such as if we are on a special diet or have food intolerances/allergies) or if we have restricted our food to the point where our nutrient intake falls, then super-concentrated superfoods may be useful once again, providing what we need in a concentrated form so we don't have to eat too much to get what we need. If we are just eating badly the solution is not a superfood. The solution is to eat better food.

If it was simply all about more-is-better, vegetarians would all live long lives. They don't. Vitamin supplements would be the solution to every health problem. They are not. In fact some studies have shown that those who take vitamins and other nutritional supplements often end up with worse health outcomes than those who do not.

It could be we can get too much of a good thing. Or maybe the impetus to eat fruit and vegetables is not as strong when we are already taking supplements. Either way, there is no single supplement or combination of supplements that can match a diet rich in fruit and vegetables.

Duplicity

When our kids don't eat their vegetables, there are few alternatives. Our rational adult mind feels honour bound to provide a logical explanation. We might say vegetables will help them see in the dark or make them stronger (although clearly it won't do either unless they were malnourished). Even telling them that eating their vegetables is healthy or good for them doesn't sway them.

Even worse, some studies suggest that such duplicitous phrases may actually put some children off eating their vegetables. From our kids' point of view, if something is good for their health or makes them strong, then it probably can't also be yummy as well — it's like the bitter medicine they have to swallow. And it's not just our children. In much the same way, many adults feel that if a food is positively delicious, it can't also be positively healthy. Food can't do two things at once, or at least do them well.

Anyway, it's not the added nutritional value our children are after when they eat! And they are not really starving (although they often say so). They are just doing what comes naturally: eating to please themselves.

Of all the food they eat, children typically like vegetables the least. This is mostly because of the taste. Fruit is more acceptable as it tends to be sweeter, but vegetables often have a distinctly bitter element to which our children are biologically as well as psychologically more sensitive. Vegetables also come with the added nuisance of being *required* to be eaten. Even without tasting them, if a child perceives that something looks like a vegetable and/or smells like a vegetable, it is definitely a vegetable and as such is yuk (and instantly rejected).

Instead of saying vegetables are good or healthy, a number of alternative solutions have been devised by die-hard parents to get children eating more vegetables more often. By and large, all of these interventions work simply by improving the enjoyment of the experience of eating vegetables.

For example, getting rid of the immediate pressure to eat something right now and saying 'just try it another time' seems to help. Carrot crunching competitions and vegetable experiments can be fun. Participation in vegetable-related activities like gardening, shopping and meal preparation also promotes a connection with vegetables and improves the chances of kids wanting to eat them.

Encouraging children to simply taste food, rather than eat a whole portion, also works. Eventually they will become familiar with the food and start to eat a bit more. Sharing meals and vegetables sets a good example. If your parents and big brother are enjoying their veggies, maybe they are not so bad after all.

Finally, there is always the old trick of simply disguising the vegetables. Replace half the meat in a bolognese sauce with lentils and a shredded carrot or zucchini (courgette). Substitute chickpeas (garbanzo beans) and cauliflower in a curry, with only a little of the chicken or beef. Shred the onions and garlic so finely they will never know they are there. Eventually they learn to expect them and find everyone else's meat-based cooking wholly unsatisfying.

The bottom line

Today we seldom eat enough vegetables. Less than 5 per cent of our total vegetable intake is green and leafy. It's little wonder that Popeye looks like Superman by comparison. It's little wonder a diet loaded with greens seems like we are eating superfoods or that vegetarians seem to be the healthy ones.

We do a little better with fruit. But only just. We all could use an extra apple (or banana) a day to keep the doctor away.

We don't need to eat excessively large amounts of fruit and vegetables or eat them exclusively. If we'd like to that's great, especially if we use them as a substitute for the highly processed, calorie-rich, nutritionally empty parts of our diet. But three of each every day (three fruit and three vegetable serves) is probably enough.

To pull this off we have to make a habit of eating them. And to make a habit of them, just like when persuading our kids to eat their vegetables, we all have to enjoy them. There are no end of possibilities. Fruits and vegetables are the most diverse and interesting foods we can eat. Some are sweet. Some are sour. Some are bitter. Some are almost too complex for words. They don't need to be super, or foreign or exotic. They don't need to come with a high price tag. We just need to enjoy eating them, so we will always eat enough of them.

Do I really have to ...

#10

Lower my cholesterol?

Q: Why is a high cholesterol level a bad thing?
A: High cholesterol clogs up our arteries, and gives other clogging elements something they can use to clog with.

Q: What if I don't have high cholesterol levels?
Should I still be worried about it?
A: Everyone benefits from lowering levels of harmful cholesterol in their blood, even those whose levels are not high.

Q: Should I avoid eating egg yolks and other cholesterol-rich foods?
A: Only if you have high cholesterol levels or are taking medications to bring them down.

Q: Should I be taking statins?
A: Only if your risk of heart attack is high.

Q: Can cholesterol ever be good?
A: No. But cholesterol inside HDL particles is a good marker of an efficient system for getting cholesterol out of our clogged arteries.

Q: Why does cholesterol-free sugar still increase my cholesterol levels?
A: Any excess sugar is happily converted into excess fat. This means there will be more cholesterol in our blood to transport our excess fat.

Cholesterol is the building block of disaster. It is the stuff that clogs up our arteries, contributing to their narrowing and stiffening, and ultimately blocking them off all together. When a blockage occurs in the arteries that supply the heart, it is called a **heart attack** (also known as a myocardial infarction or MI). When a blockage in blood flow to the brain occurs, it is called a **stroke** (also known as a cerebrovascular accident or CVA).

Together, heart attacks and strokes are among the most significant causes of death in humans, and the most likely reason that most of us will not reach a hundred. If we don't want to die any time soon, keeping the blood flowing to our heart and our brain is top of the list. And one way to do this is to keep our blood cholesterol levels in check and prevent this from blocking off our arteries.

Scientists have been routinely measuring cholesterol levels in human blood for about the last fifty years. It turns out that if we keep our blood cholesterol levels low throughout our lives, the chances of remaining healthy and surviving to a hundred are significantly increased. In addition, our chances of surviving other common problems of being overweight, having high blood pressure or diabetes, are also improved.

By contrast, if we have high cholesterol levels in our bloodstream, this raises our risk of having a heart attack or a stroke. In addition, all the other bad things that cause narrowing of our arteries (like diabetes, high blood pressure, smoking and stress) do this through triggering the excess build-up of cholesterol in the walls of our arteries. This cholesterol in our arteries comes from the cholesterol in our bloodstream. So having high cholesterol levels in our bloodstream just makes it easier for everything else to kill us.

The road to ruin

Blood vessels function in our bodies just like the roads in our cities, allowing for a steady flow of traffic along freeways and major arterial roads, and then venturing off into smaller and shorter streets until we reach our destination.

Like any transport system, the health of the roads is critically important for maintaining the healthy flow of traffic on them. If the surface of the road stays smooth, traffic can flow easily and get to where it needs to go. Smooth roads also don't offer much resistance, so wear and tear on the vehicles travelling along them is also kept to a minimum.

Over time, changes inevitably occur to the surface of any road due to fatigue and abrasion. A road will typically thicken in some places and become thinner in others, creating an uneven, bumpy surface. This roughness increases wear and tear on any vehicles that passage along its uneven surface, as well as making the sound of the traffic distinctly noisier. As the years go by, the road surface gets stiffer and less flexible. Eventually, small bits might even get eroded and flake off.

Underneath the surface, the base of the road is just as important. It takes most of the pressure load of the passing traffic and usually outlives the surface, which can be continuously replaced. But over time, the packing of the soil beneath the pavement begins to weaken, while at the same time it is put under even more pressure by the stiff upper crust. If no maintenance is undertaken, eventually potholes will form in the road, and traffic will be disrupted.

Importantly, these changes do not occur equally in all parts of the road. The sections that easily become damaged and form potholes the fastest usually have the extra pressure of heavy vehicles or have the added force of breaking and turning the corner. By contrast, a conventional car driving on a well-maintained straight road does very little damage.

Almost the same process of progressive deterioration that happens to our roads also occurs in the arteries and blood vessels of our body, where fatigue, abrasion and general wear and tear lead to changes known as **atherosclerosis**.

As with the city roads, these changes do not occur equally in all parts of our blood vessels. Our largest blood vessels, like our largest roads, are under the greatest pressure and so are most vulnerable to atherosclerosis. Equally, in those sections of blood vessels where blood flow divides and needs to quickly turn a corner, the extra shear on the road surface increases the wear and tear and the risk of forming potholes.

As the years go by, the surface of our arteries gets stiffer and less flexible, just like our roads. This is simply known as **hardening of the arteries**. Our blood vessels may thin in some places but thicken in others and may even start to bulge a little bit. This is known as **plaque**, because from the surface it looks like a commemorative plaque jutting out from a smooth wall. As will be discussed later in this chapter, this plaque is made mostly of cholesterol.

This bulging plaque creates turbulence in the blood flow, makes the ride rougher and creates resistance for all the blood cells that normally roll over it. Just like traffic on a rough road, this turbulence also creates more noise, sometimes enough to be heard by a stethoscope (called a **bruit**).

Just as the softening of the road base ultimately leads to potholes, accumulating cholesterol-rich plaques in the walls of large arteries softens their resolve, and reduces their resistance to the stresses of regular use. If no pre-emptive maintenance is undertaken, the plaque becomes progressively unstable. But while the road surface remains intact, the traffic keeps flowing, so there are no symptoms to know that problems lie ahead.

But then one fateful day, a load stresses an unstable artery past its breaking point. The surface of the weakened artery becomes suddenly eroded and a pothole is formed. This is exactly what happens during the sudden event of a heart attack or stroke.

The life and death of John Hunter

 John Hunter was a Scottish surgeon and one of the most influential scientific figures of the 18th century. His motto was 'Don't think, try the experiment'.

This brought him fame, but also got him into trouble. In a legendary experiment he inoculated himself with pus taken from a prostitute with gonorrhoea, a sexually transmitted disease. He aimed to prove that syphilis and gonorrhoea were actually different symptoms of the same illness. And when he got both, his fame was assured. Unfortunately, it later turned out that the prostitute also had both syphilis and gonorrhoea, so his acclaimed conclusion was actually wrong.

In his later years, he suffered greatly from chest pains. When he became upset, a frequent problem for this temperamental Scotsman, his heart began to race and soon after he would experience crushing pain in his chest. He keenly observed that his 'life was in the hands of any rascal who chose to annoy or tease him'. This time, he was fatally accurate. On 16 October 1793, following a heated meeting with the hospital board of governors, he left the room, groaned and dropped dead.

The problem with a hole in the surface of an artery is the same as if we accidentally cut ourselves. Blood can get out! Fortunately the pothole is usually quite small and repair crews quickly move in to make a clot and stop any blood leaking away. But just like a single accident at peak hour on the freeway, the flow of blood through a damaged artery can quickly turn into a parking lot.

And this is an even bigger problem because blood is supposed to flow. When it doesn't flow it clots. It's not like traffic that can get going again when the lights turn green. Stopping means sticking and this is a disaster for the heart and the brain, as everything downstream of the accident that depends on that blood flow will suffer and eventually die. Unlike our skin, hearts and brains cannot grow back. Any significant loss of blood flow always means some loss of heart or brain function.

To get things moving again after an accident, the road must be opened up. The quicker this can be achieved, the more likely any permanent damage can be prevented or at least kept to a minimum. This is usually accomplished by rushing to hospital in an ambulance where surgeons will thread a thin balloon through the blocked artery, and carefully blow it up to restore blood flow once again. This is known as **angioplasty**.

Another way to quickly restore blood flow is to dissolve any clot using clot-busting medication, like using a tow truck to drag away the debris of an accident and open things up again as quickly as possible. This is how many strokes are also managed in hospitals.

Clot busting

 It is well known that chance favours the prepared mind. But sometimes people just get lucky. Scientist William Tillet was working late in his laboratory one night. He was trying to prove the *Streptococcus* bacteria he was working with could be used to prevent the clotting of human blood. It couldn't. So he walked out frustrated, leaving his test tubes in the rack without bothering to clean up. Much to his amazement, when he later returned, the clots he had seen form in the tubes that contained bacteria had miraculously dissolved. He had accidentally discovered a clot buster, which he later named **streptokinase** after the little bacteria from whence it came.

Although it was well known that heart attacks were caused by clots in the coronary arteries, at the time the only treatment available was aspirin. Aspirin could prevent new clotting but did not make what was already there go away. Consequently the clot-busting streptokinase became an instant hit. When given to a person within a few hours of having a heart attack the chance of dying was reduced by 25 per cent. Clot-busters in many different forms continue to be used today to unblock arteries following heart attacks or strokes.

Sometimes surface erosions are very small, and have only a limited and temporary impact on traffic flow in our arteries. These tiny potholes are not big enough to trigger a blockage or a heart attack. But as the scars of each little erosion are left behind, the roadway is progressively narrowed. Just like with a freeway, if we lose a lane or two, it's not a major problem most of the time. However, things come to a head at rush hour, when more traffic needs to use the road.

The same occurs in our heart. A little narrowing of arteries is not a big problem most of the time, as there is still enough blood flow to get by. But when our heart needs more blood flow, such as when we exert ourselves rushing about or experience other stresses that get the heart racing, things come to a head. In such circumstances, any narrowing in the road to our heart can suddenly become a limiting factor for our heart to get the blood as quickly as it needs. This is usually experienced as chest pain (known as **angina**) and is often a forerunner of more complete and more serious blockages in the future (i.e. heart attack or stroke).

What is cholesterol?

Cholesterol is universally portrayed as the bad guy. It is not intrinsically bad. At least, it doesn't start out that way. Cholesterol is a waxy substance that is made by all cells but especially by the liver. It is actually a vital component of healthy cellular function. Every time our body makes new cells we need cholesterol to build them.

Cholesterol is used by our cells at their surface a bit like a sealant, to stop things getting in or out of their own accord. This means the only way into or out of a cell is through the right channels. And channels can be regulated, opened or shut as required, so a high degree of control can be exerted to keep things safe and stable.

Like any household sealant, cholesterol is also flexible. This means that cell membranes enriched with cholesterol are not only waterproof but can bend too, allowing the cells in our body to change shape or even move about as required. This is unlike (low-cholesterol) plant cells, which have a rigid outer coating, so seldom go anywhere in a hurry.

Each cell of the human body has enzymes to manufacture cholesterol as required. On average, the human body makes about 1 gram of cholesterol each day, about half of which is made by the liver, and then transported out to where it is needed.

It's a delicate business to move cholesterol around our body to where it is needed for sealing and construction. This is because cholesterol is a type of fat. Like other fats and oils, it doesn't dissolve in water. Cholesterol would just congeal like oil, floating on the surface, where it would be completely unusable as well as toxic to the environment. This is in contrast to other essential elements such as sugar, which can simply dissolve in our blood and be transported to all the far-flung corners of our bodies as needed.

To get around this very specific oil-and-water problem, our body uses special waterproof container trucks known as **lipoprotein particles,** so named because they are particles that contain lipids (like cholesterol), and proteins, which are the truck drivers. The specific proteins in each lipoprotein particle confer specific functions to these particles, directing where they go and what they do when they get there. In this way some lipoprotein particles are quintessentially bad for our health. Some others can be good for us. And others are just plain ugly.

The 'bad' cholesterol

Most of the cholesterol that circulates in our bloodstream is contained in small LDL particles. The main job of LDL particles is to transport cholesterol out from the liver where it is made or collected and truck it out, like building supplies, to any areas in the body that need it to build. Places that are damaged or inflamed need more cholesterol to rebuild themselves, so they capture LDL particles and stockpile it for their needs.

This is particularly the case for blood vessels. When they are stressed, damaged or inflamed for whatever reason, they accumulate cholesterol (which they largely take from LDL particles). This accumulation of cholesterol progressively leads to plaque formation along the walls of large blood vessels and instability, which ultimately leads to heart attacks and strokes.

The cholesterol that is contained and moved in LDL particles is called **LDL cholesterol**. Consequently, LDL cholesterol is generally considered to be the 'bad' cholesterol. This is because high blood levels of LDL cholesterol, and especially years of exposure to it, are associated with an increased risk of heart attacks, strokes and other diseases involving blood vessels.

This association was first recognized many years ago when it was found that some people and their families had extremely high levels of LDL cholesterol in their blood, up to ten times higher than normal. As a result, they had an enormously increased risk of heart attacks, even occurring as early as five years of age, and a sadly short life expectancy. At the same time, it was also clear that some people born with much lower concentrations of LDL cholesterol than normal in their blood had a lower risk of heart attacks and strokes, and increased chances of longevity.

Cholesterol free

Given cholesterol's clear association with heart attacks and strokes, the obvious solution was to tell everybody to stop eating cholesterol. Why would we want to add to our burden by eating more? So the message went out in the seventies and eighties that cholesterol-rich foods were off the menu.

Cholesterol-rich foods

 Animals and all the products made from their fat are rich in cholesterol. Consequently, the major sources of cholesterol in our diet include:
- meat and poultry, especially those parts that are visibly fatty, the skin, brain, kidneys and liver, sausage, bacon, mince, pâté, etc.
- egg yolk (there is no cholesterol in egg white)
- full-fat dairy products (especially cheese, butter, whole milk, ghee, custard, and ice-cream)
- crab, shrimp, lobster, oysters

- fish eggs (caviar, roe, etc.).

Plants contain only tiny amounts of cholesterol, at concentrations at least a hundredfold lower than in animals, and a hundredfold lower again than products made from their fatty parts, like butter. This means that plant products like margarine generally have a lower cholesterol content.

Under this new order, many 'cholesterol-free' products like margarine became highly marketable, and made major inroads into everyday diets. We all wanted the healthy low-cholesterol alternatives. Cholesterol in food was the bad guy even though it was LDL cholesterol in our blood that was really the problem. But in the end it turned out that what we ate and what was in our blood was not as closely linked as was originally thought.

For the vast majority of people, eating a little more butter or going 'cholesterol free' in their diet has little or no effect on their blood cholesterol levels. This is because the human body makes most of the cholesterol it needs: about 1000 milligrams (1 gram) of cholesterol each day. On top of this we usually take in about another 200 mg from our diet. But if we didn't eat any cholesterol at all (e.g. if we were fasting or vegan), our body would simply make up the difference by synthesizing a little more cholesterol to ensure everything runs like a well-oiled machine. Equally, if we ate twice as much cholesterol as we'd usually eat (e.g. if we eat a lot of butter on one day instead of our usual no-cholesterol margarine, or have caviar for a special occasion) our liver would simply make a little less cholesterol that day.

This is why there is only a weak link between the cholesterol in our food and levels of cholesterol in our blood. Only about one in every five people is sufficiently sensitive that eating more or less cholesterol makes any significant difference to their blood concentration of LDL cholesterol. This is mostly due to their specific genes that control cholesterol absorption and handling.

But public health is all about the greater good. Even if only one out of every five people will actually benefit from a low-cholesterol diet, persuading everyone to go 'cholesterol free' lowers the average LDL cholesterol levels by 2 to 5 per cent. On a large scale, 'cholesterol free' ultimately adds up to slightly fewer heart attacks and strokes.

But while benefits of a low-cholesterol diet are small in the general population, it is a very different story if the liver has no way to get round it and simply make up for the shortfall. This happens when we take a medicine that inhibits cholesterol synthesis known as a **statin**. And this is precisely what millions of people do.

Statin quo

The most widely used class of medication to lower LDL cholesterol is the **statins**. There are a number of different formulations, doses and agents available. Each of their chemical names ends in the suffix 'statin' (e.g. simvastatin, atorvastatin, rosuvastatin, pravastatin, pitavastatin, etc.). But everyone knows them as just statins.

Statins work by partly inhibiting the manufacture of cholesterol by the liver. To make up for the shortfall, the liver then actively takes back harmful cholesterol from the bloodstream and tissues. As a result, in people taking statins LDL cholesterol levels fall in the blood by a third to a half, and the risk of heart attacks and strokes falls with it. This is at least ten times better than a low-cholesterol diet.

For every 1.0 mmol/L (40mg/dL) we can decrease the LDL cholesterol levels in our blood using a statin, the risk of a heart attack is about 20 to 25 per cent lower. For people born with high cholesterol levels this is a life saver. However, even in people with relatively normal or low levels of LDL cholesterol in their bloodstream, statins will still lower their risk of a heart attack or stroke by the same amount. Obviously this makes a lot of sense for those at a high risk of having a heart attack or stroke, like those with diabetes, kidney disease, high blood pressure, the elderly and some Indigenous populations. Consequently, these (high-risk) people are often put on a statin regardless of what their cholesterol levels are, as any less cholesterol in their blood means less cholesterol in their arteries and a more stable road into their future.

Breaking the mould

 Fungi like yeast, mould and mushrooms produce some of the most potent poisons in the world. They do this largely to protect themselves from their adversaries. For the most part, these are not humans, but rather other microorganisms. The antibiotic penicillin was accidentally discovered when it was found a mould that grew on stale bread made a particular poison that fortunately only killed bacteria. And if it worked once to discover penicillin, thought Akira Endo, a young Japanese microbiologist, then maybe another fungus had other secrets worth interrogating.

In particular, because cholesterol is just as essential for bacteria as it is for humans, It made sense to Endo that some clever mould would take advantage of this weak spot and make a poison that stopped bacteria from generating the cholesterol they needed to survive.

After examining thousands of different strains, Endo found what he was looking for: a unique blue-green mould produced a specific chemical to block cholesterol synthesis in bacteria. This gift from nature became the first statin, used to lower cholesterol in humans.

Other natural statins were subsequently discovered in red yeast rice as well as oyster mushrooms. However, none of the statins used today is natural. Rather, they are synthetic relatives that have been further optimized for their effect on LDL cholesterol, as well as safety and tolerability in people.

It could be that slowly growing in the cracks of your bathroom is a mould that contains the secrets to ageing. That could explain its longevity? Or not?

Statins work best in combination with a low-cholesterol diet. For the reasons detailed above, when we don't get cholesterol from our diet our liver makes more cholesterol to make up the shortfall. But these same cholesterol synthesis pathways are inhibited by statins. So if we were on a statin, and also cutting out cholesterol-rich foods in our diet, the achieved levels of LDL cholesterol in our blood will be even lower, and as such, this approach is almost always recommended by doctors.

Statins are not without their problems. In particular, some people cannot take a statin because of troublesome side effects. The most common of these are muscle aches and pains, which are experienced by up to a third of people taking statins, especially those on high doses. These symptoms can be bad enough to not only make them feel miserable but also reduce the amount of healthy physical activity they can do. Recent studies have also suggested that the use of statins may increase the risk of diabetes by an amount equivalent to drinking a can of soft drink every day.

These problems mean that taking a statin is probably only worthwhile for people with a high risk of a heart attack or stroke. For the average person with a low risk of having a heart attack, the cost, safety and tolerability issues of taking a statin are probably worse than the small absolute benefit that could be obtained from using one. It may be a miracle drug like penicillin but, like penicillin, it shouldn't be put in the drinking water.

Knock on

Although the cholesterol in our diet usually has only a small effect on the cholesterol in our blood, that doesn't mean butter and cheddar are completely off the hook. The amount of LDL cholesterol made by our liver and then pumped into our blood is also influenced by the amount and types of many other things we eat — as a kind of knock-on effect — even if they are completely cholesterol free.

For example, people eating food naturally high in unsaturated and monounsaturated fats (e.g. those eating a Mediterranean-style diet) generally also have lower levels of LDL cholesterol in their bloodstream regardless of how much cholesterol they are also eating. By contrast, people regularly eating a diet high in saturated fat and/ or trans-fat generally have higher levels of LDL cholesterol in their blood. In essence, these fats irritate the liver into making more cholesterol, even when our bodies don't need it. The importance of these different fats on our health is discussed in detail in Chapter 6.

Fibre also matters. We get fibre when we eat plenty of cereals, fruit and vegetables in our diet. This fibre has a number of health benefits, which are further discussed in Chapter 9. However, one of the key advantages of eating lots of plant fibre is that it reduces our LDL cholesterol levels. It is thought that fibre causes the liver to increase its production of bile acids, chemicals that help keep digestion working properly. But to make bile acids, the liver uses up cholesterol as a substrate, which means there is less available to make LDL cholesterol for the blood, which goes down slightly as a result.

A little competition

Although plants contain only a little cholesterol, they do contain lots of chemicals that are very similar. These are called (phyto)sterols or stanols.

They are highest in whole grains, legumes, nuts and seeds, but can be found in most plant-based products.

Unlike cholesterol, sterols are not directly useful to human metabolism, are less easily absorbed and rapidly pumped back into the intestine when they are. But because of their similarity to cholesterol, plant sterols effectively compete with it for access to the pathways used for absorption and cholesterol packaging by our intestine. This means that in a mixed meal containing both plant and animal products (e.g. meat and vegetables, wholegrain bread with cheddar cheese), the plant sterols effectively outcompete the animal cholesterol, so less of it gets into our blood.

A number of companies have deliberately enriched their foods with plant sterols, including margarines, yoghurts, salad dressings, cheeses, breads and even orange juice. This is mostly a marketing tool.

As discussed earlier in this chapter, our liver is normally quite capable of compensating for the cholesterol we now don't absorb, simply by making a little more. So eating sterol-fortified foods or taking supplements will have very little or probably no effect on blood cholesterol levels in most people. It's not cholesterol absorption that is usually the limiting factor.

However, as with a cholesterol-free diet, if we are on a statin that inhibits the production of cholesterol by our liver, then taking high doses of sterols (>20 g/day) can be enough to modestly lower LDL cholesterol levels in the blood. And this is how advertisers can ethically make their pitch for sterol-rich margarine or eating more nuts.

Good cholesterol

Not all cholesterol in our blood is bad. About a quarter of all cholesterol travelling in our blood is transported in small dense packages known as high-density lipoproteins. These particles have a high density because they are mostly protein and very little fat. Any cholesterol inside them is called **HDL cholesterol.**

Although both LDL and HDL contain cholesterol, HDL is very different from LDL because of the proteins it also carries. These proteins direct HDL particles to soak up excess cholesterol from where it is importunately deposited and transport it back to the liver for excretion, storage or recycling. This is known as reverse cholesterol transport. And obviously, this is a good thing if we want to reverse the unwanted cholesterol deposits in our arteries.

HDL particles are also able to transfer some of their helpful proteins to other lipoprotein particles, which change them from cholesterol dumpers to cholesterol retrievers, allowing them to bring their fatty cargo safely back into the liver, rather than get stuck in our blood vessels.

These helpful actions partly explain why HDL cholesterol is often considered the 'good cholesterol', and why it might be good to have more of it in our blood. Certainly, people with consistently high levels of HDL cholesterol have lower risk of heart disease and strokes, and greater longevity. By contrast, those with low HDL cholesterol levels often have more problems with cholesterol deposits in their blood vessels. So measuring the levels of HDL cholesterol in our blood, and particularly its relationship with bad LDL cholesterol (e.g. the LDL/HDL cholesterol ratio) is a powerful way to gauge the balance of our risks for having a heart attack or stroke.

HDL particles are used up faster when trying to deal with the other changes in fat metabolism, such as excess weight or diabetes. So HDL cholesterol levels often fall by half in these conditions, and the severity of this fall is a good marker of underlying problems in our overall health.

The problem is there is no clear evidence that increasing our HDL levels on its own also changes our risk for heart disease. This is probably because, unlike LDL cholesterol, it's not the cholesterol in HDL that causes heart disease, but rather HDL's functions that are important. And these can't be easily estimated just by measuring HDL cholesterol levels. Consequently, HDL cholesterol levels in our blood are best considered more a marker of risk than a mediator of it.

This doesn't mean that things we're usually told to do to raise our HDL cholesterol, like losing excess weight, increasing physical activity and stopping smoking, don't work. They certainly do. It's just that we don't get their benefits simply by increasing levels of good cholesterol in our blood.

Panacea

 In Greek mythology, Panacea was the goddess of universal remedy. Her power came from a cure-all potion which healed the sick. Not surprisingly she became the favourite of doctors. Her sister, Hyegeia, had superpowers too, as the goddess of hygiene, dispensing preventive health advice. There was no obvious animosity between siblings, as the absence of disease was not the same thing as good health, and there was plenty of work to go around.

Alcohol has long been regarded as the quintessential panacea, especially by the intoxicated. But even sober scientists can be swayed by its charm. The most common theory is that drinking booze, any booze, is able to raise good (HDL) cholesterol levels in the blood. So booze can't be all bad (hic).

Sadly, it's not that easy. It is perfectly true that alcohol triggers the liver to make more of the proteins used to form HDL particles. So HDL cholesterol levels are modestly increased in those who drink regularly compared to non-drinkers. And the more we drink the higher go our HDL cholesterol levels. People who drink like a fish often have fantastically high levels of good cholesterol in their blood, but it is not enough to clean out their arteries. Any more than a glass a day, and the risk of heart attacks and strokes goes up, not down.

As the great poet Homer Simpson rightly identified, alcohol is both the cause and solution to all of life's problems. In doing so, he opened an irrevocable schism between the two sisters Panacea and Hyegeia, who have fought wildly over what is good for us ever since.

The ugly cholesterol left over

As discussed in Chapter 4, any calories that come into our body that are not used up by physical activity or metabolic processes are stored as fat against a time we might need them again. This energy store is largely in the chemical form of **triglycerides**, which we bank in our fatty tissues chiefly under our skin and around our waistlines. When we are eating, these fat stores are built up. When we are not eating, these same triglyceride stores are slowly broken down to provide fuel for activity and metabolism.

Most triglycerides are made by the liver, which converts excess energy in our diet into triglycerides for fuel and storage. As with cholesterol, triglycerides are an oily fat, so they don't easily dissolve in blood or water. So to truck triglycerides out from the liver to the storage sites in our fat, they must be moved in large triglyceride-rich transport trucks. As these particles are mostly transporting triglycerides, they have a very low density. They are therefore called very low-density particles or **VLDL** for short.

When we digest a meal that contains fat, the released triglycerides also need to be moved out of our intestines, and trucked to storage sites in our fatty parts. So our intestines use their own very, very low-density transport particles. These are known as **chylomicrons**.

Because these different fat transport particles are all triglyceride rich, the easiest way to work our how many there are in our blood is to measure the blood triglyceride levels, which is routinely done as part of the standard blood lipid test.

The problem is that all these triglyceride-rich particles also need some cholesterol for water proofing. So high levels of triglyceride-rich particles in the blood also means that there will now be lots of cholesterol, not in good HDL, not in bad LDL, but instead stuffed into these large ugly triglyceride-rich transport particles. This is often called **remnant cholesterol**, and is easily calculated by measuring the total cholesterol levels in the blood and then subtracting the cholesterol contained in LDL and HDL. The remnant cholesterol is essentially what is left over. It can also be estimated by just measuring the triglyceride levels.

In healthy people, this remnant is only a very small component of their total cholesterol. In others it can constitute over half of all the cholesterol in their blood. And this *is* a problem.

Due to their particularly ugly size, these triglyceride-rich particles are just small enough to get into the walls of our arteries, but too big to easily get out again. The fatty particles and the cholesterol they carry often gets left in the walls of our arteries. In fact, in extreme cases, these particles can deposit all of their load, forming ugly fatty-yellow lumps under the skin (known as xanthomas).

Raised levels of triglyceride-rich particles often go hand in hand with low concentrations of HDL (good) cholesterol. It is thought that HDL particles are used up when trying to deal with an excess of these fatty trucks and return their contents back to the liver. So as blood triglyceride levels rise, levels of our good cholesterol usually fall.

Of all the different things that can go wrong with our blood cholesterol levels in this day and age, the most common problem is having far too much remnant cholesterol. Therefore having too much remnant cholesterol is also often the main offender in many premature heart attacks.

On average, for every 1 mmol/L (88 mg/dl) increase in the triglyceride levels in our blood, we double the amount of remnant cholesterol and consequently double the risk of an early death.

Conversely, if we can reduce our triglyceride levels by 1 mmol/L (88 mg/dl), then our risks will halve.

Fortunately, of all the cholesterol problems we can possibly have, this one is also the most easily fixed. The most common cause of high levels of remnant cholesterol is having too much (triglyceride) fat already deposited around our waistlines. In other words, all the storage sites are already full, so these fat-rich particles have nowhere to go. By losing weight and keeping it off, we can also keep our cholesterol levels under control, chiefly by reducing remnant cholesterol. Even in people who are not very overweight, eating moderately and being more physically active will lower their remnant cholesterol.

Diabetes can also trigger the over-production of these ugly triglyceride-rich particles by the liver. And to make matters worse, the fat and muscle which normally take up any excess refuse to do this in diabetes, as they become increasingly resistant to the signals that would promote this. Consequently, high triglycerides in the blood are the most common lipid problem in people with diabetes, and further increase their risk of heart attacks and strokes, and a generally foreshortened life expectancy.

Fructose is the new fat

 Sweet things can also be a cause of rising blood cholesterol levels, even when they are completely cholesterol free and contain almost no fat. In fact, the excess sugars we eat probably have a far greater impact on our blood cholesterol levels than all the cholesterol we eat.

Our bodies are designed to make hay while the sun shines, or rather, make fat in times of plenty. So in those brief times when fruit became ripe, sugary and wonderfully abundant, humans have historically gorged themselves, and converted excess sugar very efficiently into fat for the leaner times ahead.

Of course, today we eat sugar all the time. Not just in fruit. Almost everything processed we eat now has some sugar to tickle our tastebuds. This makes it seem to our Palaeolithic physiology that fruit is in season every single day. And so we make copious triglycerides, and transport them in triglyceride-rich VLDL trucks to our abundant fat stores, hoping they will have enough room so they can unload their cargo. But in modern times, there is often a delay or limited space, so they ramp up into the blood, causing our blood triglyceride levels to rise, and with it, remnant cholesterol.

People who regularly drink (alcohol) heavily often have elevated triglyceride levels. This partly reflects the extra calories that come with each drink as well as the direct effects of alcohol on their liver. This effect is reversible so people with high triglyceride levels are often advised to cut down any excessive intake of alcohol. The many health benefits of moderating our alcohol intake are discussed in Chapter 2.

Finally, it is often recommended that a healthy regular intake of fish has benefits for our cholesterol levels and therefore our health. This is chiefly because fish (and oily fish like salmon, tuna, herring, mackerel, anchovies and sardines, in particular) contain high amounts of special polyunsaturated fatty acids (known as omega–3 (-3). The many benefits of omega–3 are discussed in detail in Chapter 6, but one particular advantage is it can modestly lower triglyceride levels. Sadly, the amount of fish we would need to eat to achieve this is usually prohibitive, unless we are fishermen and/or don't mind smelling like them.

The bottom line

Lowering the levels of (bad) LDL cholesterol and (ugly) remnant cholesterol in our blood is the simplest way to not clog our arteries and die from a heart attack or stroke.

Our levels don't need to be high. It doesn't take much cholesterol to provide the substrate for the many other unhygienic things that damage our blood vessels — high blood pressure, smoking, diabetes, obesity, stress — to start building cholesterol-rich plaques along the walls of our blood vessels. Obviously, having too much cholesterol makes it easy for them to wreck the health of our arteries. However, regardless of how much cholesterol we currently have circulating in our bloodstream, if we had less of it, then any plaques we had would be smaller and less likely to break apart under pressure.

We don't all need a statin to live to a hundred. But as we get older and our risk of having a heart attack or stroke increases, many of us will. Until then, the best way is to deal with the things that use cholesterol to make potholes in our arterial roads. This makes cholesterol isolated and less important which, when dealing with baddies, can prove just as useful as taking them out.

Do I really have to ...

#11

Lower my blood pressure?

Q: Why is high pressure a bad thing?
A: Ask a balloon.

Q: How high is too high?
A: A maximum (systolic) blood pressure above 140 mmHg means that your blood pressure is probably high enough to warrant treatment.

Q: Then I'm okay so long as I am below 140 mmHg?
A: No. Any pressure above 115 mmHg causes tension in our arteries.

Q: How low is too low?
A: It depends on what you are used to.

Q: Is there anything special I need to do to keep my blood pressure from rising?
A: Read this book.

Q: Should I avoid eating salt?
A: Only to suit your taste.

When we go to the doctor for a health check, the first thing they are likely to test is our **blood pressure**. Doctors seem to love testing blood pressure. It's easy, fast and cheap to measure. But most of all, it's worth their while.

High blood pressure is one of the most easily prevented and most easily treated risk factors for dying earlier than we would want to. In fact, the World Health Organization lists high blood pressure as the number one preventable cause of a premature death in human beings. And if all these experts are so obsessed about preventing and treating high blood pressure, then maybe we should be too.

Under pressure

In order to move all the blood around our body once every 4 to 5 minutes, blood must flow fast and never, ever stop. The force of our flowing blood is the **blood pressure**.

This pressure is not insubstantial, as anyone who seen too many horror movies or any recent TV shows will easily appreciate. Today, we can't have a medieval battle scene or grizzly murder without seeing blood spray out in absolute torrents.

The kind of pressure that exists inside our arteries can be appreciated simply by breathing in very deeply and then blowing out as forcefully as we can, as if we were blowing up a balloon. The maximum force of that breath out is about the same as the maximum force generated when our beating heart squeezes down to pump out blood. Our heart spends about one-third of its time squeezing inwards to push blood out (known as **systole**). The other two-thirds of its time is spent in a relaxed state (known as **diastole**), slowly filling up with blood in preparation for the next heartbeat.

Pools of blood

 To keep us alive, our heart squeezes out 5 litres of blood (about 10½ pints) every minute. Over a lifetime this would be enough to fill 100 Olympic-sized swimming pools.

For most of the last millennium, the heart was thought to be just the pool heater. Without a beating heart dead bodies are dead cold. And with one, live bodies are commensurately warm. Consequently, the heart was logically viewed as the vital source of body heat. So if we were ever to fall in love or get frustrated, or we felt a little hotter under the collar, we'd have only our heart to blame. And what are those very calm, indifferent people but simply cold hearted?

It was initially believed that blood was made by the liver, brewed from the vital nutrients found in food and drink. This is why Christian religious ceremonies, where wine is changed into blood or bread is transformed into flesh, were not viewed as mystical at all. That was exactly what most people believed happened in humans every day.

After being made by the liver, it was thought that blood was enriched with heat (from the heart) as well as other vital spirits from other vital organs, before being delivered throughout the body via arteries and veins. It was assumed that blood was then simply consumed by the body; transmuted into flesh and bones. The reason that blood flowed was because it was ordered to do so, like food flowing fresh from the restaurant kitchen in the type and amount requested by the customer.

It seemed like a good explanation at the time, and held sway for over 1500 years. But at 100 Olympic-sized swimming pools a lifetime, that's a lot of takeaway. Today, we know blood circulates under constant pressure, so we don't need to refill the blood pool all the time. And our heart is definitely the pool pump, not the heater.

Measuring blood pressure

Blood pressure can be measured simply by placing a pressurized cuff around our upper arm. As air is pumped into the cuff, the pressure inside it slowly builds to progressively constrict our arm. Eventually there comes a point at which the constricting pressure of the cuff is higher than the maximum pressure that is generated by the flow of blood, and blood stops flowing into our arm. The pulse at our wrist completely disappears, and our arm starts to tingle.

Then the pressure inside the cuff is lowered by letting air slowly out. Eventually, there comes a point at which the pressure in the cuff now becomes less than the maximal pressure generated by the blood pressing forward in the arteries of our arm, so blood begins to flow again.

The person taking the blood pressure can gauge the return of blood flow by feeling for a pulse in the arm or listening with a stethoscope pressed over an artery. This is because when the blood first returns to the arm, with each little turbulent spurt of blood that can be felt coming down the artery, a kind of tapping noise can also be heard, in time with each pulse. The pressure point at which this noise first occurs as the pulse returns to the arm is called the **systolic blood pressure**, as it corresponds with the maximal pressure generated as our beating heart contracts (in systole) to pump out the blood.

The systolic blood pressure is usually somewhere between 120 and 140 mmHg in most adults. This literally means the pressure in our blood is sufficient to push up a column of liquid mercury 12 to 14 centimetres (about 5 inches) into the air. Since mercury is fourteen times heavier than water, a similar column of water would need to be at least as tall we are (on average between 160 to 190 centimetres, or 5 to 6 feet, in height) to measure human blood pressure. This is why doctors still use a column of mercury and mercury-based numbers and not water to measure our blood pressure. It also explains how our heart can generate enough pressure to push blood all the way to our toes and back again.

The circle of life

 The idea that life is a circle is ancient. The circle is a symbol of wholeness, integrity, security, divine perfection, perpetual, without beginning or end. Well before the Lion King, many civilizations had their circle of life; think Stonehenge or the Bhavacakra, the Buddhist Wheel of Life.

Like a circle, nature is also viewed as perfect and perpetual, like the cycle of the seasons, the sun and the moon. Everything rolls and everything comes back. In 1626, physician William Harvey began to question the then prevailing view of blood flow being just a one-way street. Seeing God in nature, and believing the motto 'as it is above, so it is below', it seemed to William Harvey that too much blood would need to be instantaneously transmuted from food and drink to explain how fast it flowed. Moreover, if God's nature normally worked in circles and man was created by God in his own image, then maybe the prefect and perpetual integrity of blood also flowed in circles, there and back, in and out, consumption and enrichment. Harvey named this pattern **circulation** and he became the first person to describe the circular way that blood flowed around the body.

The lowest pressure in any artery is known as the **diastolic blood pressure,** as it corresponds to the time when the heart is relaxed, dilated and filling during diastole in order to get ready for its next contraction. Diastole is a very important period for the heart as blood can only get into it when it is relaxed.

Diastolic blood pressure is also detected using a cuff. As noted above, when the cuff around our arm is pumped up very tight, blood flow only gets through intermittently if and when the pressure in our blood exceeds the pressure in the cuff. This intermittent turbulent flow of blood can be heard as tapping sounds using a stethoscope. But as more air is let out of the cuff, and the constricting pressure around our arm falls, at some point, the pressure in the cuff falls below the lowest pressure of our blood, which is the diastolic pressure, usually around 70 to 80 mmHg.

Below this level the constriction of the blood pressure cuff is insufficient to prevent the continuous smooth flow of blood into the arm and so the tapping sounds of intermittent turbulent flow in blood vessels go away. Diastolic pressure is therefore gauged by the sound of silence in our arm. For this reason it is much harder than systolic pressure to measure accurately, especially in noisy environments like medical practices or shopping malls.

When recording the blood pressure, it is common for doctors and nurses to report the blood pressure as the systolic over the diastolic blood pressure. So when they say the blood pressure is 120 over 80, it means a maximum (systolic) blood pressure of 120 mmHg and a minimum (diastolic) pressure of 80 mmHg. This is like the daily weather forecast that provides the maximum and minimum temperatures, and in the same way is used to tell us what the future may be for our health.

Pressure control

Exactly how much pressure there is inside our blood vessels is determined by a number of different factors, all of which are closely regulated by the healthy human body.

Firstly, how much blood we have in our body is an important determinant of how much blood pressure can be generated. Just like air in a balloon, if we let it all out, then pressure inside goes down. So when people lose large amounts of blood, like after an accident, their blood pressure is also often low. 'I feel a weak pulse,' the paramedics cry on television. But what they are really saying is that the systolic blood pressure that generates the pulse is low. They will usually try to fix this by pushing a large volume of fluid quickly ('stat') into blood vessels via a drip, while attempting to stop any bleeding. Once blood volume is restored, so will be the pulse of the systolic blood pressure.

For the same reasons, if there is too much blood/fluid in our body, just like overinflating a balloon, the pressure inside will inevitably rise. Normally each of us has approximately 5 litres (10½ pints) of blood, one-third of which consists of cells that use the blood for transport. The other two-thirds is salty fluid in which the cells all flow. So if the body holds onto more salty fluid than it should, it can drive up our blood pressure. This may occur when those same systems which regulate blood fluid levels are compromised by disease, such as in kidney, heart or liver disease.

Blood-letting

 Throughout human history, one of the most popular treatments for just about any ailment was to make a hole in a blood vessel or two and let out about 500 mL (1 pint) of blood. The reason people actually believed that this could work was because they also believed that bad blood was the root of all evil. Just like in *Game of Thrones*.

It was also believed that the better health and longer life enjoyed by women was because they regularly lost blood during menstruation and this purged them of bad blood. And what is good for the goose is good for the gander.

Blood-letting became so popular as a treatment that it became an industry in itself, carried out independent of doctors by skilled barbers. The classic striped pole outside the barbershop actually symbolizes the letting of red blood followed by the wrap of white bandages to stop the bleeding.

Of course, blood-letting has no benefit for sufferers of ill health, and probably helped many sick people to an early grave. Even so, those healthy people who regularly give blood do generally have better health and longer lives. But this is probably because blood donors are usually altruistic individuals, who do many other things to look after their health apart from giving blood.

The strength of a heartbeat during each contraction of the heart also partly determines the pressure of the blood in our arteries. This is something like the strength of each puff we'd take to blow up a balloon. The stronger and faster we puff, the higher the pressure we can generate. Same with our heart. Equally, if our heart is damaged and is pumping weakly or slowly, our blood pressure can be low, such as in some people with heart failure.

Another determinant of the pressure inside a balloon is the balloon itself and, in particular, how elastic it is. Blood vessels have strong elastic walls, which literally balloon out in response to the sudden increase in pressure generated by the beating of the heart. We can sometimes actually see this 'bulging', in the big blood vessels in someone's neck or arms.

As blood vessels bulge outward under pressure of the pulse, it creates **tension** in the elastic walls. This is something like having a small rubber band around your wrist. When you apply some pressure to stretch it bigger and pull it away from your wrist, this generates tension in the rubber band. The more pressure you apply the more tense it gets. When you let the band go it snaps back onto your wrist re-using the pressure you used to stretch it out. This is elastic recoil.

The same thing happens after every pulse along our elastic arteries. When healthy blood vessels distend as the pulse comes through, just like stretching a rubber band, the walls get tense and try to push back. This recoil generates a considerable inward squeeze. If our arteries were just hard lead pipes, with no recoil at all, blood flow would have to stop and start because the heart is a stop–start pump, squeezing out blood only a third of the time, and relaxing to fill itself up for the other two-thirds. But because of the elastic recoil adding its own squeeze to the blood as it snaps back like a rubber band, the flow of blood in our arteries never stops.

Hardening of the arteries

 As we get older we get less compliant, less able to bend to the will of the world, more stuck in our ways. This is especially the case in our normally elastic arteries. This is called hardening of the arteries.

When the force of pulse pressure flows in an artery, it should distend outward, making more room for the passing blood. An elastic artery also takes away some of the tension in the wall, converting it into elastic recoil.

But an old hard artery is like an old rubber band; it doesn't take much pressure and can't snap back. So the tension in the walls of old arteries is higher and systolic pressure is higher.

On average, systolic blood pressure levels slowly go up by about 1 mmHg every two to three years of our adult life, chiefly because our arteries get harder. By the time we retire, on average the systolic blood pressure is usually at least 20 mmHg higher than when we were in our twenties.

By contrast, the diastolic pressure is not increased or may be lower as we get older. This is because the elastic recoil that generates it is reduced in our age-hardened arteries.

One key difference between the pressure problems of static air in balloons and blood in our blood vessels is that our blood is flowing, like fluid along a pipe. This means that hydraulic (flow) factors also influence the pressure inside our arterial pipes. For example, imagine a tap connected to a hose. It's easy to get water out of the hose if the diameter of the hose is big. But to run the same amount of fluid down a series of smaller tubes is much harder, and can only be achieved by turning up the tap, increasing the pressure in the system. What makes it harder for liquid to flow down small pipes is known as **resistance**. The higher the resistance, the higher the pressure needed to overcome it to ensure continuous flow at the correct rate. The lower the resistance, the less pressure we need to generate to ensure that flow continues at the same rate.

The body keeps our blood pressure levels relatively constant throughout our busy days. This is achieved chiefly by balancing the output of the heart (how fast and how strong), the volume of fluid in our blood and the resistance to its flow. The latter is achieved simply by changing the diameter of our blood vessel hose pipes (known as resistance vessels).

If our blood pressure was falling, we'd activate pathways to increase the output from the heart so it would beat stronger and faster. Our kidneys would be called on to retain fluid to increase the volume of blood. At the same time we'd also constrict blood vessels supplying non-essential organs, like the skin, making us look pale. This acts to increase overall resistance to flow in our pipes and prop up the blood pressure supplying essential organs. Equally, if our blood pressure was rising, the opposite pathways are activated to tame the heart by removing excess fluid and dilating our blood vessels. The failure of these control mechanisms is the most common cause of abnormally high or low blood pressure.

Blood pressure is generally considered to be too low when the systolic blood pressure is below 90 mmHg. But it really depends on what we are used to. For some people, and especially the elderly with hard arteries, a pressure more than 120 mmHg may be required to feel well and safe, especially as they stand up. On the other hand, low blood pressure is quite normal for some people, and not a problem at all. If anything, these people are generally very healthy.

Stand up, drop down

 In most people their blood pressure is a little lower when they are standing up than when sitting or lying down. This is because blood pools in our legs when we are standing, so slightly less blood is able to get back to the heart, fill it up and provide the volume to pump up the blood pressure. This pressure drop is usually small and no more than 5 to 10 per cent. This is because standing up immediately triggers reflex responses to cause the constriction of resistance blood vessels and an increase in our heart rate to prop up the pressure.

In some people, their blood pressure can drop very significantly (by over 20 mmHg) when they stand up. This is known as **postural hypotension** and is sometimes experienced as dizzy spells or even fainting.

A big drop in pressure on standing up is usually because something interferes with the reflexes required to keep the blood pressure up. For example, people who are dehydrated (have a low blood volume) or overly hot are more likely to feel dizzy when they stand up, because the protective reflexes have nothing left to give. Some medications, specific illnesses like diabetes or Parkinson's disease and even ageing itself can also interfere with these protective reflexes, and make dizzy spells in standing more likely.

High tension

High blood pressure is usually a silent killer. There are no obvious symptoms of excess tension on the walls of our arteries. And unlike balloons or rubber bands, our blood vessels seldom break under the pressure of being filled, unless they are abnormal to begin with. However, all the pressure applied to our blood vessels inevitably causes some tension in their walls. This stress and strain progressively leads to damage or loss of function in our blood vessels, and any organs that depend on blood flow through them in order to work properly. This is called **vascular disease**, and results in problems like heart attacks, strokes and poor circulation to legs or the kidneys. High blood pressure is the most common modifiable risk factor for vascular disease.

The point at which the tension/stress on the walls of our blood vessels is too great and requires treatment is called **hypertension** (literally too much tension). It can be broadly defined as:

- a systolic (maximum) blood pressure of 140 mmHg or higher
- a diastolic (mimimum) blood pressure 90 mmHg or higher.

Using these criteria, about one-third of all adults will have too much tension in their blood vessels. Over a lifetime at least three out of every four adults will eventually develop hypertension or need medication to prevent it, mostly after the age of sixty.

This does not mean that if our systolic pressure is 139 mmHg when we see our doctor, our blood vessels are fine and under no tension at all. In fact, there is a continuous relationship between the level of pressure in our blood/tension in our arteries and the likelihood of bad things happening to our blood vessels, like having a stroke. The greater the pressure in our blood vessels, the greater the tension in their walls, so the greater the risk of vascular disease.

The risk of vascular disease is actually lowest when the systolic blood pressure is about 115 mmHg. As blood pressure levels rise higher than this, our risk of problems increases roughly proportional to the blood pressure. But by the time we get to above 140 mmHg the risk of bad things happening in our blood vessels is significantly greater than the cost and side effects associated with using treatments to do something about it. So doctors will generally call it hypertension at a systolic blood pressure above 140mmHg. However, in older or frail people, 150 mmHg may be a better point at which treatment benefits exceed the downsides.

Neither threshold for the diagnosis or drug treatment of hypertension means that we should do nothing about our blood pressure before this level. There are many things we can do in our diet and lifestyle to get our blood pressure lower and keep it there. This is just as important if we have don't have hypertension. At least a third of all deaths due to excess blood pressure occur in people who do not have hypertension.

It has been estimated that if we all reduced our systolic blood pressure to about 115 mmHg it would reduce heart attacks and strokes globally by about half, and add nearly ten years to average life expectancy. What's not to like?

Boys and girls

 There are many obvious differences between women and men. These go without saying. But there are many others that are not so obvious, but just as important. One of these is blood pressure.

Prior to the menopause, women have slightly lower blood pressure levels than men. After the menopause, these differences reverse, so that older women are more likely to have high blood pressure than older men. Around three-quarters of women over 60 will develop hypertension, compared to two-thirds of men of the same age.

These differences in blood pressure between men and women partly explain why damage to blood vessels caused by high blood pressure (such as having a stroke) is also more common in older women than in men.

Keeping control

There are many simple things that we all can do to prevent or slow the development of high blood pressure. A clue for what sort of things we might do can be found by looking at people around the world and comparing their blood pressure levels with their diet and lifestyle habits.

Although most people progressively increase their systolic blood pressure as they get older (mostly through hardening of the arteries), some people don't. For example, people who don't put on excess weight, vegetarians, individuals not exposed to stress, and those who don't eat too much salt, generally all have little or no increase in blood pressure as they age. So we probably have to do some or all of these things to have some of the benefits rub off on our blood pressure too.

As discussed in a previous chapter, an increasing waistline has a number of effects on our health, including raising our blood pressure and making it difficult to bring down on our own. High blood pressure is twice as common in people who are obese. Increasing waistlines are probably the main reason why blood pressure levels are also rising across the world. By contrast, losing a few kilos or pounds can make a real difference to many aspects of our health, including our blood pressure. For every kilogram (2.2 pounds) of weight we lose, our systolic blood pressure will go down on average by approximately 1 mmHg (e.g. losing 10 kilos, or 22 pounds, in weight will usually lower our blood pressure by 10 mmHg, which is as much as achieved by taking blood pressure lowering medications).

Blood pressure and the pill

 The first time most women get their blood pressure taken is when they want to go on the pill, and repeatedly thereafter if they want to stay on it.

This is because taking medicines is all about weighing up risks, like doubling the stakes in backgammon. Taking the pill doubles the risk of having a stroke. This is not a big increase in absolute terms, given that young women generally have low blood pressure and a very low risk of having a stroke in the first place. So even if you double your risk by taking oral contraceptives, it is still a very low risk (i.e. double a one and you still only have two). It is also often less than the health risks associated with being pregnant.

Because high blood pressure increases the risk of having a stroke, doubling an elevated risk further by then taking the pill is not a good idea (i.e. double a four and now you have a risky eight). This is why before prescribing the pill, doctors will always check your blood pressure first, as well as checking for other risks for stroke like being very overweight, smoking, having diabetes or a history of blood clots. Any woman found to have high blood pressure can then be recommended to use progestogen-only pills that don't affect the blood pressure or some other form of contraception.

If our blood pressure is normal, regular physical activity can reduce the chance and the degree to which it will rise as we age. In those people with high blood pressure, getting regular exercise can lower their blood pressure and improve their response to blood pressure lowering medications. By contrast, regular couch-potatoes have higher rates of hypertension, and it is more difficult to manage.

Smoking also raises the blood pressure levels. The nicotine contained in tobacco acts to constrict blood vessels, so during each cigarette, blood pressure levels rise between 20 to 30 mmHg. Even though levels may fall again afterwards, these surges in blood pressure are extremely damaging to the blood vessels and to the heart.

A diet rich in fruit and vegetables can also help reduce the risk of developing high blood pressure. Lifelong vegetarians have lower blood pressure levels. At this point in time, exactly what part of fruit and vegetables it is that helps lower blood pressure is unclear.

Our blood pressure is usually higher when we're stressed. Stress makes our heart race and beat more strongly, while the resistance vessels constrict. This can sometimes lead to a surge in blood pressure when we are under the pump. For example, our blood pressure when seeing the doctor usually rises to be 5 to 10 mmHg higher than what it is when we are comfortably at home. This can sometimes make it appear as though we have increased blood pressure to our doctor, even if we don't really have high blood pressure at home. This phenomenon is known as **white-coat hypertension**, even though most doctors don't wear white coats anymore.

Chronic activation of some stress response pathways also leads to a chronically higher blood pressure. In those who live largely stress-free lives (such as secluded cloistered nuns), increases in blood pressure with age are seldom seen. This suggests that accumulated effects of a stressful life may be at the very core of many blood pressure problems. In fact, interventions to reduce or manage stress in our lives can significantly reduce elevated blood pressure levels. The importance of stress management to the health and wellbeing of some people cannot be underestimated (see Chapter 16).

The salt wars

While there are many practical things that can make a difference to our blood pressure levels, the only one most people really remember is something about eating less salt. So much so that the 'low salt' option has become synonymous with the healthy eating alternative. Almost no one shakes salt on their food any more, for fear of appearing unhealthy (as heretical as anyone striking up a cigarette or adding teaspoons of sugar to their coffee).

Most diet guidelines now tell us to limit our intake of salt to less than 100 mmol (or 2.3 grams) every day. This is about half of what most adults will usually eat each and every day. The vast majority of this salt is hidden inside the tasty processed foods we eat, such as bread, spreads, sauces, cheese and fast foods. Even without the salt burden, we know we should be eating less of these things anyway!

The rationale for reducing salt in our diet is very straightforward. Our daily intake of salt is correlated with our blood pressure levels. The more salt we eat, on average, the higher our blood pressure will be. And because high blood pressure damages blood vessels, which leads to heart disease, strokes and death, if we ate less salt, our blood pressure would be lower, and the risk of heart attacks, strokes and death would, in theory, be reduced.

But while such logic is appealing, especially as a low-cost dogmatic public health message, the actions of salt in the human body are much more complicated, and certainly extend beyond blood pressure regulation.

On average, eating less salt will lower systolic blood pressure a little, maybe 2–3 mmHg and only in the short term. Whether this is sufficient to make any real difference to our health prospects is debatable. Even though people who regularly eat more salt have slightly higher blood pressure than those who do not, long-term studies have failed to confirm that these salt eaters are the same people who actually go on to develop high blood pressure or need treatment for it.

Why eating less salt isn't the simple solution it first appears, probably stems from our evolutionary origins. About a billion years ago, the first known organisms emerged from salty oceans. To achieve this exodus, these sea creatures (our ancestors) needed to take the ocean with them. So today, our inner salty sea and its balance is a fundamental part of our physiology. By weight the human body is about two-thirds salt water.

Although we can eat our salt and vinegar chips or drink gallons of fresh water, the salt concentrations inside every human being hardly change. We have survived and continue to survive by keeping things constant.

Our kidneys are the chief regulators of this balance. They continuously filter our blood, allowing over 5 kg (11 lb) of salt to fall into the urine every day, along with any toxins dissolved with it, before selectively reabsorbing over 99 per cent of the salt back, leaving the toxins to be lost into the urine. Overall, less than 0.5 per cent of the filtered load of salt ends up in our urine. In healthy individuals, this loss equates almost exactly with the daily amount of salt we'd eat (5–6 grams).

Consequently, if we eat a packet of salty chips (and that's 1 gram of salt by the way) it's not a major effort to tune reabsorption down slightly and expel the extra gram of sodium out into our urine. Equally, if we didn't get much salt during the day (for example, if we were fasting), it's not very hard to increase reabsorption very slightly to maintain the salt/water balance.

Our salt balance is under very tight control, involving a range of chemical signals between kidneys, the heart, the adrenal glands and, of course, the brain. If salt intake is reduced, these pathways signal the kidneys to hang onto more salt. If salt intake is increased, these pathways are suppressed to increase salt excretion and offset increases in blood pressure that would otherwise occur. This is why we don't blow up or deflate like a balloon.

A grain of salt

 In ancient times there lived a king called Mithridates. He was famous for his unbelievable resistance to being poisoned, a common problem for rulers of that era. His superpower was attributed to a unique cocktail he drank containing over fifty different elements. Many of these were known poisons, although not dangerous in the tiny doses he used in his famous antidote. The last of the listed ingredients was the addition of a single grain of salt (*addito salis grano*).

Many were convinced by his longevity, and his recipe remained the popular panacea of apothecaries for almost 2000 years. However, some were sceptical of the story and found the idea a colossal boast. As a result, the phrase that something should be 'taken with a grain of salt', like Mithridates' antidote, came to mean something considered with great scepticism.

Many of the medicines we use today come from low doses of poisons. The most popular blood pressure-lowering drugs (ACE inhibitors) originated from the venom of the Amazonian pit viper (*Borthorps jararaca*). The blood thinner warfarin is also widely used as rat poison. Maybe Mithridates was onto something. Or maybe his whole story should be taken, like his antidote, with a grain of salt.

This is the rub. These same balancing pathways that keep our inner sea in perfect balance are also implicated in the development and progression of human disease, from cardiovascular disease and diabetes, to cancer and mental illness. Indeed, the wide use and effectiveness of drugs that block these pathways stand as testament to the importance of these pathways, beyond simple actions on salt regulation. But if this is true then, by implication, our salt intake must also have multiple consequences beyond those on blood pressure.

Many studies have looked at the association between salt intake with heart disease and the risk of premature mortality. Some have shown that high salt intake is associated with poor health, some have found no effect at all, while others have found that individuals with a low salt intake have worse clinical outcomes. This is despite trials clearly showing that salt restriction lowers blood pressure.

This inconsistency forms the basis of the so-called 'salt wars', an unscientific and often vitriolic war of words between salt reformers (who want all added salt in food banned) and salt sceptics (who think there are more important things to change in our diet).

The salt reformers argue that everything else that has been shown to lower blood pressure is beneficial in terms of heart attacks and strokes. Why should salt intake be any different?

The salt sceptics argue that this is not always true. A parable once told by Michael Alderman (a notable sceptic) goes something like this. Elevated blood pressure is dangerous for women during pregnancy. So once upon a time, all pregnant women were advised to limit their weight gain in order to reduce their risks from hypertension during pregnancy (known as pre-eclampsia). From a blood pressure-centric point of view, this worked very well. But while pre-eclampsia was reduced and blood pressure lowered, mortality in babies was dramatically increased. So no one now recommends weight restriction for women during pregnancy.

In the same way, the salt sceptics (such as the author) argue that while eating less salt can lower blood pressure, that's not all that it's doing and its cumulative effects may be far from positive. In fact, one problem about going on a low-salt diet is that it will trigger pathways to retain more salt, and activation of these pathways can be damaging to our health. Indeed, there is some concern that putting otherwise healthy people on a low-salt diet will not make them healthier, but rather the opposite.

Clearly for some people and populations who usually consume a large amount of salt (e.g. more than 2 teaspoons a day), maybe as part of their traditional diet (e.g. because they are using salt as a food preservative) or because that are eating a crazy amount of processed food, there is a good reason to suggest their salt-laden diet is bad for them.

In addition, some people develop high blood pressure as a result of their bad genes. Most commonly these bad genes interfere in some way with their salt balance. For example, some bad genes prevent the kidneys from getting rid of as much excess salt as they should. If we are born with these bad genes and we don't eat much salt in our diet, then it's not a problem. It's only if we eat too much of it that there's an issue here. So in these special cases it appears that eating too much salt is a problem. But in reality, eating salt is simply unmasking the real issue with the genes.

This also partly explains why salt in the diet increases blood pressure by much more in people who are old, have diabetes or are overweight. People with these conditions are said to be **salt sensitive** and reducing the salt they eat is often more actively recommended in these settings.

But for the rest of the world, there is probably little need to restrict the amount of salt that most of us eat (roughly the equivalent of a teaspoon a day) for the sake of our blood pressure. Our kidneys should do the job just fine.

The bottom line

High blood pressure is bad for our blood vessels and that means that it is ultimately bad for our health. Controlling our blood pressure is one of the most practical ways to keep our blood vessels supplying the blood required for good health. Many of the things we have discussed will help, like reducing stress, losing weight, and being physically active. But knowing what our blood pressure is, by getting it regularly checked, and acting on its advice, is probably the simplest and cheapest way to make sure we are on track for a hundred.

Do I really have to ...

#12

Breathe fresh air?

Q: Is air pollution bad for me?
A: Is smoking?

Q: Will having house plants help?
A: Only if you keep them alive, and then only for decoration.

Q: Should I move to the seaside?
A: Not only for the sea air.

Q: As a non-smoker, why should I care about smoking?
A: Because smoke gets in your eyes, too.

Q: How can this room still smell so bad?
A: Because chemicals can stick around, and still jump back into the air months later.

Q: What about electric cars?
A: There is no exhaust. But the wheels on the electric car still go round and round.

Ever since we were kids, we've been encouraged to go outside and get some fresh air. This is more than our parents simply wanting peace and quiet, or moving the kids away from the breakables. It is also more than just getting some sunshine or even physical activity. Most people believe getting some fresh air into their lungs will do them good. So much so that 'getting some fresh air' is widely recommended as a cure for almost all ills.

Today, we spend most of our lives stuck in cars, offices and living rooms, breathing processed and conditioned air. Consequently, getting some (fresh) air has also become synonymous with any change from the status quo, usually for the good.

It is easy to understand the logic. Sick and frail people go outside less often, so get less fresh air. But this is because they are sick and frail, not because the air will miraculously heal them. Healthy people often go outside and get more fresh air. But this is simply because they are healthy, not that the air has made them so.

Fresh air isn't even fresh. Most of the air we breathe in has been circulating for millennia. Each breath we take theoretically contains at least one molecule breathed previously by at least one other individual.

In fact, there is nothing in pure fresh air that specifically impacts our health. But that is the point. It's just air, made up of 78 per cent nitrogen and 21 per cent oxygen. There is no more oxygen in the fresh air outside than there is inside the house. Consequently, attempts at remediation by opening windows, improving ventilation, buying house plants or planting trees in our neighbourhood will not significantly change the chemistry of 99 per cent of the air we breathe.

Keep the aspidistra flying

 Indoor plants are a popular addition to any household. Providing we remember to water them, they will pay us back with aesthetic living beauty.

The aspidistra is among the most famous examples. Not because of its style, but rather its extreme tolerance of neglect, poor light and air quality. It is also known as 'the cast-iron plant'. So much so that in Victorian Britain, the aspidistra came to characterize an unbreakable middle-class chutzpah.

Indoor plants are said to make us happier and more relaxed. At least while we keep them alive. House plants will also absorb and break down some harmful airborne chemicals as well as collect particulate matter. However, their impact on indoor air quality, though significant, is actually quite small compared to, for example, regularly throwing open all the windows and doors or thoroughly cleaning the house more than once in a while.

Each day, we inhale about a dozen cubic metres of air. This is about the same amount of air contained in a small office. Even if we were locked in that unventilated office, with no way for air to get in or out (like in a hermetically sealed bank vault or in an air-lock on some science fiction movie), we'd have enough oxygen in that space for at least a couple of days.

Fortunately, continuous ventilation in houses and offices means that, in reality, we never change the concentration of oxygen in our air, even if we are chained to our desk with the door firmly closed, breathing heavily.

So, rather than the things *in* fresh air being beneficial for us, what's actually more important is what is *not* in fresh air. This is pollution. And it is the real killer. The combination of air pollution and smoking results in more deaths in humans across the world than any other single cause. So it's hardly a wonder that we ask our kids to go and get some more 'fresh' air.

Sea change

Fresh air has long been sold as the best tonic for all ills. Even before we could just hop on a plane and head for New Zealand, people would head for the hills, or go down to the beach to take in the air. This was not just for a good time. It was also for our health. Mountain retreats or seaside spas did and still do a roaring trade doing just this — providing a little clean air and better health to their customers.

Obviously, when compared to living and breathing in a highly-populated metropolis that was continuously burning fuel for warmth, cooking, transport and industry, the bracing open air of the seaside seemed as unpolluted as Eden. So the sea air seemed good for them, chiefly because the air at home was not. But were the fabled curative effects of 'taking the salt air' any more than just a change of scene?

Some studies have shown that people who have ditched their office job and moved to live by the coast do seem to have better health on average than those who stay put. Of course, there are many reasons for this benefit. For example, it may have more to do with the reasons we'd want to live by the sea or that we possess the mobility and resources to make a change. It may have nothing to do with the fresh air.

The smell of the sea

 Long before we finally get to the beach, it is possible to smell and taste the sea air. It is distinctive: tangy, slightly sulphurous and pregnant with memories of ice-cream and suntan lotion.

The distinctive smell is due to gases released from marine organisms, the most well-known being dimethylsulphide (DMS). In high concentrations it reeks more like a rotten cabbage, but in low levels, such as by the sea, it smells just like a beach.

The sea smell is not just a waste product. It is also one way other sea life can identify areas rich in food supplies. DMS also helps to make clouds over the sea, which can act like a hat on a sunny day, to keep microorganisms from catching too many rays.

These responses act to keep the ecology of the sea in balance. Indefinite blooms of sun-loving algae would be a bad thing. So, as algae stocks grow, the increased release of DMS brings in the clouds and the algae-eating predators to keep growth in check. Equally, too little algae is bad for the sea. So when stocks are low, the lower levels of DMS help keep the clouds and predators away, helping the algae to flourish again.

Sea salt does not dissolve in the air, but the surf generates **sea spray**, a fine mist of water particles that are scattered into the air by the wind and the waves. In these water droplets there is salt, some iodine, magnesium and other elements. But while these are all useful in the human body, there is not enough of these elements in sea air to make any difference to our health when breathing them in. And we can easily get plenty of minerals in the food we eat.

Human bodies are about 0.9 per cent salt. Sea water is approximately four times as salty (3.5 per cent). Although we are advised to drink in the sea air, drinking sea water is off the menu. Even if we were dying of thirst and there was (salt) 'water, water, everywhere' there'd be 'not a drop to drink'. If we did, it is more likely we would perish.

Because salt water is more concentrated than our own salty body fluids, deliberately inhaling salt water (which is known as **hypertonic saline**) drags water from the body onto the surface of the lungs. This can make it easier for people with bronchitis or other lung problems to break up thick mucus clogging their lungs and move it out during an infection. In the same way, hypertonic saline sprays can also help clear blocked noses resulting from colds or allergy. As most people do not have sick lungs, chronic coughs or blocked noses (especially when they plan to go to the beach), salt air offers no particular assistance to them.

If the weather is windy, it's often believed that the air must be fresher. And the seaside is usually breezier than inland areas. This is because water absorbs and releases heat at a slower rate than land, creating temperature differences in the morning and evening that trigger the flow of air (known as sea breezes).

But while strong winds certainly can help blow away local air pollution, winds can also bring in pollution from elsewhere, where it can become trapped in seaside eddies or undergo a chemical reaction with sea spray and sunlight that increases its toxicity. So a wind-swept beach may not have the clean fresh air we were hoping for after all.

Dust-bowl blues

Dust has long been the bane of miners, farmers and anyone else who works the soil. In the 1930s, a combination of drought and loss of native vegetation saw thousands of metric tons of topsoil simply blown away, turning the Great Plains of the United States into a virtual dust bowl. It was not simply farms and livelihoods that were lost. Dust particles also got into people's lungs, killing thousands.

This wasn't the first time something like this had happened in the world. The same disastrous effects of pollution on human lungs were also seen with the unregulated burning of coal in London in the 19th and 20th centuries, creating a black and sulphurous pall over the city. This became known as **smog**.

Humpty Dumpty's theory

 The word smog is a portmanteau, a fusion of the words 'smoke' and 'fog' usefully packed up into one word (like a two-compartment case, also known as a portmanteau) and perfectly captures the characteristics of both.

The *Los Angeles Times* first used the term smog in 1893 in an article about the very thick and 'pea-soup' fogs of London. However, it wasn't until 1905 in a paper variably describing smoky fog or foggy smoke over London that Dr Henry Des Voeux brought the term smog to public attention. Hence, the quirky term smog never features in the stories of Sherlock Holmes, or the writings of Hardy, Wilde or even Dickens, though they all comment on its peculiar features.

In the preface to *The Hunting of the Snark*, Humpty Dumpty argues that a portmanteau word like smog comes about if you 'make up your mind that you will say both words, but leave it unsettled which you will say first … but if you have the rarest of gifts, a perfectly balanced mind, you will say (them both together).' Is it breakfast? Is it lunch? Oh I can't decide, it's a bit of both really. So we'll call it brunch.

In conflict over whether to ask for the President to refute (i.e. contradict) or repudiate (i.e. reject) suggestions of racism, Sarah Palin used them both together and coined a new term **refudiate**. However, she failed to quote Humpty Dumpty as evidence for her perfectly balanced mind.

One toxic element in smog is really just dust, also known as particulate matter. There are different kinds of particles in the air we breathe. Big particles get efficiently trapped in our nose, mouth or throat. These can cause allergies and tickle our throat, but they don't get much further so don't cause much damage to our lungs.

Some particles are much smaller, thinner than a single silky strand on a spider's web. This makes them dangerous. Because of their very small size, the particles can bypass our defences and penetrate deep into our lungs, along with the oxygen we breathe. And once in our lungs, they act like an irritating splinter, triggering an inflammatory reaction. Some tiny airborne particles can also act as transport for hitchhiking toxins, chemicals and metals. Ultra-fine particulate matter (over twenty times smaller than a spider's web) can also cross our lungs and enter our bloodstream.

As discussed elsewhere, where you have inflammation going on, there is also the potential for collateral damage. In the case of air pollution, fine particles trigger inflammation in the lungs. So being exposed to air pollution increases the risk for other lung diseases as well as lung cancer.

Inflammation in the lungs can also kindle inflammatory processes occurring elsewhere, such as those associated with heart disease. Consequently, the concentration of fine particles in the air we breathe every day (i.e. the quality of our air) is strongly associated with our health, and particularly that of our lungs and our circulation.

Many of the fine particles we breathe come from the burning of fuels by vehicles and industry, and the chemical reactions set off in the atmosphere as their by-product. Consequently, our daily exposure is largely determined by how close we live to traffic and industrial sites, as well as prevailing wind and climate conditions that serve to either concentrate or dissipate their exhaust emissions. In some places, significant air pollution also comes from natural sources like fires, volcanic eruptions, windblown sand and soil.

All of this pollution comes from outside our homes, in the supposedly fresh air. Why then would we recommend that our kids go outside and breathe in more pollution?

Historically, the reason was that the air quality inside our houses used to be far worse than outside. Back when we had open log fires, candles and burning torches for light, staying indoors was positively toxic. Indoor air is easily contaminated, chiefly because it is less efficiently ventilated. So throwing open the windows and doors or getting out of the house (aka getting more fresh air) was lifesaving commonsense. Even today in the developing world, the burning of solid fuel for cooking and heating fills living spaces with fine particulate matter and probably kills as many people around the globe as smoking itself.

However, even without an open flame, our kitchens can be an air pollution hazard. Particulate matter from cooking is thrown up into the air. This is how we can smell what is for dinner at the other end of the house. More fine particles fly off when we cook with meat and the volatile animal fats therein. This is why the bacon or the roast beef can smell so great through the house, compared to simply roasted potatoes. Also, the hotter we cook (e.g. frying, sautéing and broiling), the more fine particles we throw off into the air. Using a gas cook top, especially for long periods, also puts more particles into the air than a flame-less electric element. And of course, if we burn our food, it doesn't matter how it got burnt, those particles go into the air too and we can smell them all through the house.

The potential health impact of airborne particles generated by cooking can be estimated by looking at lung cancer rates. Everyone knows that smoking causes lung cancer. But lung cancer sometimes occurs in people who have never smoked at all during their life, with women potentially at greater risk than men. This may be partly attributable to the extra time women often spend in the kitchen breathing in fine particles thrown off from their cooking (especially when using oil for stir frying/deep frying in Asian cuisine).

Most modern kitchens have a range hood over the oven or stove that aims to trap most (but not all) particulate matter, as well as odour and moisture released from our cooking. These would work quite well if we remembered to turn them on, or could tolerate the incessant whir of the extractor fans. But while they can help the house, many are not sufficiently placed over the front burners anyway to have much effect for the cook.

Smoking kills

The single most practical way to lose years off your life is to inhale tobacco smoke. Half of all long-term smokers will die prematurely of tobacco-related disease, reducing their life expectancy by ten years, on average, and taking many more quality years besides, due to the first-hand effects of smoking on their health, on their lungs, on their heart, on their breath, and even on their appearance.

However, for much of its history, tobacco was considered a medicinal cure-all, like coffee or alcohol, used for almost every known ailment. It was even used to raise the dead.

A smoking revival

 In the 18th century, there was no mouth-to-mouth resuscitation. Instead the resuscitation of persons apparently dead from drowning was undertaken using tobacco smoke. But as the dead obviously did not breathe, smoke couldn't be inhaled. So instead it was applied internally as an enema.

Interestingly, it might actually have worked. In some people, holding their breath and putting their head under cold water can trigger a reflex that changes the rhythm of their heart. In rare cases, this reflex may stop the heart altogether. This is one possible explanation for inexplicable 'drowning' deaths that occur in seemingly strong swimmers or in shallow waters close to shore.

However, the heart can sometimes be restarted again if a large amount of hot air is being blown up your backside. As the hot gas suddenly distends the bowel, this sends an urgent signal back through the nervous system to the brain that is literally strong enough to wake the dead.

The restorative benefit of smoke has nothing to do with the nicotine or any other chemicals contained therein. This is because blood does not flow when we are dead. So (without modern CPR to push it along) blood cannot move medicinals to reach our heart or brain, even if they are injected directly into a vein. This is probably fortunate, because nicotine is a toxic poison that can only be safely used by the recently deceased.

Much like the defibrillators of the 21st century, the smoke-enema treatment became so well regarded that enema stations (with a pipe to instil the smoke and a bellows to blow) were set up at all the common drowning spots like life rings, with lifeguards smoking at the ready to administer first-aid.

Given that it was widely understood that smoking was able to bring the dead back to life, it was impossible to imagine any harm coming from it. Undead zombies and even Frankenstein had not yet come into the popular imagination. So, at the time, the notion of bringing people back from the dead proved to be the biggest gimmick since the raising of Lazarus. But still, despite its recognized success, this indelicate procedure eventually fell out of practice, not least because it was demonstrated that the principal active agent in tobacco smoke, nicotine, was actually poisonous. And now with the weight of evidence we have, it is hard for any enlightened non-smoker to understand how it is possible that any sane person still smokes.

Although rates have declined from nearly half the population fifty years ago, approximately one in every seven adults continues to smoke and five out of every six of those on a daily basis. These people are not insane, reckless or indifferent (or even undead). It is just hard for them to imagine a life (or even a day) without a smoke and the consolation that each cigarette provides. They are addicted.

If you are a smoker then the single most important thing you can do for your health is to stop smoking. Please, return this book and buy one on how to quit and stay smoke-free.

However, most likely you are not a smoker. And why should you care if others want to smoke? It's their own damn fault, isn't it? Live and let die!

The fact of the matter is that smoke eventually gets into our lives, too. Every day, smokers and their smoke interact with non-smokers in their shared environment. And some of the hundreds of toxic chemicals that smoke contains can be passed on through the air to non-smokers. About one in five non-smokers has detectable levels of chemicals derived from the breakdown of inhaled nicotine in their blood. This is called **second-hand smoke**.

Second-hand smoke

Second-hand smoke is a major risk to health. Rates of some cancers, heart disease, stroke, depression and many other life-shortening illnesses are clearly increased by exposure to second-hand smoke, even for a person who never smoked themselves.

The size of this effect is not small. For example, the risk of a heart attack or stroke in non-smokers repeatedly exposed to second-hand smoke is increased by between a quarter and a third. This is the risk equivalent of smoking five cigarettes a day, even though the exposure to smoke is less than 5 per cent that of a five-a-day smoker.

Because of the clear risk to health in those indirectly exposed to tobacco smoke, smoking in public places, both indoor and outdoor, has been banned or heavily restricted. Some countries now ban smoking in cars. Along with declining numbers of smokers, the evolution of smoke-free legislation has reduced exposure to second-hand smoke by over two-thirds of what was breathed in thirty years ago, when it was even still possible to smoke on a plane.

And no smoking, please

 Today, the idea of flying through the toxic clouds of someone else's smoke is almost inconceivable, let alone the risk it runs of setting fire to the air-fuel and oxygen in the central tanks and blowing up the plane!

In the seventies, 40 per cent of all adults were regular smokers. At last in the majority, non-smokers pressed for their own rights. Not surprisingly, airlines were reluctant to lose 40 per cent of their market through banning smoking. To reduce the discomfort for non-smoking clientele and the potential for on-board confrontation over the issue, passengers were segregated on planes into separate sections: 'smoking or non-smoking'.

In 1987, Australia became the first country in the world to ban smoking outright on all domestic flights. Recognizing that it would actually save them money through easier seating allocation (e.g. no more smoking or non-smoking sections) as well as reduced cleaning costs, all the airlines quickly got on board. The potential benefits to the flight crew were also obvious to the Federal Treasurer of the time and future Prime Minister, whose wife had previously worked as a flight attendant.

The Australian government did not ban smoking on international flights initially for fear that it would disadvantage the local (then government-owned) carrier. Many were concerned that it would have been too much to ask smokers to abstain on the very long flights to and from Australia. It took another eight years before smoking was banned on all flights to and from Australia.

Although first proposed in 1969, it wasn't until the year 2000 that the US legislated that all flights, both domestic and international, should be smoke free across America.

Today, all aircraft and many workplaces are smoke free, especially indoors. This is important because simply separating smokers from non-smokers, as was tried on planes, doesn't work as tiny airborne particles of smoke permeate everything, even things that are relatively far from the action.

The most common solution is simply to send smokers outside, which is why smokers now huddle outside of many buildings. This moves the problem, but doesn't eliminate it. Anyone and anything within proximity of a smoker, indoors or outdoors, will still be exposed to their air. And we all have to get in or out of the building sometime, so we will frequently pass through their toxic clouds.

Third-hand smoke

Sometimes we come into a room or space where a smoker has been and it reeks! We instantly recognize the lingering pungent odour from cigarette smoke. This smell is caused by aromatic fumes emanating from dust particles and tar which coat not only carpets, curtains and sofas but also clothes, hair and even the skin of smokers.

These particles can remain in place for many weeks after the cigarette has been extinguished and the fog of (second-hand) smoke has cleared. However, over time the residue of smoke leaches its volatile organic chemicals back into the air, giving rise to the characteristic smell of a room that has previously hosted a smoker. This airborne residual is sometimes called **third-hand smoke**.

Unlike smoke in the air, which tends to dissipate over time, the toxins in third-hand smoke build up with each cigarette smoked in a room, cumulatively contaminating the environment. The more cigarettes that are smoked in a room, the more it will smell. This is especially the case in small, hot spaces, such as inside a car.

The important thing about third-hand smoke is that it is just as toxic as puffing on a cigarette. Third-hand smoke is made up of the same toxic chemicals that fall in and out of the air until they are breathed in or blown away. All of the same diseases that are increased by smoking exist in higher rates in people exposed third hand to someone else's smoke.

The other important feature of third-hand smoke is that it is notoriously resistant to conventional cleaning. Airing out the room, turning on the fan or vacuuming until we collapse can never fully eliminate the distinctive smell of smoke. This is because the tar in smoke literally sticks to surfaces, which then continues to slowly emit smelly and toxic chemicals for days or even months after.

The ongoing contamination of indoor air with the re-emitting pollutants is not unique to cigarettes. Many other chemicals can create a toxic residue that continues to emit over many months. A classic example is the new-car smell of cars that can persist for over a year after the car is first sold.

That new-car smell

 New cars smell different from old ones. Even the used cars that have been rebuilt and refurbished, as good as new, don't smell the same as a freshly minted brand-new vehicle.

A lot of chemicals go into making a car. There's a lot of plastic, glue, rubber, solvents, vinyl, carpet and sometimes leather. And just like when cooking a burger, some of these chemicals become airborne when heated and we can catch their aroma, especially when it is concentrated by the narrow confines of the interior. Even months later we can still catch a whiff of new-car smell on a hot day, as the heat draws out the last residues of newness.

Although comparatively pleasing, the new-car smell is definitely not good for us. Think glue sniffing.

Eventually, that new-car smell melts and blows away or becomes overpowered by impregnated body odour, flatulence and the food scraps that the kids have lost down the back seat. But for a good long time, the car felt and smelled new.

Other things in our houses also continue to emit fumes into our air, including paints and varnishes, cleaning and disinfecting products, sweaty shoes, body odours and even the residue of pets — long after the paint has dried or the source has left the stage. These offensive gases are obviously concentrated indoors because of less ventilation, so it makes sense to throw open the windows and doors as much as possible and allow them their escape.

Another popular way used to fix the problem of persistent fumes is the **bake-out**. This involves raising the temperature as much as possible for a few days to the point that most of the volatile substances hiding in the house become airborne. Then we can open every door and window, turn on every fan and blow the fumes away.

Exhausted

Burning of fossil fuels by cars, motorbikes and trucks remains a major source of air pollution. Exhaust pipes spew out a range of toxic chemicals and small particles, which are thrown up into the air by the turbulence of passing vehicles and create the visible smog that shrouds many modern cities.

At least three times as many lives are lost every year due to the noxious chemicals created by vehicles than are caused by car accidents. Most of these deaths occur due to lung problems, especially in vulnerable individuals with pre-existing lung disease. But even in otherwise healthy people, and even at levels below the commonly used air-quality guidelines, the closer to a major road we live and work, the greater our risk of heart problems, stroke, dementia, some kinds of cancer and even reduced fertility as a result of our exposure. In numerical terms, the effect of eliminating all car exhaust on human survival would be greater than curing melanoma.

It is easy to understand that car exhaust can be harmful. We have all read about or seen on television and film people taking their own lives by breathing in exhaust fumes from an engine. Although the catalytic converters in modern engines and other safety features make it difficult, it still remains the second most common method of suicide. A simple cabin sensor would seem an obvious solution to prevent this. These have been in operation in planes for years, with automated oxygen masks that drop down in the case of (low oxygen) emergency. In truly smart cars, a cabin sensor would just shut off the engine when tripped. This would save thousands of lives each year, at least as many as airbags.

But for those of us simply walking down the sidewalk beside a busy road in an airless concrete canyon of a modern metropolis, there is no simple alarm or oxygen mask that drops from the ceiling. Most exhaust gases are odourless and invisible. They only look like smog when they react with sunlight and other chemicals in the atmosphere.

Bad ozone

 We normally think about ozone as the good guy. Floating around 22.5 kilometres (or 14 miles) up in the ozone layer of our stratosphere, it works like sunscreen protecting the earth against the harmful effects of sunlight and its ultraviolet radiation. But at ground level, where it is not supposed to be, ozone has a dark side, especially at the contact points of our lungs and our skin.

This 'bad' ozone is created when vehicle and industrial emissions like nitrogen dioxide and volatile hydrocarbons react together with sunlight and oxygen in the troposphere where we live and breathe. Ground level (bad) ozone levels are highest in the summer smog of industrial cities like Los Angeles and Beijing.

The problem with ozone is that it is highly reactive. This is why it forms such a good protection against ultraviolet light in the upper atmosphere. But when it gets into our lungs it can react with surface fats to trigger inflammation and injury. The same sort of thing happens when we inhale cigarette smoke, and you know how that turns out.

~~~~~~

While most of the particulate matter comes from incomplete combustion of burning fuel (especially diesel), the wearing of brakes, tyres and the road surface itself also generates small airborne particles. Think of the visible smoke created by the fast and furious spinning of tyres and screeching of brakes in the movies. Although we never travel quite so fast, each spin or brake creates its own tiny wake of smoke. Multiplied by the many times we spin our wheels or use the brakes to stop them, as well as the many millions of cars doing this daily, the so called 'non-exhaust' particles that are generated in this way now represent a major source of pollution. One day we will all have electric cars. But while they will have no smoking exhaust pipe, they will still generate emissions from their brakes and tyres.

Recognizing the preventable risks posed by air pollution, a number of countries have adopted 'clean air' legislation designed to reduce emissions, including tighter vehicle standards, reducing road use through public transport alternatives, fuel taxes, green alternative energy production and improvements in technology, including better fuels, low-pollution engines, catalytic converters, and start–stop systems to shut off the engine when it would otherwise idle. Some countries have even adopted anti-idling regulations, to limit idling to no more than 3 minutes every hour. While it may all seem excessive now, in the end we will all live a bit longer as a result.

The bottom line

We can throw open the doors and send the kids outside. We can escape to the seaside. But that would be mostly for our sanity. The air is no fresher out there than it is here inside.

Pollution gets into the air. And in a well-ventilated world, air gets everywhere; there is no escaping it. It is clearly worse closer to the source, next to a smoker, along a busy road or over a cook top. But even safe in our non-smoking home, the density of fine particles and chemicals in the air inside is much the same as it is outside.

Smoke is bad for smokers. Pollution is similarly bad for everyone who breathes. But change is also in the air. As with smoking, the greatest driver of change is public opinion and social acceptability. Today, we recoil in horror from a fuming exhaust pipe on an old car or a factory spilling black smoke, as much as we would if a smoker lit up beside us. We now prefer to buy the electric car or heater we believe to have the best emission standards. This is not just simple economy. It is life and death.

Do I really have to ...

#13

Get more sunshine?

Q: Why does sunshine make us stronger?
**A: All our super powers ultimately come
from the radiant light of a yellow sun.**

Q: What is wrong with staying indoors?
A: Ask any prisoner. Sunshine is an escape.

Q: I'm okay so long as I don't get too much?
A: Or your wings will get burnt.

Q: Why can't I just take vitamin D?
**A: It's not the same. Just like fruit juice will
never replace an apple or an orange.**

Q: Won't I just get more wrinkles and spots from the sun?
A: Not if you take care of your skin.

Q: How do I take the weather with me?
A: You already do.

Q: Can sunshine make me high?
A: Ask Icarus.

If there was a symbol for health and happiness, it would be drawn like the sun and carry a wide beaming smile. By contrast, misery and sadness would be like looking out on a gloomy day, with raindrops steadily falling from a black cloud in the shape of tears.

It is common to want to group things that are alike in our minds. Sunshine and happiness have much in common. They are both moods and have their seasons. They both feel warm on our skin. Often simultaneously. They are both essential for good health and have persistent effects on its outcomes, even long after they have gone away. Both give us the energy to go and do the things that need to be done.

Man and Superman

 Superman is really not that different from us. He is not so super without sunlight. Indoors, trapped inside his dark office at the *Daily Planet*, he becomes Clark Kent, his weak, myopic alter ego. But take him outside on a sunny day, his athleticism and long-distance vision are unstoppable.

Superman gets all the energy required for his extraordinary super powers from the radiant light of a yellow sun, which he then stores up in his copious muscles for later use.

This is just like green plants which use the sun's radiant energy to generate stores (of sugar) that can be burnt later when specific actions are called for. This means that plants (and Superman, for that matter) can still work in the dark, unlike a solar panel.

While humans do not gather the sun's energy directly, all our strength to get up, up and away just like Superman also originates from the radiant light of a yellow sun. It's just that we get it indirectly by eating plants, eating the things that eat plants or eating the things that eat other things that eat plants. In this way, all our super powers ultimately come from the sun.

The sun has been worshipped as a deity not just by pagan cultures, but by almost every civilization at one time or another. For many people, the sun is considered the ultimate source of their being. And in a roundabout way, it really is.

Yet today there aren't many sun worshippers left. Most people spend less than 7 per cent of their time outside in the sun. And even when we get outside, we are usually covered from head to toe. We need to change this. For our health's sake, it's about time we went outside and got some sun.

Radiating

Sunlight takes just over 8 minutes to travel from the surface of the sun to the surface of the earth. The sun's rays are a complex mixture of different kinds of light across different wavelengths. Each part has some effect on our health.

Just less than half of the sunlight reaching the earth is at a (visible) wavelength that our eyes can perceive. Visible light is composed of all the different colours (wavelengths) that we can see in a rainbow.

The other half of the light reaching the surface of the earth is infrared radiation. All hot things give off infrared radiation, including humans and Superman's eyes. But as the sun is half a million times hotter, it gives off much more infrared.

Infrared light is mostly invisible to human eyes (unless we are wearing night-vision goggles). However, even if we can't see it, we can still feel its radiant energy as it penetrates and warms our skin. Clouds will reduce the intensity of infrared radiation that reaches our skin so it feels a little cooler when the sun is hidden behind a cloud. However, infrared radiation can penetrate through glass, so we can feel the warmth of the sun just by sitting near a window, even without going outside.

Greenhouse gas and global warming

 Hot things give off infrared radiation which works to heat anything that it comes in contact with. The hot sun's infrared radiation heats up the earth. The warmed earth also gives off infrared radiation, but not as much as the sun, because it's not as hot.

The atmosphere around the earth acts a bit like a blanket on our bed. It stops some of the infrared radiation of our body heat being lost into the night and keeps us cosy and warm. This is also called the greenhouse effect, because glass or plastic over a greenhouse also works in the same way: keeping the heat in when it gets cold outside.

If the earth had no atmosphere it would feel like sleeping naked under the stars instead of being tucked up in bed. Our world would be frozen in an eternal winter, like in the movie, with an average temperature of about −18°C (0°F).

Carbon emissions released into the atmosphere after coal, gas and oil are burnt inefficiently increase the trapping of infrared radiation. In essence, the earth is now wrapped up in a really thick double blanket, even in summer. So even though the heat source isn't warming up, it's getting much hotter in bed. This is one of the major reasons why our world has become significantly warmer over the last century.

The remaining 2 to 5 per cent of sunlight is ultraviolet radiation, or UV for short. As with the visible light in a rainbow, there are also different wavelengths of UV light. All of them can cause sunburn and damage our skin.

The majority of ultraviolet radiation reaching the earth's surface and our skin is UV-A. The intensity of UV-A light is relatively constant throughout daylight hours, regardless of cloud cover and the seasons, as our atmosphere hardly blocks out any UV-A light. By contrast, the protective ozone layer in the upper atmosphere blocks out at least 95 per cent of UV-B. This is fortunate, because even though the dose is fifty times smaller, UV-B is a thousand times more potent for causing sunburn and skin damage than UV-A. Even though the atmosphere does a great job as our sunscreen, the total amount of UV-B getting through can vary over four-fold depending on the place, the time of day and the season. And the times when UV-B is at its highest are when we burn the easiest.

For example, under a clear sky close to the equator, the UV-B levels are much higher than they would be on a sunny day in northern or southern latitudes where sunlight comes through the earth's atmosphere on an angle, and has a much thicker ozone layer to penetrate before it reaches us.

Similarly, when the sun is highest in the sky, shining straight down in the middle of day, there is less atmosphere between the sun and our skin, so there is relatively more UV-B in the midday sun. Thus it is often recommended that we should avoid exposure of unprotected skin to sunlight during peak hours for UV-B radiation (generally between 10 am and 3 pm) when only 'mad dogs and Englishmen' go out. By contrast, the greater slice of atmosphere traversed by sunlight at the beginning and end of the day means that UV-B levels can be less than a third of those in the middle of the day. For this and many other reasons, these are the best times of day to be active outside. In the middle of the day we can take a siesta.

Siesta time

 In many countries, it is customary to retire indoors during the ultraviolet peak of midday and take a siesta.

It's not just because of the heat. Even in cooler climes, it is common to feel a temporary drop in alertness and an inescapable desire to take it easy for a while. This snoozy sensation is particularly amplified after having a large meal and maybe a glass of wine, rapidly followed by a large dessert. Remember Christmas or Thanksgiving? It's not the excess turkey, it's just the excess that amplifies our natural biology. So afterwards it's hardly surprising that it feels like a good time to go and lie down for a while.

Siesta-time is about more than just avoiding the UV rays, digesting the meal or escaping the in-laws after a festive lunch. Those who nap habitually and briefly (less than 30 minutes) have lower rates of high blood pressure, diabetes and heart disease and a slightly longer life expectancy. Whether this reported benefit is actually because these people are taking a nap is unclear. It may just be that those people with the time and space to take a nap in the middle of the day aren't the ones always rushing back to work or fighting their post-lunch dip with caffeine and stress.

Unlike infrared radiation, clouds have only a small effect on UV-B. So even on those cloudy days in summer, when our skin feels cool, the UV-B levels can still be dangerously high to unprotected skin. By contrast, standard glass blocks the transmission of UV-B, so although we feel the radiant warmth of the sun, we'll never get sunburnt while we are inside the glass bubble of our car or the office unless we open the window and let the sun hit our skin directly.

The higher we climb, the less atmosphere there is between us and the sun. So direct exposure of our exposed noses to UV-B can be a third more when we are skiing up in the high mountains than when we are sunbathing at sea level. Ultraviolet light is also able to bounce off highly reflective surfaces like snow, doubling again the UV-B exposure to skiers and other alpine enthusiasts. This why those mountaineers always look so tanned and eventually so wrinkled. At sea level, reflected sunlight off sand and water can also modestly amplify exposure, although a tenth of that achieved with fresh snow. But the problem is that at sea level we usually show ten times as much skin.

Over the last century the widespread use of chlorofluorocarbons (CFCs) in industry has resulted in depletion of the ozone from the upper atmosphere. Ozone is one of the important things in our atmosphere that keeps out UV-B. So declining levels of ozone in the upper atmosphere over the last fifty years have allowed more UV-B to penetrate to ground level, and has significantly shortened the time it takes to burn our skin in direct sunlight. Depletion of ozone has not made the world hotter, and is not a cause of climate change. But ozone depletion and global warming are both caused by human activity and are both dangerous for human health. They are also preventable as the recent stabilizing of the 'hole' in the ozone layer over Antarctica demonstrates following wholesale changes in our use of CFCs.

D-day

Our skin also absorbs the radiant light of a yellow sun. And just like Superman, we also use it to generate something that makes us stronger and faster. This is **vitamin D**. Most adults get over 90 per cent of their vitamin D simply from the sun on their skin. Without vitamin D, we can become weak and fragile; as different from an athlete as average human beings are from Superman.

Ultraviolet light is destructive, like fire. But it is also possible to harness fire to do our cooking. In the same way, our skin uses some of the damaging UV-B radiation that penetrates it when we are exposed to sunlight to cook up a precursor of vitamin D (called vitamin D3 or cholecalciferol), using excess cholesterol as a substrate.

This vitamin D3 is then shipped to our liver where it is converted to a storable form of vitamin D. It is then released into the blood, where it circulates for a few weeks before being finally tucked away in our fat. This stored vitamin D is liberated only when it is needed, when the sunshine goes away. This may be tomorrow when we have to go back to work inside our office after our long sun-drenched vacation. Or it could be many months later, as summer light fades into cold dark winters, sending us indoors or cozied up with hardly any skin showing through. The vitamin D stores generated in the warm light of summer literally have allowed us to live our lives in very cold climates.

Black and white and fish

 Although we are all pretty much the same on the inside, on the outside, humans come in many different colours. Most people think that this is probably due to sunlight.

Our ancient hairless ancestors were probably all dark skinned. High levels of skin pigment, melanin, protected them against the ravages of UV-B out on the sun-baked equatorial savannah. In this case survival of the fittest was survival of the blackest. Had they been pale-skinned, they would have soon died off from skin cancer and reduced fertility, due to the destruction of skin folate by UV-B.

However, as our ancestors spread out into darker, colder climes, this same dark skin became a liability. Less sunlight and less UV-B per unit of sunlight meant much less vitamin D could be made. So the only ones who could survive were now those with lighter skin. In this case survival of the fittest became survival of the whitest. So over millennia, across Europe and Asia people became slowly whiter.

The food with the highest levels of vitamin D is oily fish. This is possibly why some indigenous peoples of the Arctic who eat a lot of oily fish have remained dark-skinned, despite making little vitamin D through the winter. However, the Scandinavians' love of herring was not enough to undo their pale genetics.

Our skin is very efficient at making vitamin D. So it doesn't take much exposure of our skin to the sun to make it. Just 10 minutes of summer sun on our face, arms and hands can meet our daily requirements for vitamin D. The more skin we expose and the longer we expose it for the more vitamin D we can make, sometimes enough to get us through a winter where our skin sees little sunlight for weeks on end.

When we get a vitamin D blood test, it only measures the circulating form, so it mostly just tells us how much sun we've had in the last few weeks. Because most of us spend so much of our lives indoors, over half of all adults now have circulating levels of vitamin D that are considered low. Obviously, low vitamin D levels are an even more common problem for sedentary couch potatoes, the obese, the institutionalized, the frail, and the elderly, who don't get out much. But even the seemingly fit office-workers labouring from dawn to dusk inside are at risk from not making enough vitamin D to get them through.

The problem with not having enough vitamin D in our lives is that vitamin D is used by our body to regulate levels of key minerals including calcium, iron, magnesium, phosphate and zinc. If our vitamin D levels are too low, our mineral balance also changes. To make up for the shortfall, our bones start being broken down by our body at a slightly faster rate than usual and the rate at which new bone is laid down is slightly slowed. This releases extra minerals that are stored away in our bone. However, in the long term, this is why low levels of vitamin D also leads to progressive thinning of our bones, increasing the risk of them breaking.

But getting enough vitamin D is more than just a means to strong bones. Many other parts of our body also respond to vitamin D. This may be why low levels of vitamin D have also been associated with an increased risk of health problems including heart disease, diabetes, multiple sclerosis and dementia, as well as some cancers. It is hard to know whether these different things are really caused by low vitamin D levels or if it's just that people who are inactive, frail or always indoors are more likely to have health problems as well as low levels of vitamin D.

The fate in our stars

As the Bible says, 'To everything there is a season, a time for every purpose' — this is particularly true for human health and disease, which each have their turn.

The ancient Babylonians tracked the annual course of the sun through the sky, and divided it into twelve parts, known as **signs of the zodiac**. People born at particular times of the year were said to be born under particular star signs. Many people still believe that the time of year at which they were born (i.e. their star sign) has made a big difference in determining the kind of person they have become.

But rather than our fate being tied to distant stars, this division may be more about the weather around certain times of the year, and its effects on our diet and lifestyle. For example, babies born in autumn have developed in their mother's womb through the warm plenty of spring and summer, so may be endowed with a slightly more robust health than those developing through the dearth of winter, only to be born in spring. This may be why the season of our birth is also associated with many aspects of our subsequent health, including the likelihood of developing mental illness, heart disease, epilepsy and dementia. In fact, studies show that babies born in spring actually live slightly shorter lives than those born in autumn, and are less likely to become centenarians. This is not a big effect. We are not bound by our zodiac sign. But we are influenced by it.

And if the season we are born in is so important as to influence our health, it is not surprising to find that it can also (weakly) influence other traits, including personality, mood and what hand we use to write with. In fact, it is even possible to predict what the weather was like at the time of our birth with some accuracy using a brain scan.

It is also true that at some times of the year we often feel low and more commonly get sick, while at other times we are filled with superhuman vitality. Ask anyone why this should be and they will probably blame the weather.

Certainly, the weather outside can significantly influence how we feel inside. Not by as much as most people think, but enough to make some people feel just a bit more invigorated on a warm sunny day. Of course not everyone gets a boost from the sunshine. Some people actually love a rainy day. And the majority of people don't respond either way. This is probably because they spend most of their time indoors.

Warmer weather definitely puts us closer to our comfort zone, which is usually around 20°C (68°F), a temperature at which we neither need to perspire to keep cool or move and shiver to keep warm. The further we get from this comfort zone — hotter or colder — the less comfortable we feel, and this plays on our emotions and the health that results from them.

But seasons are more than just temperature. Sure, summer is mostly hot and winter is mostly cold. But in spring and autumn the weather is predictably unpredictable. This kind of unsettled weather can be vaguely discontenting. And the bigger the change, the greater the problems.

An ill wind

 Many cultures have a saying that describes 'an ill wind that blows no good'. This is more than just a figure of speech. Some places in the world experience strong winds and extremely rapid fluctuations in temperature.

For example, in some special places, cold, moist winter air travels up a high mountain range, leaving residual warm, dry air to rapidly flow down the other side. The most famous examples are the Föhn wind in Europe and the Chinook of the Rocky Mountains. Here, the fastest ever change in air temperature was recorded, with the temperature rising from −20°C to 7°C (or −4°F to 45°F) in just 2 minutes.

Not surprisingly these hot winds are also infamous for making people feel unwell (or at the very least feel that they are wearing the wrong clothes).

At least half of all adults claim to experience changes in their health with changes in the weather, including more frequent headaches, joint pain, tiredness and even catching more colds. Of course, colds are caused by viruses, not the weather (see Chapter 14). But as the air temperature changes around us, so does the feeling of stuffiness in our nose. Even though our nose does not actually block, a change to hotter and humid air will make it feel more congested, like when we're in the shower. But once we step out of the shower, the blast of colder, less humid air makes our nose suddenly feel more open, creating that fresh 'woo-hoo' sensation in our head. The same thing happens in reverse when we move from the air-conditioned dry cool indoors to the humid heat outside: our noses and heads may feel more blocked and stuffed up. So we blame the weather.

The vast majority of people with arthritis or chronic back pain really do feel more discomfort on stormy, cold or damp days and feel better on warm days. Whether this is a direct issue (e.g. the joints or nerves change with the weather) or indirect one (e.g. related to the effects of weather on our mood, behaviour, diet, physical activity, mobility, participation, perception of illness or pain) is unknown.

Allergic conditions like hay fever, dermatitis and asthma attacks are more common in spring as pollen and dust are whipped up by stronger winds and act as an irritant. The moist air associated with seasonal storms can also concentrate and break up pollen and pollution into smaller particles that are more easily inhaled deep into the lungs and can trigger asthma attacks. Warm and moist conditions also promote the release of fungal spores that can set off allergies in some people.

Finally, breast cancer is also more commonly diagnosed in spring and early summer, and this association is more pronounced the further we get from the equator, where seasonal change is most dramatic. A similar association exists for prostate cancer diagnosis in men. But this is not because cancer is caused by the seasons. Spring is traditionally the season we try to get things in order, like spring cleaning. So spring is also the time we get round to finally going to the doctor.

Allergic to sunlight?

 Ever walked outside the house during the day and the first thing you do is sneeze? For at least one-third of all adults, looking suddenly at a bright light actually makes them sneeze. It is definitive proof that sunlight is hardwired into our brain.

Classic examples are going outside on a bright day, throwing open the curtains or emerging into light after driving through a tunnel. Some people sneeze if a flash from a camera catches them in the face.

What causes this reflex is still a mystery. It is probably also the same reason most of us also involuntarily shut our eyes when we sneeze (an all too frequent cause of traffic accidents).

Blue skies

The seasonal weather is more important to our health than just hot and cold sensations on our skin or its ability to generate vitamin D. The amount and intensity of visible light that gets into our eyes definitely also affect the functions of our brain and way we feel. This is thanks to special light sensors at the back of our eyes. These sensors are different from the ones that we use to see. Instead, we use these ones to help us feel how we should feel.

These light sensors are hardwired into parts of our brain that control our body clock. All animals have a clock that keeps the body's functions appropriate for the time of day. It's not just to regulate when to fall asleep and when to wake up (the so-called sleep cycle), but also a whole host of other daily biological rhythms including our mood, alertness and reaction times, and things like our temperature, our blood pressure and our appetite.

Getting our eyes out into the sunlight is one important regulator for our biological clock. This is obvious to anyone suffering jet lag, who then goes for a walk outside and returns feeling refreshed as though they are now at last in the right time zone. In particular, light in our eyes stimulates our brain to become a bit more alert and focused in its thinking. It's daytime, so wake up! This is a bit like the 'buzz' response to a cup of coffee. And like coffee, too much light at the wrong time (such as using a bright computer screen in the evening) can also keep us awake at night.

Interestingly, it not just any light that can do this. Although any visible light is stimulating to our brain, compared to working in darkness, it seems to be the blue wavelengths that really stimulate our light sensors and therefore our brain. The light we see doesn't need to be all blue or look blue like the sky. Blue light is contained in most white light (e.g. fluorescent bulbs, TV and computer screens) though not nearly as much as in sunlight.

Blue light is especially dominant in our eyes at dawn. So maybe this particular response to blue light is one way our eyes can get us to jump start our day, just like a morning cup of coffee.

Red sky at night

 Red sky at night is supposed to be the delight of shepherds and sailors alike. Everyone knows this old saying.

Sunlight contains all the colours of the rainbow. Most of these colours pass through the earth's atmosphere, like light through a transparent window. But the chemical elements in our atmosphere are able to scatter the sunlight coming in on a blue-violet wavelength. This is a bit like a diffuser on a fluorescent light that spreads light all over our workspace, except that the atmosphere just scatters the blue light. And so the daytime sky looks blue.

The sky only looks red in the evening and morning precisely because the sky is blue during daylight hours somewhere else. The sun we see on the horizon as a hot orange ball in an iridescent red sky, is precisely the same sun that looks pale yellow on a bright blue background at high noon, another quarter turn around the earth.

At dusk and dawn the angle of the sun is so low in the sky that its light cuts through much more of the atmosphere. As a consequence, half a day of blue sky light is being removed before it reaches our eyes. Take away all the blue and the sunlight appears orange-red. Hence red sky at dusk and dawn.

Why a red sky at night is auspicious for shepherds and sailors is simply because if they can see a red sunset in the west, the air must be clear in this direction. And since the prevailing weather usually comes from the west, tomorrow will probably be a bright sunny day.

Conversely, red sky in the morning leaves everyone feeling half asleep (through want of blue light in their eyes) and ominously anticipating the cold front following the clear air exiting to the east where the sun was rising.

Another explanation for this phenomenon is that we began our evolution under the sea, where blue is the only colour of light that penetrates deep down. So we could only tell day from night by sensing blue light.

This is also one reason why deep-sea fish are mostly red. Without any red light reaching into the deep down below, red fish are as good as black. So the clownfish would be okay. Blue fish, like Dory, on the other hand, would stand out in the gloom and be especially vulnerable to being eaten in deep waters.

For many reasons, we all feel a little low in winter, a bit stir crazy, sleeping more and interacting less with others. However, some people are especially prone to cabin fever during winter, when sunlight levels are at their lowest. Perhaps the most famous example is the character of Jack Torrence in *The Shining*.

The Shining

 Jack takes a job as winter caretaker in an isolated mountain hotel. Like the previous caretaker before him, Jack succumbs to cabin fever, becoming increasingly irritable, violent, psychotic and ultimately an axe-wielding homicidal maniac. There might have been ghosts and a possessive hotel too, but they were mostly in his head.

Working away on his typewriter in the half-dark, Jack wasn't seeing much sunlight through the day. This might have started to play tricks with his fragile mind. Getting out a bit more could have helped him (if the hotel was not so snowbound). Maybe a bit of ice-skating or skiing? But all (inside) work and no (outside) play made Jack into a monster. Had he been busy spending his days working under the shining bright glare of a computer screen, things might have turned out differently.

Sunshine and glasses

Many people have difficulty seeing things in the distance. They can see close up things just fine, like when reading a book or using a computer. But, like Clark Kent, they need glasses to bring distant objects into focus. This is called short-sightedness or **near-sightedness**. It is the reason why most people wear glasses, and is the most common disability to affect human beings.

It has been estimated that at least half of all adults in the world are near sighted. It never used to be this way. A hundred years ago it was maybe 10 per cent at best. But today, the people who don't wear glasses are in a minority. In some Asian countries over 95 per cent of all young adults are now near sighted.

Think back to your childhood when there was only one optician in the whole town. Today, there is a glasses shop in every shopping centre, and often two or three, all doing a roaring trade. The best sign of a significant problem is a growing commercial interest in it.

The reason for this dramatic change in our collective vision is not clear. Many people think it has something to do with the way we now use our eyes. Like Clark Kent, our daily planet is often a low-light environment, trapped inside concrete canyons of urban life, isolated from the visual stimulation of distant landscapes. Today we spend most of our lives inside, focused close-up on the computer screen, phones and even reading books (thank you, reader). All this time spent looking at things up close and in the dark actually makes our eyeballs grow longer.

We are adapting to our environment. But our adaptation is making us more suited to computers. At the same time we are becoming less able to focus on the distant hills or the screen at the front of the lecture hall. (Fortunately, we have the notes close at hand on our iPad.)

Rather than the cause of our near-sightedness being straining our eyes with too much near work, it may simply be that the outside sunshine we are now not getting is just as important for the size of our eyeballs. Even under a hat, sunlight outside is at least twenty-fold brighter than the lights we have on indoors. Although we can see inside just fine, the extra brightness of our yellow sun is probably important to keep our eyeballs under control, particularly as we are growing up, balancing out all the maladaptive effects of all the close-up time indoors. Certainly, kids who get outside lots have a significantly lower rate of needing glasses as they get older.

Don't look at the sun

 We were always told not to stare at the sun, lest we go blind. Even at dawn and dusk when most of its intensity has faded, staring too long at the sun can leave a lasting impression.

This is not because sunlight will actually fry our eyeballs. Our lens does not act like a magnifying glass that focuses sunlight to burn little black holes in the back of our eyes. At most, the temperature increases only three to four degrees, about the same amount as when we have a fever.

So it's not the heat of the sun that will scar our vision. Rather it's the chemical reactions set off after staring at the intense light of the sun that can be enough to permanently damage the light-sensing cells at the back of our eye.

Fortunately this almost never happens. Most times when a light is too bright for our eyes, we'll look away just by reflex before any damage is done. At worst, sometimes a residual after-image persists for a few minutes.

During a solar eclipse it's common to want to take a long look at what's going on in the sky. But even though the sun might not seem too bright, looking at even a sliver of sunlight provides enough intensity to damage our vision. After watching an eclipse without any eye protection, it can take many months before your eyesight will return to normal, if at all.

As we get older, our eyes also wear the effects of continuous exposure to sunlight in a different way. The most important changes occur in the lens, whose job it is to focus light coming into the eye by changing its shape/curvature, so that any image that reaches the back of the eye is sharply defined, with clear edges and contrast.

A healthy lens is normally very elastic, allowing it to quickly and efficiently flex to change shape. When looking into the distance, the lens should become long and flat. But when looking at objects close up, like when reading or sewing, the lens retracts to become smaller and rounder to accurately focus the incoming light.

The human eye has the ability to read a book up close and then look up and almost instantaneously focus on our children running on the other side of a park. If you try this with a camera, it seems to take an eternity to get into focus. The human eye does it almost instantly because of its elastic lens.

But as we get older, our lenses become progressively stiffer. And stiff lenses cannot as easily change shape. This means the ability of our eyes to focus on nearby objects reduces as we age. This is known as **presbyopia** (or far-sightedness). All of us will eventually have this annoying problem to some extent as we get older.

The progressive stiffening of our lens is a very slow process, so it may be hard to notice it happening. Sometimes people only realize when they notice they are holding reading materials further and further away in order to focus on them. This is often called 'short arm syndrome' because as our lens becomes stiffer we always need to hold the object just a little bit further away. Eventually, our arms become 'too short' and some extra help is needed to focus on things at close range.

Lens stiffening does not always result in poor vision. Some people find their eyesight actually improves as they get older and they don't need their glasses anymore. This is sometimes called second sight. This does not mean that lens stiffening has not occurred. In fact, there's usually another factor at work, such as the fact that they were near-sighted to begin with.

The same changes that make the lens stiffer can also make the lens less transparent as we get older. This is known as a **cataract**. Early symptoms of a cataract include objects appearing less vivid and having less contrast, especially in low light, as the cataract scatters the light entering our eye. Some people with cataracts also have difficulty telling colours apart, like blue and green. And less blue light getting into the eyes may affect sleep and mood, as well as thinking. Their brains feel as though they are, literally, living in the dark.

Those with cataracts may also experience glare when looking at bright lights, such as when driving at night. Eventually, cataracts can obstruct the passage of light into the eye and block our vision. At least half of all adults will eventually experience some degree of vision loss due to cataracts. Typically both eyes are affected, but usually one side is worse than the other.

As well as old age, excess exposure to ultraviolet light can also cause cataracts. Consequently, wearing sunglasses, a brimmed hat and avoiding direct sunlight at the peak hours of ultraviolet radiation are important ways to reduce our risk of cataracts, not to mention skin cancer and crow's feet.

Burnt by the sun

Skin cancers are easily the most common form of cancer in the world. They are more common than all the other cancers combined. On average, skin cancer will occur in two out of every three white-skinned individuals as they get older, most commonly as they reach advanced age.

Most skin cancers are caused by too much time under the sun. In fact, they almost always occur in areas of our skin chronically exposed to the sun (e.g. our face, ears, neck, shins and the back of our hands). The most important cancer-causing element in sunlight is excessive UV radiation. This is why preventing excessive exposure to UV-A and UV-B is the most important way to prevent skin cancer as well as sunburn.

However, excessive exposure to sunlight is only part of the story. Our skin has natural defences against sunlight. The most important of these is the brown skin pigment, melanin. Melanin absorbs and dissipates damaging ultraviolet energy. In essence, melanin is designed to take the bullet, so that other parts of the skin are spared.

People with fair skin, especially those with hazel or blue eyes, (natural) blondes and redheads have less melanin in their skin. This means that for the same sun exposure, much more UV radiation enters their skin than in those people with dark skin. So skin cancers are at least twice as common in people with fair skin as in those with dark skin enriched and protected with melanin.

A healthy tan

 Tanning is a defence mechanism used by our skin to protect against damage from ultraviolet radiation. Any excessive exposure to sunlight increases the production of (brown) melanin in our skin, so our skin looks more tanned in colour as a result. The increase of melanin production keeps going for a few weeks after a burst of sunshine, so our tan keeps developing for a while after exposure to the sun.

Tanning is not a perfect solution. In fact it is no more protective for our skin than using an SPF-4 sunblock. Getting a tan does not obviate the need to protect ourselves from sun damage. If anything, tanning is a warning sign that we are getting too much sun and need much more protection.

In times past, having a tan was unfashionable, symbolic of those (lower class) people who had to do rough, outdoor manual labour. By contrast, fair skin represented the wealthy who could afford to either stay indoors or wear bonnets and carry umbrellas to retain their pale complexion.

Tanning probably only caught on by accident, when in 1929 the French fashionista Coco Chanel saw too much sun on her vacation. On her return to Paris, she shrugged nonchalantly and proclaimed, 'a girl simply has to be tanned'. And so tanning was given legs.

Most deaths from skin cancer are due to melanoma, in which the specialized skin cells that provide pigment to the skin (melanocyte) become seriously derailed and start to grow autonomously. To become a dangerous melanoma, melanocytes must go through a number of changes, beginning with the formation of a mole. Moles are unsightly but limited growths on the skin that remain largely the same for decades.

However, sometimes a mole can throw off the shackles and become a (melanoma) cancer. This is why watching out for moles or unusual freckles that have changed in shape, size or colour (e.g. dark brown to black, blue-black or red) is an important way to identify those spots in which growth is no longer restricted and a cancer may be forming. The earlier a cancer is identified and treated, the better the chance of avoiding surgery, disfigurement and/or death.

What is still not understood is why, if it is our faces that get most regular sun exposure, do melanomas mostly occur on the body, especially on the torso and legs. One theory is that it's intense intermittent sunlight exposure on naturally pale spots (like the torso and legs), leading to sunburn, that is the real villain.

Certainly people who have experienced sunburn during their childhood or adolescence have a higher risk of developing melanoma than those who never got burnt. Yet even adults who get burnt by the sun also carry an increased risk. Despite this fact, we are often careless and get needlessly sunburnt at least once every summer.

Weathering

Excess sunlight is also responsible for almost all visible changes in skin's appearance that occur as we get older. This may be easily appreciated when looking at the sun-exposed skin on our neckline and comparing it to adjacent areas of non-exposed skin on the chest. Sun-damaged skin is distinguished by wrinkles and crinkles, irregular pigmentation and a thick leathery appearance, like the peel of an orange. This is quite different to the other skin (for example, over the breast) that has been protected from the sun, which although it is exactly the same age, is usually smooth, unblemished and relatively thin by comparison.

When we despair about wrinkles and lines, rough skin and unwanted pigmentation in our advancing years, we need not look further than our time in the sun for their foundation. Four out of every five wrinkles and most of the unwanted freckles on our faces are due to our sun exposure.

Wrinkles and crinkles

 Wrinkles happen in very specific places, because of the way the skin has been folded and creased repeatedly, year after year. Although ageing affects all areas of our skin, it is most pronounced in our face. This is partly because of its unrestricted exposure to sunlight, but also because the muscles in our face are the most active in the whole of our body, repeatedly stretching and folding our skin.

We are told that we shouldn't squint or make faces, in case this expression gets stuck on our face. However, it may well be that years of mirth and laughter have given us laugh lines or years of worry have given us frown lines. Our faces reflect how we repeatedly use them, so wrinkles are therefore as unique as the face that wears them.

Because expression lines occur when our face is expressing something, they mostly disappear when the muscles are at rest, like when we are asleep. This is one reason Sleeping Beauty looked so beautiful. However, the same effect can now be achieved with Botox injections, which essentially put the facial muscles into a coma and so achieve the same beauty that we possess when we are fast asleep.

We get wrinkles because the skin that is repeatedly folded eventually refuses to bounce back. For example, if we screw up a piece of paper and then try to flatten it out again, it is almost impossible to iron out the creases because the paper is inelastic. If you screw up a rubber swimming cap in the bottom of the bag, it looks just the same when you take it out again — because rubber is elastic.

Our skin get less rubbery, and more papery, as we get older. This is partly because all elements of sunlight (UV, infrared and visible light) progressively damage the organized elastic elements deep in our skin. Although this sets off a healing response, the healing is never perfect (and increasingly less perfect as we age). Every day in the sun leaves in its wake just a little bit more disorganization and a little less elasticity, ultimately becoming visible to the naked eye as wrinkles, drooping and other changes of ageing.

As we get older, it's also common for dark blotchy changes to appear in areas of our skin that have been consistently exposed to sunlight, such as our face, shoulders, hands and arms. These are known as **sunspots,** or sometimes **age spots.** Sunspots may affect any skin type but are a particular problem for Asian women. This is why so many carry an umbrella on a sunny day and habitually avoid the sun. Their greatest fear is getting darker or blotchy skin.

Although they look like freckles and are triggered by sunlight, age spots are very different. With more sun, we get more and darker freckles as (melanocytes) pigment cells in our skin make more (melanin) pigment in response to sunlight. But when we stay out of the sun, our freckles will go away, like our tan. This doesn't happen with age spots.

As we age, the number of pigment cells in our skin slowly declines (by about 10 to 20 per cent every decade). But this process can be patchy. Some areas do better than others, leaving islands of pigment cells desperately trying to make up for the losses elsewhere. This leads to some areas looking darker than the surrounding skin, and the appearance of blotchy old skin or sunspots.

Sun block

There are many practical things we can do to prevent our skin getting exposed to too much sun without staying indoors all the time. The most obvious one is to use a sunscreen.

A sunscreen with a Sun Protection Factor (or SPF) of 15 filters out approximately 93 per cent of all incoming UV-B. An SPF 30 keeps out 97 per cent and SPF 50 keeps out 98 percent of the UV-B. By contrast, standard make-up provides an SPF of about 4, approximately the equivalent of sitting in the shade or under an umbrella and blocking out maybe half of the UV-B radiation.

SPF refers only to its actions against UV-B and a high SPF does not equal protection from UV-A and infrared rays. So many sun-blocking products now tout themselves as having broad spectrum coverage, or at the very least care enough about UV-A to put data about it on their label. To block visible light, sunscreens have to be opaque.

The key limitation of sunscreen is that it only works if we remember to put it on before we go into the sun for extended periods. Moreover, if we put it on, most people use less than half the amount that was used to determine the SPF, so the real SPF that we are getting is probably only a quarter or half that listed on the label.

To get the full effect we can try to remember to apply the appropriate (larger) amounts. However, a simple trick is to reapply the sunblock again 15 to 30 minutes after the first application. This means we get the full effect and are less likely to accidentally miss any areas.

The first sunscreen

 The dangers of excessive sunlight on skin are flamingly apparent for anyone who has got sunburnt. The obvious solution of hats and lots of clothing are stifling in hot places, like Australia. And what if you wanted to throw off your clothes or go down to the beach?

The solution came to Milton Blake, an Adelaide chemist, after reading a German technical trade publication that described a chemical that possessed the property of absorbing the burning ultraviolet rays of the sun. From his home laboratory, he synthesized and refined the product that became the world's first sunscreen.

He was not the first to think of sunscreens. Fifty years earlier, Austrian scientist Otto Veiel had used tannin to protect skin from ultraviolet rays. But tannins, like those found in coffee and tea, badly stain the things they come in contact with. We would end up looking tanned anyway and so would our clothes.

Physical barriers like a wide-brimmed hat, sunglasses and tightly woven or specifically designed UV-protective clothing also work well. A good wide-brimmed hat (with a brim over 7 centimetres or 3 inches) will provide the equivalent of sun protection factor 7 for the nose, 3 for the cheeks, 5 for the neck, and 2 for the chin. By comparison, a narrow-brimmed (bucket) hat will give us a 2 for the nose at best, and not much elsewhere. Not quite the equivalent of a 30+ sunscreen, but every little bit helps.

A great pair of sunglasses can make the hat look even better. But, more importantly, sunglasses protect the sensitive skin around our eyes that can be hard to reach without sticking suncream painfully into our eyes. This is also the one area that most people hate getting wrinkles (known as crow's feet) because everyone looks at their eyes. The best protection from UV is achieved by sunglasses with a wraparound style or side shields. If light gets around the sides then it wrinkles our skin.

All types of fabrics can disrupt solar radiation to a certain extent. A typical cotton shirt provides an Ultraviolet Protection Factor (UPF) of about 10 (analogous to the SPF used to rate sunscreens). Tightly woven fibres, thick fabrics, wool and polyester materials let the least amount of UV through. Dark-coloured fabrics also have greater UPF than light-coloured fabrics. But no one is going to wear dark wool on a scorching summer day. Fortunately, it is now possible to buy clothing with a high UPF (15 to 50) that still feels light and comfortable for summer. This is particularly important when we are swimming, as getting normal fabric wet halves its UPF.

Many people are concerned that the regular use of sunscreens, hats and clothing will mean that our protected skin loses the UV-B it requires to make vitamin D. While this is perfectly true for very short-term sun exposure, the point of sunscreen is to allow us outside in the sun for longer where we usually expose far more skin. Even the most conscientious of beachgoers makes more than enough vitamin D to get them through their weekday inside the office. Only those who always stay indoors out of the sun seem to be at risk of vitamin D deficiency.

Icarus

 King Minos was an island-nation despot who persecuted and punished his subjects for their misdemeanours. He even fed them to his pet Minotaur. Icarus and his father, Daedalus, were political criminals trying to flee from this tyrannical regime. Initially, they had helped Minos trap the Minotaur in an inescapable labyrinth, but now they were a liability. In fact, they had leaked the plans of the labyrinth to the rebellion, and now the Minotaur was dead. It seemed that their days, too, were numbered.

From the dark tower in which they were imprisoned, Daedalus hatched a daring plan of escape. He and his son would fly out into the sunlight on wings constructed from feathers and leaves that had been blown in by the wind. These would be bound together with wax from spare candles.

The plan was not without its risks. Fly too low and the feathers would become heavy, cold and damp in the sea fog. Fly too high and the sun's heat would melt away the wax. Taking the middle road, exposing himself to neither too much sun nor too little, Daedalus flew to his freedom.

Of course the exuberance of flight was too much for Icarus, who soared upwards and melted his wings, before crashing down and drowning in the cold dark sea.

In the end, Minos got his just desserts. Daedalus saw him boiled to death in his own bath, killed by both heat and water simultaneously. For Daedalus, revenge had no middle ground. No chance of escape for Minos.

The bottom line

Sunshine is our favourite means of escape. Released from our lives spent trapped in office towers, spending time outside on a sunny day can seem like freedom from bondage. Like Clark Kent, we throw off our myopia, our weakness, our moodiness and our clothes and thrive in the glow of a yellow sun, using its power and storing its vitality to get us through dark times to come.

But it is a narrow road of escape. Often we so relish our freedom that we ignore the warning signs and get burnt, wrinkled or blinded. At least a third of all adults get sunburnt every year. In those under thirty, it is more like half. It is not because we are stupid, ignorant or drunk. But, like Icarus finding his wings, sunshine is intoxicating. So once again, moderation is the obvious and only solution.

Do I really have to ...

#14

Not catch cold?

Q: *Can I catch a cold by getting cold?*
A: **Only if you come back indoors.**

Q: *Why is there no cure for the common cold?*
A: **Because our symptoms are how we fight it.**

Q: *What do you get when you kiss a guy?*
A: **You get enough germs to catch pneumonia.**

Q: *Can I catch a cold on a plane?*
A: **Only if someone with a cold sits near you**

Q: *Should I use a tissue or a handkerchief?*
A: **Yes.**

Q: *What about a hot toddy?*
A: **Cheers.**

Q: *Will taking supplements help my cold?*
A: **A little at best.**

It is often said that good health is not the same thing as not being sick. But every time our nose is blocked, our throat is sore and we're feeling miserable, the mere absence of any illness seems just as a vital. Rain, rain, go away!

The one illness that will influence our lives and health, more than any other, is not cancer or diabetes. It is the **common cold**.

It spares no one. It is more contagious than the plague and there is no vaccine. And although innocuous and mercifully self-limiting, more lost work days, missed parties and general misery can be pinned on the common cold than on most other diseases combined.

Of course this is chiefly because the common cold is so very common. On average, we will get three to five colds a year. Our children will usually experience at least twice as many more. Each cold will last about a week to ten days, although it will probably only be bad for two or three days at most. Yet, multiplied by eighty-plus years, the all-too-common cold will take nearly eight years of our hard-won life and productivity, and turn it into sniffles, snuffles and rubbish bins of crumpled tissues. And then, of course, there are all those days at home looking after the kids.

This book is supposed to be all about the practical things we can do to extend our life. It turns out that one of the most practical things we can do is to not catch (a) cold, just like our mother said!

Sharing germs

Colds are caused by viruses that infect our nose, sinuses and throat. Viruses are very different to bacteria, as different as ants are to antelopes. Sure they are both microscopic germs and both can cause infections. But any similarity stops there. So antibiotics (which just kill certain bacteria) don't work on viruses or on colds.

There is not just one special (common cold) virus that causes a cold. In fact, the same all-to-familiar illness we call a cold can be individually caused by hundreds of different viruses, with few or no common elements. Furthermore, the viruses that cause a cold also frequently undergo mutation to change their chemical composition and alter the ability of our immune system to recognize them. Taken together, this is why we can't easily vaccinate against a cold like we can against measles, which is just one virus that has changed only very little over the last thousand years. It is also why year after year we can get cold after cold, even though we may have only just recovered from the last one.

To get into our nose and throat, viruses must travel from someone else's nose or throat. Unlike ants, viruses don't have legs and can't move on their own. Traditionally, it has been thought that sneezing or coughing sprays tiny droplets of virus-rich mucus secretions (yuk) into the air, much like an aerosol from a spray can. These droplets are then inhaled by their next victim, or land on something another victim will later touch and bring to their nose, eyes or lips. As the happy jingle reminds us, 'coughs and sneezes spread diseases'. So we feel a little queasy when someone is coughing next to us on the bus and can fully understand why some people wander around with surgical masks on.

However, most colds don't just blow in on the breeze. More commonly, our runny nose ends up on our hands as we wipe or touch our nose, or cough or sneeze into them. The germy passengers are then transferred to the things we touch, until someone else inadvertently touches the same spot with their hands and then brings them to rub their eyes, touch their mouth or pick their nose. And hey presto, there goes another cold.

Viruses can survive about a day on a hard surface (like a door handle) and a few hours on a soft one (like a hanky). Should someone touch one of these contaminated hotspots and then bring the virus into their nose, on average about two days later, a third of people will have a cold. However, in a household, a school or a workplace we often share many hotspots, meaning that most colds run through them like a hot knife through butter.

Boy germs

 Kissing is great fun. Our lips are extraordinarily sensitive to touch. And the high we experience from using them is unparalleled by any drug. Kissing is also an important part of bonding and intimacy, the merits of which are discussed in the final chapter of this book.

But there is a catch. When kissing, couples not only exchange saliva but hundreds of millions of bacteria as well. Girls get boy germs and boys get girl germs.

Almost all of the bugs naturally found in the human mouth do no harm whatsoever. However, many of the viruses that cause colds and throat infections can be readily transmitted through kissing an infected partner, whether or not they are experiencing any symptoms.

Why humans are the only species to kiss and exchange saliva in this way is unclear. If it was only stimulation there are many other better places to touch to excite a response. One theory has it that it is best for a girl to exchange saliva with any prospective mate early in the relationship, and get infected with anything he might give her as soon as possible, while she is still strong and can handle it. Glandular fever, EBV, CMV, let's get them over with. Later on, if you become pregnant, is not the time to become infected because it risks (infecting) the baby. So kissing and exchanging germs should usually come first, before the sex.

Symptomatic

While colds are caused by viruses, the unpleasant symptoms that come with them — blocked and runny nose, cough, sneezing, sore throat, headache, etc. — are largely triggered by our body's reaction to them, rather than any damage caused by these voracious bugs.

For example, the watery, runny nose (which is often accompanied by sneezing) is caused by an increase in secretions from glands in our nose trying to clear the virus away. There can also be seepage of serum (the yellow cell-free part of blood) into our nose. White blood cells, which are part of our body's defence system, also find their way in. These cells release a green protein (myeloperoxidase) that causes the gunk coming out our nose to turn yellow/green. This change in colour is not caused by bacteria and should not be taken to mean we need to take antibiotics. It just means that our white cells have been called into action.

The blocked nose we experience with a cold comes about as the large veins in our nose dilate, squashing the space available for air to flow, especially in the early and middle phases of our cold. Our nose is literally blocked. This is why blowing our nose never seems to give the relief we expect, despite all the effort and all the stuff that ends up in our tissue or hanky. Only during the final phases of a cold, as the volume of secretions increases and their clearance is diminished, will a good blow do the trick.

Curiously, one nostril is usually more blocked than the other at any one time during a cold. And it's not always the same one! In fact, which nasal passage is most blocked usually alternates from one to the other over a period of several hours. This so-called 'nasal cycle' is thought to be a defensive response, possibly to keep one nostril open to breathe while the other one is being pumped full of protective fluids.

Even one nostril at a time, a blocked nose changes how our voice sounds when we have a cold. Some speech sounds use airflow through the nose and sinuses (such as the letters 'm' and 'n'). Other sounds use only our mouth (such as 'ss', 'p', 'b' and 'k'). So our cold makes only some words and some letters sound funny (or nasal, as it is often described). Show ne the unny!

A blocked nose also makes it more difficult to breathe through our nose, so we have to breathe more often through our mouth instead. This further contributes to our dry, sore throat. It also makes our breathing noisy, keeping us and our partner awake through the night.

The severity and type of cold symptoms varies among individuals and with different viruses. Not every infection will result in symptoms. Sometimes we will feel just fine while others in our family are hit hard.

When given the same dose of the same cold virus, men and women come down with a cold as often as each other. However, women are generally more likely to be exposed and catch a cold because of greater contact with contagious children (who get twice as many colds as adults do).

The symptoms of a cold are also objectively the same in men and women. There is no such thing as a 'man-cold'. However, men and women perceive symptoms differently, so from a male perspective a cold can seem a bigger issue. It's not that men are wusses. But they actually are.

Catch (a) cold

These days, we use phrases such as 'having a virus' to describe our sniffles because we have a fair idea of their origins. For exactly the same reason, the term 'common cold' has been widely used since at least the 16th century. Most people really thought that the cold temperature really did have something to do with it. For example, in traditional Chinese medicine, a cold is caused by inhaling the cold wind (a *yin qi*). It's still widely imagined that we can actually breathe in the cold, to literally catch it, so that even when we come back indoors the 'cold' stays with us.

If we think about it carefully, many of the symptoms are very similar. If we go out on a cold and frosty morning and inhale deeply through our nostrils, we do get a tingle in our nose. We may even sneeze. Take a deep breath of cold air in through our mouth and our throat feels dry and rough. Sometimes, it will even trigger a cough. If we stay out for too long in the cold, we may start shivering, our hands will be cold to touch and our fingers turn white. So *a* cold is just like *being in the* cold.

As our immune system begins its fight against the cold virus, it resets the brain's control of body temperature. So instead of running at close to normal body temperature, the immune system releases temperature-increasing chemicals (called pyrogens), which turn up the heat and establish a new slightly hotter temperature at which the body should run. This is usually experienced as feeling chilly or cold because, from the brain's point of view, we are colder than it wants us to be. So it makes us shiver and breathe faster, and shuts down our peripheries to warm us up in exactly the same way it does when trying to cope with cold weather.

A number of theories have been put forward to explain how cold weather could actually influence our susceptibility to viral attack. Some studies have suggested that short-term exposure to cold weather or getting chilled alters the immune system of the nose's defences. Some viruses can also be killed by ultraviolet light, which is in shorter supply on cold wet winter days than clear summer ones. However, neither of these stacks up to rigorous investigation.

Cold facts

 Because of the enormous human and economic costs of the common cold, many studies have tried to get to the bottom of it. The most famous of all were performed at the Common Cold Research Unit (CCRU) in Salisbury, England, that operated between 1946 and 1989.

Over this time, more than 20,000 healthy volunteers were paid to come in for ten days, to be infected in different ways, with different viruses and in different settings, and then closely observed to see whether they eventually caught a cold.

For example, in one experiment, subjects were drenched with water and left out in the cold before receiving a dose of infected mucus.

Although much was learnt about the illness, being wet and cold appeared to have little to do with it.

Advertisements for volunteers presented a stay at the CCRU as an unusual vacation opportunity. And in austere post-war Britain, it became oddly popular as a kind of paid package holiday, doing your civic duty, getting away from it all, with room and free meals thrown in. Many students also found it a quiet place to study while being paid.

But just because we can't literally catch 'the cold' doesn't mean we shouldn't wear our winter woollies. Perhaps the most important reason to dress warmly on a cold day is simply because it allows us to venture outside and be active for longer and not have to come back inside where our friends and family can share their infectious mucus droplets with us. Most viruses are transferred and amplified in heated indoor areas and the risks of catching cold are greatest in colder months when we share confined indoor spaces. Equally, colds are less common in summer, when we spend more time outside. So indirectly, your mother's advice to put on a coat or a scarf when going outside did reduce the risk of us catching (a) cold.

Stressed and tired

Stress is known to be a risk factor for infectious diseases, including the common cold. The more stress we are under, physical or psychological, real or perceived, the greater our susceptibility to them.

Why stress impacts on the frequency or severity of our colds is complex. It is partly that unhappy, stressed people don't get out much, preferring to stay sedentary and indoors where rates of virus transmission are enhanced. People who deal with stress more effectively in their lives also cope better with the stress of having a cold, because they already have the tools. Equally, those prone to or under stress find colds more demanding.

However, there is also some biology involved. For example, it is known that stress has significant negative effects on the immune system and its ability to fight off infections. How this happens is discussed in detail in Chapter 16.

Bugs on a plane

 People often complain about catching a cold after travelling on a plane, especially on long-distance flights. However, these symptoms are mostly due to reactive changes following prolonged exposure to a low-humidity and low-pressure environment, rather than any virus.

Viruses can be transmitted during a flight when someone is coughing or sneezing in the seat next to us or within a few rows in front or behind. But no further.

The ventilation system on modern planes is very efficient. Air only moves from overhead to under the floor. Before any air is recirculated, it also passes through high efficiency filters, which effectively remove any particles and bugs potentially contained within them. Taken together this means that the spread of any airborne particles along the cabin of the plane is highly unlikely. If we do catch a cold it is more likely we got it in the terminal, after our hands came in contact with something sticky.

Other enclosed public spaces, such as trains, buses, trams or cars do not have such efficient modular ventilation. These have not received the same attention as planes but as we use them much more, they are probably more significant sources of airborne bugs.

Night-time sleep is another important contributor to daytime health. And after a night of broken sleep it's easy to understand why. We just don't look or feel the same in the morning. Lack of sleep is also associated with an increased risk of catching a cold, probably because sleep quality and quantity also influences immune function and resistance to infection.

To prove this, the CCRU documented the sleep habits of a group of people over a period of two weeks and then gave them a dose of cold virus. If they were getting less than seven hours of sleep a night, or if their sleep was of poor quality (which was measured), getting a cold from the virus was much more likely.

Wash your hands!

Sending our kids off to wash their hands is probably the simplest thing we can do to protect their health. It is also one of the most valuable. When performed frequently and efficiently it really does reduce the risk of getting or spreading many important infectious diseases, including the common cold.

The principle of hand washing is simple. Disease-causing germs get onto our hands from the things we touch. They subsequently transfer to our mouth, nose or eyes and can sometimes lead to infection, depending on the type of organism, the dose, our individual susceptibility and where we stick our sticky fingers. About 40 per cent of people with a cold will have the virus that caused it detectable on their hands at any one time. This can then easily transfer onto other surfaces or other things that we touch.

Although we might wash our hands until they are free of dirt and they look clean enough, water alone is not particularly effective in getting rid of any of the viruses that cause the common cold. We really do need to use soap. Most germs are embedded in the surface layer of the skin, formed by acidic fats, oils and other debris. To effectively dislodge them means alkalinizing and/or dissolving this layer, then mechanically rubbing them off.

Water is still important, but only because it helps the soap get onto our hands and then off again. Water is essential to liquefy a hard soap bar. Most liquid soaps also need a small amount of water to help them spread across the surfaces of our hands, where massaging, rubbing and friction is used to create a lather of tiny soap bubbles that allow otherwise insoluble grease, fats and oils to disperse into the water. It is not clear whether lathering itself is required to dislodge the germs from our hands, but it is an excellent marker for having done the hard work required to dislodge them.

The other reason for turning on the tap is that the soap/detergent (in which many germs are now suspended) needs to be fully rinsed away from the skin surface. This is best accomplished by putting our hands under a reasonable flow of running water, followed by efficient drying.

In hot water

 Whether we use the hot or cold tap to wash our hands has nothing to do with how well it works in getting rid of germs. It's not as if the average hot-tap temperature will kill disease-causing germs. After all, they happily grow at body temperature!

Placing our warm body parts under warm water is certainly more comfortable than running them under the cold tap. Just try taking a cold shower! So because it's a bit more comfortable (and we are, after all, largely creatures of comfort), people who wash their hands spend slightly more time rinsing under a warm tap than a really hot or really cold one. However, the time spent rubbing and scrubbing with soap, away from the water, is far more important for germs on our hands than the time spent running them under the tap.

Hot water has its downsides too. There's the power/gas bill. If we're not paying for solar, there is the carbon footprint. There's also the risk of scalds and burns. Water temperature can also affect how irritating the soap is to our skin. So, unless you are trying to warm up your hands on a cold day, the hot tap is a waste of water, and a cold rinse would do the job just fine.

Antimicrobial soaps or gels are not generally required and don't do a better job than old-fashioned soap when it comes to dislodging cold viruses. However, for other infectious illnesses (like diarrhoea) and in special situations like hospitals or in people with reduced immunity, these special soaps can have a useful role.

Antibacterial wipes can be handy if we're out and about and don't have access to soap to wash our hands. However, evidence for the success of alcohol-based hand sanitizers is modest at best. And while they certainly work for some infections (especially vomiting and diarrhoea), trials have not shown that using alcohol wipes alone can stop us from catching a cold.

Use a tissue or hanky?

The contagious virus that causes a cold is contained in those yucky secretions coming out of our nose. What we do with those secretions is a large determinant of whether other people will catch it too. Obviously, wiping them away with our hand is unhygienic. Even using the back of our hand that we don't use that often for touching doesn't work. This is because we seldom wash it effectively and frequently touch it with the font of the other hand.

Most modern mothers would just tell us to use a tissue if our nose is running. Disposable (*washi*) tissues have been used in Japan for hundreds of years. However, they were only introduced to Western culture in the 20th century, ostensibly as an easy means for women to remove facial cream. They soon caught on as a simple alternative to a handkerchief for blowing noses. Indeed, the chief marketing strategy was to denounce the humble handkerchief with the slogan 'Don't Carry a Cold in Your Pocket'. So today, hankies are widely considered to be decorative, unhygienic and old fashioned.

Hankies were popularized by King Richard II of England, who was possibly sick of wiping his royal nose on his robes. He was, after all, only ten years old when he came to the throne. Hankies have been found in and around places for almost as long as people have been weaving fabric. However, handkerchiefs became so popular in young King Richard's time that they were given away as a keepsake or token sign of favour by chivalrous knights, or displayed proudly in a pocket as a sign of ostentation. Today, there are few microbially conscious people who would want to see someone else's hanky, let alone willingly accept one belonging to someone else. When Othello found his wife with another man's handkerchief, well, he just knew Desdemona was sharing his germs!

The mother of inventions

 Necessity is often the mother of invention. So in desperate times we must use what's at hand. And not just to wipe our nose.

In 1913, New York socialite Mary Phelps Jacob was ready to go out on the town. She had recently purchased a sheer evening gown for one of her gala events. The standard undergarment to go with it should have been a corset, made out of whalebones. But the bones just didn't work under the sheer fabric and stuck up unfashionably from her plunging neckline. The obvious solution was to ditch the corset. But she also couldn't go around with everything showing through from under her sheer dress.

So Mary experimented. And ingeniously she discovered that tying two silk handkerchiefs with some pink ribbon could effectively do the job of the unsightly corset. And so the modern bra was born!

But while hankies are literally and figuratively green, the environmental credentials of disposable tissues are also problematic. The environmentally conscious would argue that the millions of trees pulped to make our tissues, and their subsequent removal into landfill, is a complete waste. Unlike most other paper products, tissues don't get recycled. Disposable tissues are (supposed to be) for single use only. By not carrying a cold in our pocket, we are happy to discard it far and wide into waste receptacles.

But it doesn't always pan out this way. We blow our nose in a tissue. If we are nearby a bin, it's easy to discard it. But if we're not near one there's a problem. We can't just drop it. Littering is socially and environmentally irresponsible! So it goes back into our purse or our pocket, where it dries out, and becomes partly usable again (how frugal!).

But which one is ours and which one belongs to our child? Do we remember to keep them in different pockets? Often they never leave until they are completely saturated and start to fall apart. Sometimes they only reappear in the washing machine, by which time all our clothes have a light dusting of tissue flakes. In this light, good old hankies don't really look so bad.

Cover our mouth and nose!

As discussed above, some viruses can become airborne when we cough or sneeze. One simple way to reduce the chance of these bugs spreading to others is to cover our mouth when coughing or our nose when sneezing. So if we feel the urge coming on and are about to cough or sneeze, what do we do? If we happen to have a clean disposable tissue close to hand, the best thing is to grab it, catch the sneeze and then throw it away.

However, sneezes and coughs are a reflex. They can come on so fast that there is little or no time to go searching for tissues. Usually by the time we find one, we have already sneezed all over everyone else.

If no tissues are to hand the best thing to do is use our sleeve to catch a sneeze or the crook of our elbow to cough into. It is not an ideal solution, obviously, but it is better than sneezing or coughing into our hands and then unwittingly transferring the germs to door handles or taps or other surfaces. As we don't tend to rub our sleeves on too many things or on other people, it is a back-up solution. It is still advisable to throw the item of clothing into the wash at the end of the day.

While a few bugs can get caught on a breeze when we cough or sneeze, most droplets that are shot out go in the direction that we are facing. So if we turn away from others when coughing or sneezing, the chance of delivering an infectious dose can also be reduced when they are not in the firing line.

God bless you

 Sneezing has always been regarded as ominous. This was especially apparent during the plagues that swept through medieval Europe. So much so that Pope Gregory VII decreed that a short prayer should be said after every sneeze to protect against catching the sickness. Gesundheit! May God bless you (because you are going to need his help if you have the plague and so will I if you have just sneezed on me!).

In Greek legend, sneezing was regarded as a portent, a message from the gods. If any business enterprise was to be undertaken, a sneeze was considered a good sign, especially if it occurred after positive words about the enterprise were said. Multiple sneezes were believed to be the gods applauding.

Once, as the great Athenian general Xenophon urged his famous troops to battle, a soldier is said to have sneezed. Taking this as a sign that the gods had blessed their battle plans, he immediately ordered their tents and carriages to be burnt and set off to war. There was no going back. Once started, a sneeze can't be stopped! Unfortunately very few of the Ten Thousand ever made it home. This disastrous event is generally regarded as the worst-timed sneeze ever.

We often see people at heavily populated places, such as airports, wearing surgical face masks in the belief that these will stop viruses reaching them and their noses. There is no evidence that these provide any benefit in terms of cold symptoms or getting colds — particularly as most of the viruses we pick up literally come from the things we touch. So Mum's old health advice not to put your finger up your nose wasn't just for the sake of good manners. Mum was right, again! A finger up the nose is one simple way for bugs to get out and bugs to get in.

Wearing a pair of gloves at an airport would seem a better solution. But unless we are well-trained surgeons it can be hard to stop ourselves from spontaneously touching our face, even with gloves on. Which, as it turns out, is probably the only reason why the face mask might work a little bit: to stop us from touching our own mouth and nose.

Feed a cold?

We're always told to feed a cold. But when we have one, we generally don't feel like eating much of anything. This is the result of the chemicals released by our body to fight off the infection also affecting the appetite centres in our brain. These same chemicals also make us feel irritable, lethargic or just plain miserable when we have a cold. Not wanting to eat may be a natural defence mechanism to help fight off infection, just like a fever. But why should our brain want to supress our hunger if we have a cold? One reason may be that if we are feeling sick, why would we want to waste precious energy trying to find food that we could otherwise use in getting well? Of course this theory doesn't hold if Mum has just made chicken soup. But our modern brain still works much like a caveman's did. Hunker down and when you're feeling better go out to hunt or gather something?

So if our brain is telling us not to eat, how come there is the well-known phrase 'feed a cold, (but) starve a fever'? It turns out that it all began with an old English phrase that says, '*Fede a cold starb o'feber*'. It looks pretty similar, but fede means '*stoke*' (as in a fire) and *starb* means to 'die'. So it actually translates as 'if you stoke a cold you may die of fever'. In fact, if you force-feed mice during a serious infection they are actually more likely to die than if they eat only what they feel like.

But while some starving (in the short term) can keep a feverish mouse alive, whether we eat or not has little relevance to our innocuous cold. In fact, most times grown-ups get a cold they don't even get a temperature. Adults generally save fevers for bugs we've never seen before or severe viral infections, like influenza. So if there is no fever or headache, and we have a runny nose, we probably just have a common cold.

In the end, most colds are mercifully short lived and will peter out after a week or so. Whether or not we are feeding a cold or starving it probably makes little difference to the biology of our cold. But feeling healthy is much more than biology. Food is a comfort not a cure. Please, pass the soup.

Chicken soup for the cold?

Of all the homemade cure-alls, chicken soup is the best known and most loved. The term 'chicken soup' has become idiomatic for all things restorative, benefitting every possible problem from the head to the soul.

In many different cultures, chicken soup is a traditional treatment for symptoms of the common cold. Chicken soup is widely known as 'Jewish penicillin'. Some of this may reflect the traditional use of chicken soup as a Sabbath meal and, by implication, the perceived importance of piety with respect to health outcomes. Nonetheless, it's a staple among Jewish grandmothers worldwide, and especially their grandchildren.

Even before the Olympics, Greek grandmothers may also claim they invented chicken soup for the common cold. Avgolemono (Αυγολέμονο) is a thick egg and lemon chicken broth widely administered for the symptoms of cold and flu, or for their prevention on wet winter evenings. Although a quintessentially Greek dish, it is likely that its therapeutic use has its earliest origin in Sephardic tradition. Adding the 'all important' lemon may have been the Greek contribution.

Not to be outdone, most Chinese grandmothers are ready and primed to produce chicken soup at the first sign of a sniffle. In traditional Chinese medicine, illness is perceived as a state of imbalance between yin and yang. Yin represents the darker, cooling forces, while yang embodies the lighter, warmer forces. In this paradigm, the treatment for cold is obviously hot, and eating chicken soup is a prime example of restoring the yang forces and balancing the cold of yin.

But what could there be in chicken soup that is so miraculous? Certainly, the steam from any hot drink may be able to dissolve nasal mucus to open blocked noses and sinuses, providing relief for a few minutes at least. In this respect, sipping hot chicken soup is really no better than a hot bath or shower.

Beyond the steam, there is no chemical or biological reason for having chicken soup when we are sick with a cold. However, the psychology can't be overlooked. Chicken soup is a comfort food on a day when we would really like some comfort. With the expectation of efficacy, the succour of being cared for, the taste of home on an otherwise dull day, there's a good reason for a bowl of chicken soup for the soul.

Need a hot toddy?

When we get a cold and start looking miserable, someone will probably say at our low ebb that we need a '**hot toddy**' (or tottie). In fact, this myth has become so popular that the term toddy has now become a ready euphemism for 'tonic' or 'pick-me-up'.

A hot toddy is the name given to a hot drink that contains alcoholic spirits, water, citrus, something sweet and something spicy. Everyone has their own favourite recipe. Most people use whiskey or brandy as the spirit. The sweet component is usually made up of liberal amounts of sugar or honey. The preferred spice in our toddy varies widely with the recipe, but usually includes the Christmassy ones like cinnamon, cloves, ginger, cardamom and/or nutmeg.

In Latin, totie (*totus*) means something that was 'brought all together, fused or amalgamated'. For example, Pope John-Paul II's motto was '*totus tuus*' (meaning all together with you). The euphemistic name 'tottie' perhaps refers to the way its spices are infused into the alcohol, slowly bringing the otherwise incompatible ingredients and flavours together over a low heat. It is customary not to boil the mix (probably as this reduces its alcoholic content as well as overly concentrates the taste as water evaporates).

The hot toddy is very different from the beverage made across Asia from the sap of palm trees (which is also variously known as toddy, kallu or palm wine). However, it is sometimes suggested that this is where the hot toddy may have appropriated its name from, as nostalgic travellers, returning from their adventures in Asia to a dour world devoid of palm trees, looked for a toddy on cold winter nights.

Improvisation

 Recognizing what we want, but not having the right ingredients to do it in exactly the same way as they do on TV, we sometimes have to make use of the resources we have to hand. This is sometimes known as bricolage or MacGyver-ing, after the famous TV character who often got out of a jam by using his ingenuity, available objects and a lot of duct tape.

Frugal innovation was the byword of the Calvinist ethic. You didn't have much to work with, so you often had to improvise.

The toddy recipe is remarkably similar to mulled wine (also variously known as hot wine, glögg, Glühwein, vin chaud), in which red wine or port (tawny) plays essentially the same role as the spirits in a toddy. Both are mixed with sugar and spices, and both are similarly used on chilly winter nights for the same revitalizing purposes. Toddies joined the drink cart only in the 16th and 17th century. But the tradition of mulled wine is millennia older, dating back to Ancient Rome.

It may be that on a bitterly cold night in Scotland, fondly remembering sipping mulled wine on the Continent was enough to push one McKenzie or MacGyver over the edge. There were no grapes in Scotland. Any red wine was reserved for the sacrament, imported and/or prohibitively expensive. So you had to improvise. And whiskey was to hand as an eager substitute. And so the hot toddy was born.

Another explanation for the name 'toddy' may be the spring called 'Tod's Well' which was the main water supply to Edinburgh, Scotland. Indeed, the murky peat-stained water on which the Scots subsisted probably looked much like the murky spice-laden concoction that they also called a toddy. A male fox is also called a 'tod'. Calling a new cocktail 'foxy' may be the Jacobean advertising equivalent of naming a new energy drink after a red bull.

The modern word 'whiskey' comes from of the Gaelic word 'uisce' meaning water. Whiskey was historically called *aqua vitae* (the water of life) and its medicinal properties widely recommended as a cure-all. But unfortunately, whiskey in those days was almost unpalatable (and still is for many people). Another toddy origins story suggests the 'toddy' was invented by doctors simply as a means to make medicinal whiskey agreeable to women and children (and women and children more agreeable).

Interestingly, the word 'toddy' seems to come into use in the English language about the same time (or maybe just moments before) as the word 'toddle', meaning an unsteady gait. This connection also gives rise to the colloquial term for young children as 'toddlers'.

Importantly there is absolutely nothing in a toddy that actually helps a cold. The citrus is a source of vitamin C, but we don't get enough in a toddy to do anything. Nutmeg, cloves and cinnamon have long been used to cure colds and contain chemicals with antihistamine, anaesthetic and/or anti-inflammatory properties (but again, not in the doses obtained in a hot toddy).

Actually, the only saving grace of the toddy is the alcohol, which has sedative and useful relaxant properties in low doses. It also makes us feel warm and cosy, as if wrapped in a blanket. For Alexander Fleming (who discovered penicillin) the remedy for the common cold was 'a good gulp of whiskey at bedtime', adding 'it's not very scientific, but it helps'.

Reach for the drugs?

The biology of the common cold is well understood. Drugs like paracetamol (acetaminophen) and non-steroidal anti-inflammatory drugs (NSAIDs) can reduce fever, sinus pain and headaches that often go along with a cold, but they don't ever make the cold go away. Decongestants like phenylephrine will unblock our noses a little. But rigorous studies with these agents have shown little or no improvement in overall symptoms. Antihistamines on their own also do little for colds.

Treatments combining all three modalities (e.g. acetaminophen, a decongestant and an antihistamine) work a little better than any of them alone (which work not much at all). Such combination therapies probably offer the best pharmaceutical means to temporarily relieve any incapacitating symptoms while the illness peters out of its own accord. However, more medication also means a greater risk of side effects, especially in young kids and the elderly.

Given the lack of success of regular medication, many people look to alternative therapies when they have a bad cold. One of the most popular is zinc.

An oyster a day

 It has long been known that low levels of zinc are associated with increased susceptibility to infection, including the common cold. This is possibly because the element zinc is used by the body for the function of key enzymes, including those that regulate inflammation and oxidative stress, both key processes in the battle against the common cold.

Few of us achieve the recommended daily intake of zinc from the food we eat. The best dietary sources of zinc are seafood (especially shellfish, crab, lobster). However, most of us get most of our zinc from beef and poultry. Some even argue that chicken soup is beneficial because it is naturally high in zinc, especially the bones and carcass that are used to make the broth.

Whole grains, legumes, seeds and nuts also contain plenty of zinc. However, fibre in plants may partially inhibit zinc absorption, so strict vegetarians need to take twice as much zinc every day to meet their quota.

Clinical trials in children have suggested that regular use of zinc lozenges during the cold season can reduce the number of colds they get, and whether they miss school as a result of them. Studies in adults have also suggested that zinc supplements can modestly reduce the duration and severity of cold symptoms, but only if taken within a day of their onset and in high doses every few hours.

The big problem is that most people really don't like the metallic taste of zinc. We could always try eating an oyster a day (a single oyster contains the recommended daily intake of zinc, around 100 mg). But then, not everyone likes oysters, either.

Vitamin C (also known as ascorbate or ascorbic acid) is also very popular for the common cold, both in its prevention and treatment. We commonly associate vitamin C with fruit (e.g. citrus, currants, strawberries and tomatoes) and some vegetables (e.g. kale, cabbage and broccoli). Ascorbate is also widely used as a food preservative, especially in processed juices. Unlike with zinc, most people would regularly meet their recommended daily intake of vitamin C. The regular use of super high doses of vitamin C can make colds slightly shorter in length (but not less severe) when compared to someone not on regular supplements. But it won't stop us getting the cold in the first place, and if we only take a vitamin C supplement during the cold it doesn't work at all.

Another popular treatment for a cold is **menthol**, a pungent chemical widely used in rubs, bath oils and lozenges. It is hard to think of a childhood cold without recalling its distinctive smell. Menthol is thought to work by deceiving our nose into thinking that we are breathing really cold air, which makes it feel less congested.

Menthol is also useful when used in conjunction with steam, such as from a hot bath, a hot drink or simply direct inhalation.

Recent scientific studies have found that the trillions of microbes that cohabit our body also have the capacity to influence our health in a number of ways, including effects on the immune system and resistance to infection. Many people now eat or drink 'beneficial' bacteria, known as probiotics, every day for their health. Interestingly, when we take them every day they do slightly reduce our chances of catching a cold. The most common probiotics are *lactobacilli* and *bifidobacterium* species found in yoghurt or other dairy products, but we can also get them as capsules.

Garlic (also known as allicin) supplements are also popular to ward off cold viruses, as well as vampires. High doses (we're talking the equivalent of over twenty cloves a day) do seem to reduce our chances of getting a cold. If we love garlic, we can knock ourselves out. But we'd smell like garlic. And if it doesn't smell, it probably doesn't contain the active ingredient.

Echinacea supplements are also widely used and have a pleasant flowery smell. They were first consumed by Native Americans as a medicinal. Again there is some data that taking very high doses can slightly reduce our chances of getting a cold and shorten its duration, but not once it has already started.

Soldier on

But before we reach for the drugs or even the supplements, it is worth remembering that a cold generally only lasts a few days. Like a good houseguest, a well-adapted parasite doesn't damage its host. It may make us miserable but doesn't really hurt us.

Stoic contempt

 'The only way to treat the common cold is with contempt,' said William Osler, a man revered as the father of pragmatic modern medicine.

Actually it might be wrong to use medication to treat the symptoms of a cold. Reducing our immune response to the virus (which is the cause of our symptoms, after all) can just prolong or exacerbate the very illness we are fighting off.

#14 NOT CATCH COLD?

For example, inflammation is a reaction that the body produces to control the virus. So suppressing inflammation (e.g. with anti-inflammatories) may be problematic. For example, one study suggested that taking aspirin for a cold actually increased the amount of virus shed into nasal secretions during a cold, making us more infectious to others.

In much the same way, many people believe that having a fever is a good thing, and a sign of a robust immune response. Raising our core temperature slightly acts to stoke immune function and improve virus killing. In fact, losing our fever response makes some infections more deadly.

But while this may well be true for serious infections, the common cold is more depressing than dangerous. So hang the science. We just want to feel better, now!

~~~~~~

When we have a cold we may feel lousy, we may look terrible, but we have things to do! In this busy over-committed world it's hard to take time off, especially for something as trivial and self-limiting as a cold. Should we just soldier on?

If we were to ask our doctor (or our mother) for their advice on what to do when we feel sick to our boots from a cold, they would probably say we should stay home, stay indoors or refrain from exercise. This may sound like the best medicine (or your mother), but there is absolutely no evidence it does any good. Moderate exercise when we have a cold doesn't make it any worse or persist any longer. And if anything, prolonged bed rest has been shown to be harmful.

It is also often suggested that we should stay at home as a kind of altruistic quarantine for the sake of our uninfected work colleagues. It is certainly true that we are most infectious on the days that symptoms are worst and mucus is pouring out of our nose (generally days two to four). But we were contagious within a day of being exposed, even before symptoms kicked in, and remain contagious until all our symptoms have gone, seven to ten days later (or even longer with kids). So taking a couple of days off for quarantine is totally impractical.

Having a cold is also usually considered a turn-off for sex. Of course, we don't want to share our germs (as if that hadn't already happened), but we also feel tired and may have a headache. We are supposed to be taking it easy. But there is good reason to reconsider.

271

During sex, and in particular following orgasm, changes in blood flow can miraculously unblock our nose, and make it easier to fall asleep. That's more than we can expect from most drugs, and more fun too.

The bottom line

We all know those people who never seem to get a cold. Whether they are really more robust or hygienic, or simply don't have ready access to biohazardous children is unclear. But when we are down with a cold, we really want to be them.

There is no trick to it really. All the usual advice about spending more time outdoors, dealing with stress, being more active, and getting more sleep probably has the greatest impact on our health by reducing our days off sick with a cold. Adhering to the cold-specific recommendations about regularly washing our hands, not picking our nose or rubbing our eyes, not sneezing or coughing on others, and keeping warm outdoors (so we don't have to go back inside) will also help us not to catch cold.

Sadly, we can't cure a cold. We can't even treat it that well. Even the best drugs and supplements have a modest impact at the very best. We could stay in bed for six to ten days and then recover, or we could walk around and ignore it for six to ten days and then recover. But it doesn't make any difference to the cold.

Or, recognizing that we are sick, we can ease our path by relaxing, having a nice bowl of soup or drinking a hot toddy before going to bed. It won't really make any difference to the outcome. However, it will help us to feel a little better while we get better of our own accord.

Do I really have to ...

#15

Avoid accidents?

Q: Can I avoid having an accident?
A: Yes.

Q: Why do cars kill people?
A: It most cases it is people that kill people.

Q: Is a little alcohol really that bad?
**A: Is increasing your risk of having an accident
by double or more really that bad?**

Q: Can I make my bones stronger?
**A: Absolutely, when you were younger. As we get older
we can mostly make (or not make) our bones weaker.**

Q: What about taking hormones for my bones?
**A: Hormone replacement therapy is a
much more complicated balance.**

Q: Should I not walk under a ladder?
**A: You should stop and hold the base for
the poor person on the roof.**

Accidents happen. It's one of those things about life that make it both thoroughly interesting as well as potentially injurious.

It's not that these events are random, an unavoidable fate or simply bad luck. For something to truly be an accident it has to be understood that, in hindsight, events could have been prevented had things gone differently; be unmade by different choices. Accidents have a cause; they are predictable and preventable — only we failed to predict or prevent them. That is why they are accidental.

Notwithstanding all possible precautions that can be taken, some accidents will still happen. But others may not. Or their impact may be lessened or changed. The critical question is what decisions we can take to improve the chances our lives will not be shortened or restricted by accident.

Henry H. Bliss

 On 13 September 1899, New Yorker Henry Bliss stepped down from a streetcar at the corner of West 74th Street and Central Park West, just a skip down the hill to Strawberry Fields. Just as he was getting off he was struck by a taxi. He died the following morning, becoming the first recorded person to be killed by a car in America.

The taxicab that did him in was electric-powered, as were most taxis in New York at the time, built by the Electric Carriage and Wagon Company of Philadelphia.

They were very popular vehicles as they didn't emit smoke or backfire frequently. They could start on a cold day (unlike steam cars) and didn't need to be cranked by hand to start (unlike those using fuel). They could only go about 40 miles (just over 64 kilometres) before needing a charge, but as Manhattan Island was not that big it didn't matter much.

Importantly, there were also no gears and few engine vibrations, so they were extremely quiet. The same concerns for the safety of pedestrians from' silent killer' cars running in electric-mode still exist today.

Collision course

The most common way for people to die by accident is in a collision involving a car, truck, bus, motorcycle, bicycle or pedestrian. The average lifetime risk of dying in a car crash is about 1 in 200.

Globally, vehicle collisions kill around 1.5 million people every year, many of whom are young and in the prime of their life. In numerical terms, this rate is almost the same as the total global burden of deaths from AIDS. At least ten times more suffer serious and life-changing injuries arising from road trauma each year.

Even though there are more cars on our roads than ever, the number of people killed on our roads is mercifully declining. The human factors that contribute to at least 95 per cent of crashes are amenable to change. To this end, many countries have adopted a 'vision zero' policy that aims, through the cooperation of providers, regulators and road users, to eliminate road deaths altogether. This is not pie in the sky thinking.

The fundamental basis of this movement for change is that car crashes are not really the problem. Rather, the real issue is that collisions result in serious injury and deaths to humans. So the first priority must be with life and death.

For example, there is a very logical argument to limit the speed of vehicles according to the kind of collision that could be predicted to occur and the mess it would make with any humans involved.

The human tolerance for being hit by a car is about 30 kph (or about 20 mph). Any faster and the pedestrian will probably be seriously injured or die. If we were to get hit by a car travelling at the usual speed limit on our roads of 50 kph (30 mph), the risk for being killed in the collision is more than 80 per cent. So any zones where there are pedestrians and cars potentially meeting each other (e.g. pedestrian crossings) should logically be designed to keep the speed to no more than 30 kph (20 mph). Today, many roads are restricted to this speed for exactly this reason.

Humans travelling in a well-designed modern car can safely take side impacts at less than 50 kph (30 mph), so intersections should obviously be limited to this speed. Equally a well-designed modern car can take about 70 kph (44 mph) head-on in frontal impacts, so this is appropriate for undivided roads. Only divided roads with free-flowing traffic (e.g. motorways, freeways, etc.) with low possibility of a side impact or frontal impact (risking mostly collision with distant infrastructure) would then have speed limits of 100 kph, or 62 mph. In this way, serious impacts of accidents can be both predicted and prevented.

At the same time, many other everyday aspects of driving behaviour can also reduce the risk of us dying in our car. Most are truly obvious and we do them every day without thinking. For example, obeying road rules makes our driving behaviours not only safe but predictable to others using the road, so we are less likely to crash into them, or them into us.

The precaution of wearing a seatbelt every time we drive reduces serious injuries and deaths in crashes by about half. This is one of the most common health messages we have to convey to our kids, because one day it may be important. Like most health messages, it doesn't feel that relevant at the time, it may be restricting and uncomfortable, but one day it might be lifesaving.

Controls around driving under the influence of alcohol or drugs are also obvious and essential, as up to one in three deaths on the road may be due to intoxication and the aberrant driving behaviour it causes.

Drunk driving

 Any alcohol in our blood affects our behaviour, judgement, precision and response time, all of which increases the risk of crashes and serious injuries when we drink and drive. The higher the level of alcohol in our blood, the greater the risks.

At a level of 0.05 per cent (or 50 mg of alcohol for every 100 ml of blood) our risk of having a crash is about twice that if we weren't drinking at all. At a level of 0.08 per cent the risk of having a crash is increased roughly five-fold compared to when we are not drinking.

Different countries have debated what represents acceptable risk, as well as what makes a sufficient deterrent to driving while intoxicated. In the US, Canada and England a blood alcohol level above 0.08 per cent is illegal, while countries like France, Germany, Australia and New Zealand have lower limits of 0.05 per cent.

In all countries, calls for lower limits (e.g. 0.02 per cent) or zero tolerance for alcohol consumption when driving continue to gain support.

Because the alcohol concentration in the blood is difficult to predict from the amount of alcohol consumed, a zero limit avoids the confusion of 'I think I'll be okay'. It also separates all drinking from driving and ensures drivers make other plans before starting to drink.

The counter-argument is that any further tightening of blood alcohol limits predominantly targets people who enjoy a drink but who don't have much risk of crashing to begin with. Keeping the limits as they are, as opposed to zero, represents in absolute terms only a very small increase in crashes, as the overall crash risk is very small to begin with. Even doubling an almost negligible risk is still almost negligible.

Of course if you are an at-risk driver anyway (e.g. teenager or inexperienced driver), doubling your risk of crashing looks a whole lot bigger, and a zero-alcohol policy makes good sense.

Although people are often concerned about having a crash during long car trips, most collisions occur within 50 kilometres (31 miles) of home. This is partly because most miles are spent driving to and from home. Most collisions occur in the late afternoon and evening, when everyone else is also heading home too. But even after adjusting for total time spent in our car, the traffic or the time of day, short, local trips still carry a greater burden of crashes

Some of this may be due to **auto-piloting**; that is, habitually driving the same route every day. It is so easy, we can do it almost without concentrating. Sometimes we pull up at home only to realize we have little memory of how we got there. The obvious problem with this is that lower levels of concentration can leave us unable to react as quickly as we need to if anything unexpected should happen, making us vulnerable to accidents.

Another increasing cause of road trauma is distracted drivers. Anything that diverts attention from the road has been shown to increase the risk of crashes. If we take our eyes off the road for any longer than two seconds, our risk of crashing is doubled. Count them. One. Two. That's all it takes. In alcohol terms, driving distracted is like driving with a blood alcohol of 0.05 per cent.

The most well-known distraction while driving comes from use of mobile phones, especially texting, dialling or surfing for information, as well as reaching for them to pick up a call. In many places it is now illegal. Talking on a mobile phone itself does not seem to be as problematic. This provides the simple rationale for automatic hands-free devices and other appropriate apps. Like a seatbelt, it seems pretty inconvenient and unnecessary most of the time. But just one time is all it takes.

Mobile phones are not the only distraction. Changing a radio station, searching for objects, reading (a map or directions), applying make-up, eating and drinking, and of course dealing with unruly children in the back seat can easily cause us to divert our attention from the road. None of these is illegal, but they all cause accidents and shorten lives.

Finally, it is also true that we all make mistakes when driving. Even the very best and conscientious drivers. As they say, to err is to be human. Although mistakes can be kept to a minimum there is no way that we can be expected to make the right choice every time. Based on insurance claims, on average, we will crash our car three to four times during our life. Fortunately most of these will only damage our car.

One pragmatic approach to road trauma is to embrace human fallibility by incorporating other changes (like the human-friendly speed limits detailed above) to lessen the impact of collisions when inevitably they occur. Roads and cars can be made more forgiving of their errant drivers.

And of course if drivers really are the problem, we could always get rid of them as a public health measure. Automated vehicles or fully driverless cars are now a reality and will certainly impact on unintentional driver lapses and errors, as well as other distracting aspects of driving. Technology will not eliminate human stupidity entirely but it may make it harder to make the kind of mistakes that cost lives.

Dry bones

In mythology, it is bone rather than flesh that is the source of life. In the Bible, God uses a rib to create Eve. In Mexican mythology, Quetzalcoatl does the same to create mankind. Even in Greek mythology, mankind is reborn after the flood from the bones cast by Pyrrha.

There are many reasons why bones should be considered to be generators of life. Only bones provide human form, a skeleton that we can still recognize even long after death. The lasting form of skeletons also makes them popular for Halloween costumes. Without bones we are merely ghosts or jellyfish.

The essential life-giving, life-saving attributes of our bones are best exemplified when we have an accident, and they do or do not break. Most fractures occur after some physical impact on a bone. Our bones are heir to a thousand (low-impact) natural shocks every day. Almost all are fended off by our robust health, reflexes and muscular physique. But, even so, our bones are able to take quite a beating.

Because of their specialized architecture, our bones are able to absorb some of the force of a blow, bend a bit if necessary and then return to their original shape. The amount of energy that can be absorbed by a bone before it breaks defines its resistance to fracture. If a bone is too fragile or the blow is too strong, even bending cannot stop them from breaking.

Even though broken bones can mend, it is a gradual process, sometimes taking many months of reduced mobility and rehabilitation before strength and resilience can be restored. And in older people in particular, because of their diminished reserves, a fracture might also mean the beginning of a slow decline in their health or, as some might think of it, a 'fate worse than death' if they become dependent on others for assistance with everyday activities while recovering.

The dowager's hump

 Many women outlive their men. A dowager is a wealthy widow who holds a title or property, literally endowed from her deceased husband.

Dowagers are famous the world over for their rule as much as for their physiology. The most famous of all was the Empress Dowager Cixi, the concubine who became the Dragon Empress of China.

A dowager's ears are said to be longer. This may be due to the fact that a long life will give you big ears, rather than the other way around. Especially if you can afford those enormous, heavy earrings.

Some older women also develop an excessive bend in their back, known as a dowager's hump. However, the same process also occurs in some men, regardless of their wealth.

A dowager's hump is caused by distortion of the spine (kyphosis) due to fractures of the vertebrae and degeneration of the discs between them. Instead of stacking up straight like blocks, the spine bends more like stacked wedges. This acts to push the head and shoulders forward, creating a characteristically poking chin, hunched back and stooped posture.

The hump is not just unsightly. It can also interfere with balance, walking, reaching for things and even rising from a throne.

There are two obvious ways to reduce our risk of breaking a bone: avoiding any strong blows (as might naturally occur in falls and other accidents) and maintaining the natural resistance of our bones to breaking so they can take any blows they receive.

Our bone is not a lifeless skeleton. On the outside of each bone, new bone is continuously built up, layer upon layer. On the inside, bone is continuously reabsorbed. This allows all the bones of our body to be rebuilt many times over our lifetime following roughly the same body plan. But unlike a building, we don't need to vacate the premises or put up the shutters while the work is going on.

The continuous remodelling of our bones also has the advantage of allowing them to adapt their shape and strength according to how they are being used. For example, the repeated pulling and pushing of muscles on our bones associated with weight-bearing activities like walking, running and jumping, stimulates the foundation of stronger bone. This is partly through causing tiny fractures in the bone.

It is quite normal for small cracks to occur here and there in bone, just as in any building. But this does not weaken the overall structure. On the contrary, it is thought that our bones' ability to develop microscopic cracks is one important way they are able to dissipate the force of a blow, and therefore not break apart so easily. Moreover, these tiny cracks make it obvious which parts need extra strengthening and stimulate the renewal of our bones in particular areas. Consequently, when we jog regularly our leg bones will be remade slightly thicker, from a subtle alteration of the balance between bone growth and bone destruction.

The opposite occurs if we are inactive, particularly as we get older. If we don't use it, we lose it. Every year that goes by that we don't use our strength, our bones become a little thinner from the inside out. Sometimes, this loss may become significant enough that the strength and integrity of our bone is compromised. This can lead to fragility and increased risk for fractures even with relatively minor trauma (e.g. a fall from standing height or less). This is called **osteoporosis**. The bones ('osteo') literally become more porous. Globally, osteoporosis contributes to over 20 million fractures every year.

Not everyone will develop osteoporosis or have fractures as they get older. One of the most important determinants is the starting point; that is, how thick and strong our bones are to start with.

The strongest our bones will get is usually in our early twenties. If we have laid down really strong bone in our twenties, it will usually take a lifetime before they thin out sufficiently to increase our risk of fracture, if at all. Equally, if our bones are small and thin in our twenties, like having a head start, we might reach that finish line sooner.

Men generally have a higher peak bone mass than women, probably because men are about 15 to 20 per cent bigger and heavier on average than women. This generally means a man would have to lose much more bone mass than a woman before his bones would be thin enough to fracture easily. Consequently, only one in five men aged fifty years or older will have a fracture due to osteoporosis during their lifetime. This compares to about half of all women.

The menopause

 In all women in their mid to late forties, a natural transition occurs in the way sex hormones like oestrogen (estrogen) are produced and released. Over the course of five to ten years, hormone production slows, becomes erratic and eventually shuts down altogether, as the hormone-producing reserves in the ovaries are exhausted. During the latter part of this transition, menstrual cycle lengths become irregular and menstruation eventually stops (known as the **menopause**). The process of the ovaries shutting down impacts not only reproductive functioning, but also almost every aspect of a woman's body and life.

As a woman's ovaries stop making oestrogen, one of the effects is the loss of its beneficial effects on bone adaptation and resilience. This is why some doctors recommend some (younger) women take low-dose oestrogen delivered as **hormone replacement therapy** (HRT) for their bones. However, this should be used only in the short term and its use needs to be carefully balanced against other risks from taking HRT, which can include heart disease and cancer.

How strong our bones will be at their peak is also determined, in part, by what we ate and our level of physical activity during the 'growth years' of our childhood and adolescence. Well-nourished, active kids make stronger bones, which carry them onwards into their future even though every bone in their body is subsequently rebuilt every ten years of their lives.

A regular intake of calcium is often recommended to help make strong bones. This is because our bones are mostly made from calcium. If we didn't get enough calcium in our diet (or enough vitamin D to help absorb it) when our adult skeletons were first taking shape, then a smaller, more fragile skeleton would be built, commensurate with the lower availability of calcium building bricks. No point building a big one if there will be not enough calcium to maintain it. By contrast, if we had plenty of calcium, sunshine and physical activity in our youth, then we can invest in building stronger bone, because we can expect to have the resources to look after it.

The subsequent rate of bone loss after its peak in our twenties is also influenced by many other factors, including our diet, smoking and the amount and intensity of weight-bearing activities. For example, we are often recommended to do more weight-bearing exercise (like walking or jogging) for the sake of our bones. And these will make our bones a little stronger. However, its effects are more modest once we have passed our twenties. It's easy to make changes to the plan when the big house is first constructed. It's much harder to change the design significantly during subsequent rebuilds. Nonetheless, the stronger muscles we get from exercise can also reduce the risk of falling, so exercise has indirect benefits for our bones as well.

Sadly, taking calcium, vitamin D and/or other supplements when we are older is, at best, only weakly effective in treating or preventing osteoporosis, and probably only in people who aren't getting enough time outdoors in the sunshine. None of them will make us less likely to break a bone if we fall off a ladder.

As easy as falling off a ladder

In order to break a healthy strong bone we need to be struck by a force greater than our own weight falling down. In other words, we normally need to fall from a height to break a bone. The most common way we go up is on a ladder. So this is the most common way we come down (with a thump). In the Bible, Jacob had a vision in which he saw a ladder reaching from earth to Heaven. It is an easy exit strategy.

Falling off a log

 In the days before logging trucks, floating trees down a large river was a practical way to transport them to American sawmills. To prevent misdirected logs from blocking the river and causing a 'log jam', lumberjacks would carefully balance on top of the floating logs. As the trees were round in cross section, just like a wheel, the logs would start to roll, dumping their jockey into the water. Unless, that is, they were able to move at the same rate as the spinning log to stay on top and out of the water. This is known as **log rolling**.

Some practitioners became so good at log rolling that they made it look very easy. So much so that any city slickers, seeing them literally walk on water, felt it probably took no skill at all. However, when they tried it themselves they soon found it was far easier to fall off a (spinning) log than stay balanced on top, much to the amusement of anyone watching. Not surprisingly, log rolling became a hit sport.

Today, we experience the same kind of malicious enjoyment on television watching over-confident people fall off slippery rotating obstacle courses. This emotion is known in German as *schadenfreude* (literally harm-pleasure). In *The Simpsons*, Nelson expresses it more succinctly as 'Ha ha!'

In many ways, climbing a ladder is similar to log rolling. It is made to look ridiculously easy, or at least not particularly dangerous, by children and professionals. However, it really should be left to the latter. And even then, falls from ladders are a leading cause of injury and death in workers involved in construction, mining, installation and maintenance.

In and around the home, ladders and steps are ubiquitous, so falls from using them are also commonplace. They occur more often in men than women, especially older men over 45 years of age. This partly reflects the fact that men generally use ladders more often than women, especially on their own. In addition, older men retain the DIY self-confidence of their youth. How dangerous can it be, after all?

The most common accident occurs when the base of the ladder slips out. This can easily happen if the surface below the ladder is wet, bumpy or uneven and the feet of the ladder don't grip. But the usual reason for the ladder slipping out is that it is set at a wrong angle. It's common to just plonk a ladder against something and quickly climb up. However, if the angle of the ladder is just a bit too shallow, the base is at risk of sliding out. Being set only 10 degrees shallower than the ideal (75.5 degree) angle for a ladder doubles the amount of friction required to hold the ladder base in place. Equally, if the angle of the ladder is set a bit too steep, the ladder and/or the climber may easily fall backwards.

Like log rolling, it is not easy to get the angle exactly right every time without experience. The simple solution is to have someone at the bottom of the ladder, assisting the climber and securing the base so it can't slip. It also pays to ascend slowly, which puts less stress on the base.

Folded step-ladders are always set at the right angle with the spreader in the locked position. Step-ladders are comparatively safer than leaning ladders (except for when the ground is uneven). However, it is still possible to fall off them, especially when mud, snow or water is on the rungs, or if we are trying to carry things (e.g. boxes, paint tins or tools) up the ladder and upset our balance.

The risk of falling is reduced when at least both feet and one hand or both hands and one foot (i.e. three points of contact) are on the ladder at all times. If we have something in one hand, at some points there are only two.

Finally, it is said to be unlucky to walk under a ladder. Obviously this is to the advantage of the one up the ladder not wishing to be bumped off it. Also if someone were properly holding the base of the ladder, there wouldn't be enough room and we would have to walk around. So if we were to even contemplate walking under, it is assumed that no one is there holding the base. In practical terms, if the angle of the ladder is broad enough for someone to walk under (i.e. not 75 degrees) and there is no one holding the base, there is a good chance of the ladder slipping, especially if bumped.

Very superstitious?

 We all know the story about walking under a ladder being bad luck. Most of us can even sing the Stevie Wonder song. The superstition about ladders is thought to have come about in the Middle Ages, long before occupational health and safety, when ladders were made of wood and rungs fastened only with flimsy, degradable rope. If the ladder's going to fall, very understandably, it would be obvious not to walk under it. Not very superstitious. Just common sense really.

By contrast, true superstition is a belief based on a lack of knowledge. So what is it that we don't understand about walking under ladders?

In the Middles Ages, the tallest building in each town belonged to the church, who maintained them with tall ladders. They may have deliberately left the full understanding of 'don't walk under ladders' shrouded in mystery for good reason. Leading a life of austere simplicity, they did not normally wear any underwear, even while up a ladder.

Falling down

Most injuries occur not when we are standing or still but when we are moving. The faster we move the easier it is to fall as momentum carries us forward if we slip or trip. In retrospect, it is usually easy to understand why we slipped (e.g. a wet floor, tripping over a cat) and the danger we failed to predict or prevent. This is why they are called accidents and they are usually preventable.

All animals have natural reflexes to prevent falling (lest they become injured and consequently easy prey). Humans are no exception. For example, when we trip we instinctively throw an arm out to rotate our body and push off with our trailing leg, both of which lengthen our next stride and aid to brake a fall. This takes quick reflexes, as well as muscle strength, to push off fast enough to get the next step into the correct braking position before our body topples over. These keen reflexes mean that banana peels and untied shoelaces are not the inexorable hazard they are often alleged to be.

However, if our reaction times slow (e.g. when intoxicated), our leg muscles are weak (e.g. when we are inactive or older), or our foot fails to grip (e.g. on a wet floor), the ability to brake a fall is reduced, so slips and trips occur more easily. As a result, at least three out of every ten people over the age of 65 slip and fall each year.

A common bone to break is our **collarbone** (also known as the clavicle). This is because the reflex that causes us to throw out our arm also puts the collarbone in danger if we can't stop falling. If we land hard on our outstretched arm or our shoulder itself, the force is transferred to the weaker collarbone, which bends and (with enough force) breaks. This is actually quite a good thing, believe it or not, because it serves to dissipate the force and prevent more serious damage to the much more important shoulder or spine.

Upstairs, downstairs

 It is almost impossible to have a period drama on TV or an Oscars ceremony without someone falling on the stairs. Globally, stairs and steps remain a significant cause of serious and fatal accidents, second only to cars in multi-storeyed parts of the world.

Stairs are a tremendous source of opportunistic physical activity. Imagine the reduced waistlines of the world if we always took the stairs. A building with stairs has many floors, which is a big plus as it reduces the building footprint and land costs, while improving the living space, ventilation and the view.

The downside is that stairs are tragically unforgiving to distraction, momentum, imbalance, poor vision, slipping, flamboyant gowns or misplaced objects. Irregularity in the steps by as little as half a centimetre (very common in old staircases) may be enough to throw off our stride.

The most common issue is when we overstep stair treads, often because we are rushing, not looking or distracted by thinking about chocolate cake. Some people fall at the second-last step because they think they have already reached the bottom of the stairs, or at the very last step as they think there is one more step to go.

One of the most practical ways to prevent falls is to maintain or enhance the coordinated strength of our leg muscles. This is usually achieved through regular physical activity and/or exercises that include a balance component.

The other very obvious solution to falling is anticipation. Anticipating slipping on a wet tree trunk, log rollers wore spikes on their shoes. This, along with their skill, made life as a river man look like a walk in park. In the same way, those at most risk of falling can take many anticipatory steps to reduce their risk, including, where appropriate, using handrails, handholds, non-slip shoes, mats and wet floors.

The bottom line

Napoleon Bonaparte protested that there were no accidents, only our failure to recognize the hand of fate. Of course, it was his bright idea to wage war against the Russians in winter. Another famous story is that during a coughing fit, Napoleon complained '*Ma sacre toux,*' meaning 'my damn cough', but his staff thought he said '*Massacre-tous*', meaning 'massacre all'. Accidents are not fate. They are just tragically accidental.

But this also means they are predictable and preventable. Fighting a winter war against the Russians, drink driving, walking under a ladder, wearing that gown to the Oscars and expecting to bound up the stairs — what did they think was going to happen?

Cars are 100 per cent safe ... when they are kept in our garages. But that's not what they're for. We have to get out, and it's predictable that when we do, accidents will happen accidentally. But we can have an enormous effect of how likely they are to occur and how much they will impact our lives. Not by being obsessive or restrictive. Just by paying attention and showing some common sense to make sure we stay upright and alive.

Do I really have to ...

#16

Deal with stress?

Q: I can't live without stress.
A: Yes, you can.

Q: Stress just gives me a headache.
A: If only.

Q: Why does stress kill?
A: Because it penetrates your mind and your soul.

Q: Does stress make me fatter?
A: Overeating and not exercising enough make you fatter. But stress can sometimes help you along.

Q: What about getting a good night's sleep?
A: You'll feel better in the morning.

Q: Why do some people seem immune to stress?
A: Self-esteem, optimism, confidence and calm.

Q: Why is depression such a big issue?
A: At least one in six of us will become depressed in the face of adversity at some time in our lives.

Q: Can I really manage stress?
A: Only if you can find what you are so attached to.

We can't always get what we want. And when we don't, we experience **stress**.

Hard work is not stressful. It's not stressful to climb a hill, only taxing. What is stressful is when the hill stops us from getting where we want to go or when we want to get there. If we've got all day and we can arrive at any time, then there's no problem and therefore no stress. But if we aren't sure we can make it over the hill or as quickly as we'd want to, then hill climbing becomes stressful.

On the other side of the hill, they may be getting worried too. They are not stressed just because they are sitting around. Sitting around is usually relaxing unless there are things we want to do. 'Look at the time! Where are you?' they might be thinking. 'Has something happened? Did I get the time wrong? Should I call?'

In both cases, it's not the action or inaction that is inherently stressful. Sometimes hill climbing is rather relaxing. While we're waiting around we've got time to burn. Stress only comes when we are attached to the outcomes of our actions, whether what we desire or fear is going to happen. We are not worried if we are not particularly attached to when we can turn up. Our friends are not worried if they're not particularly attached to when we get there. No worries. No stress.

Our attachment to the outcomes we want acts a bit like the strings on a puppet. When we want our puppet to stand up (but all it wants to do is fall over), we pull on the strings. When we want our puppet to do something in particular, we pull the strings again, until the desired and expected outcome is reached.

The tension that we feel when our strings are pulled is called stress. The emotional response we have to its pull is called **suffering**. And although our strings are invisible, just like a puppet we all suffer under the weight of our attachments.

The reason we put up with stress at all is not because we like to suffer, but because we are fiercely attached to the outcomes and what we desperately want to happen. We get stressed by so many different things because we have great expectations.

Sometimes we are attached to a possible future, when we will get something or achieve something that we don't yet have. This is called desire or ambition. The stress that comes with desire is well known by anyone who has ever really, really wanted something, but is not sure they can get it. For example, 'Will he want to go out with me?' 'What will I need to do to make sure I get the job?' 'Will I make it?'

Sometimes we are attached to a possible future we are afraid to lose. For example, we have a job but are worried about losing it. We have a love in our life but we worry about keeping them. We wouldn't get stressed if we weren't attached to these outcomes or simply didn't care. But we do care and that's why we can feel so stressed. It's not the loss that makes the situations stressful. We all lose things. It's our expectations and the fact we care so deeply about them that makes us feel stress when things don't go to plan.

Sometimes we are also very attached to the outcomes of past events (possible pasts) and continue to be stressed by them. We regret. 'What if?' or 'If only?' We resent others their outcomes, because they could have been ours.

Stress is a normal part of life because it is human nature to feel the wanting pull of desire and the fear of loss. We are not bad people, fearful, sinful or greedy. We just have expectations and can't get satisfaction.

The motivation of stress is more than just the pull of our attachments. The other motivation is the belief that our stress will vanish if we only get what we want: satisfaction. For example, if we are running late for an appointment, the (suffering from) stress could vanish if we could just make it there on time. So stress acts as both carrot and stick.

The attraction of certain outcomes, their desirability, is a personal thing. We all want what we want. But these things can be very different in different people. Not everyone stresses about running late. Not everyone frets about getting a high-paying job. We usually stress more about (getting or losing) the things we value most because our attachments are much stronger. The more attached we are to getting that job, having those things and being there on time, the greater the stress our invisible strings put us under. Some outcomes can seem as important to us as life and death. We suffer a lot over these.

Sometimes we also stress more about things we feel we could almost get, that are nearly within our grasp. It's harder to feel stress about the things we expect we just can't get, but while there is hope there is also stress.

We are also influenced by social norms that make us want what others expect we should want, in so far as we care what others think.

The modern reality of consumerism feeds off our wants, fears and desires and, in many cases, creates the expectations that cause us to feel stress. Shouldn't we be like that?

Sometimes, a little stress makes us stronger. In fact, when we are angry we fight harder, think more optimistically, and make more risky decisions, determined to get the job done. For many people, stress is their most important motivation, so that nothing gets done without a deadline or the pressure of expectation. But in the long term, the strings we use to pull ourselves in one direction or another can actually hold us down.

Heaven

 Most people think that if they had everything they ever wanted, they wouldn't be stressed at all and wouldn't suffer (it). This is just how most people describe heaven, a state of bliss, wanting for nothing. 'I'm in heaven,' they say.

But wanting for nothing is not the same as having everything we want. The two are often confused.

In Eastern philosophy, moksha, nirvana or other liberated states of perfect heavenly bliss are those in which we have all we need right now, freed from fear of loss and desire (i.e. no stress and no suffering). This is because when we live in the moment, just for today, there are no outcomes or expectations, so no strings of attachment.

Many religions practise non-attachment to essentially achieve the same blissful end, not by receiving everything they want but by wanting for nothing. They do not worry about tomorrow. Unencumbered by strings of attachment, 'enlightenment' is a literal term.

Having fewer attachments does not mean being disengaged or inactive in our lives, but rather doing the best we can, or the most appropriate thing at the time, and let the outcomes take care of themselves. *Che sera, sera.* What will be, will be.

Stressed out

When we suffer stress, it is a signal that we are not where we mean to be or are in danger of not being there. Stress can be a motivation to get us out of bad situations or stand and fight to stay in good ones. This is why the body's stress response is often called the 'fight or flight' response. The drive of stress is there to give us resources to fight or get out of there, to deal with a problem or avoid it.

There are many different things that this drive does to our mind and our body. One of the most obvious is that stress causes our heart to beat harder and faster and our blood pressure goes up. Imagine that you have to stand on a stage in front of a crowd of people. Your heart is probably pounding scarily fast and feels as if it could leap out of your chest. This is one of the things that stress does.

Most people think that a racing heart is just trying to fuel our muscles with the energy they need to fight for our food or run away from a lion. But our muscles already have the energy stored inside them for a burst of activity, allowing sprinters to sprint and weightlifters to lift without needing any more oxygen from their heart.

Actually, our heart beats fast and strong mostly so we can give our brain the extra energy it needs to think. Even though we can't always get the work done when stressed, our mind is really working harder trying to formulate a plan. A working brain needs more energy-rich blood to function, and this is what our racing heart provides.

While a racing heart when we are stressed is usually not a problem (really not that much different from when we exercise) there is a limit. If the heart starts beating too fast and too vigorously, blood can flow out from the heart at a faster rate than it can flow back in. If this mismatch goes on for too long, the heart would literally run out of blood to pump.

Obviously this is a dangerous situation. So there is an emergency reflex that is triggered when things are getting out of control in the heart. This reflex is like slamming on the brakes in a speeding car, and causes the heart to abruptly slow and blood pressure to drop sharply. This will make most people feel lightheaded and, in some cases, temporarily lose consciousness or faint.

About one in three adults will experience a fainting episode during their lifetime. It doesn't just happen to young women; men faint just as often. In fact, anyone can faint given the right trigger.

Fainting becomes much more likely when the flow of blood back to the racing heart is also compromised, so the brake-reflex is automatically deployed much earlier than in normal circumstances. The most common example of this is when soldiers faint after standing at attention. Instead of the blood being propelled back to their hearts through the movement of their muscles, it pools in their unmoving legs. Once their heart is going faster than the limited rate at which blood can be returned, whammo, the brakes come on and down they go. These same reflexes can sometimes be triggered in some people when their heart goes racing off due to extreme pain, straining while going to the toilet, during childbirth, prolonged coughing or even laughing (though the joke has to be really funny).

Following a fainting episode, people usually are back to normal within a few minutes. The biggest problem with fainting is the things people hit on the way down. And this means that fainting is a major cause of ending up in an ambulance or in hospital.

Playing possum

 Many animals use the trick of lying absolutely still and feigning death as a way of confusing overwhelming adversaries. The most famous example is the American Possum, so this behaviour is sometimes called 'playing possum'. Possums also let out a putrid smell, completing the unappetizing picture for any would-be predator.

Playing possum is said to work for humans who are attacked by grizzly bears defending their territory and/or their cubs. Certainly, it could be that dead things are not perceived as threatening. But equally, the options of fighting or running from a grizzly are doomed to failure (the bear always wins). So the 'playing possum' option looks as though it works by comparison. This is known as survivor bias.

When people faint they are not subconsciously playing possum. Although frozen with fear, possums are awake. They know what is happening and feel the stress of the situation. They just can't and don't move. By contrast, during a faint, for ten to fifteen seconds you are out cold.

Sometimes deer are also known to freeze when confronted with the oncoming headlights of a car. This scenario is also often used to describe the look of some people when they are startled. But rather than being frozen with fear, the highly sensitive eyes of deer (which are adapted to seeing in low light) are literally blinded by the bright headlights of oncoming cars. Unable to see anything, they stand still. The same thing would happen to us if we were suddenly to close our eyes and hold them shut. We would take a moment or two to get our bearings before being comfortable to move in any direction. However, for a deer this moment is all it takes to get run over.

~~~~~~

Broken hearted

People who (for whatever reason) suffer more stress in their lives on average will die younger than those who lead relaxed, stress-free lives. The most common reason is that stress increases the risk of having a heart attack or a stroke. For example, people reporting chronic work stress or marital stress have about double the risk of suffering a heart attack or stroke. Employees who work long hours, are overcommitted or over-invested in their work also tend to have more heart problems than other workers. Some research suggests up to a third of all heart attacks may be attributable to stress.

Why stress breaks our hearts is unclear. Obviously stressed people tend to not look after themselves as well, eat the wrong things, be sedentary, become overweight, smoke and drink more often, make the wrong choices or feel powerless to make the right ones. Often they are too busy being stressed. For example, average cholesterol levels generally rise during exam times. This could be one reason why stressed people have more heart attacks.

Stress also quickens our pulse and raises our blood pressure. The faster our heart beats and the harder it pumps the blood, the less smooth (more turbulent) the flow of blood becomes. This can easily be appreciated when we turn on a tap for filling a bath. If we turn the tap on a little, the flow is nice and smooth, making almost a straight line into the bath with hardly any noise. But if we're in a hurry and open the tap up as far as it can go, the water begins to slosh around irregularly, breaking up the smooth line descending into the bath and creating a lot of noise.

The same swirling turbulent flow happens if we open up our heart on full. However, unlike the pipes attached to a bath tap, our pipes can normally change their diameter. If flow increases to the point that turbulence is an issue, our blood vessels sense this and relax, thereby becoming somewhat larger. Bigger pipes can take much more flow before any turbulence occurs. So, no stress in our arteries.

The problem comes when this doesn't happen anymore. The most common reason is that our arteries become older and less flexible and eventually resemble a rigid steel pipe that is used for plumbing. This is called hardening of the arteries and is discussed in Chapter 11. Hard pipe-like arteries that can't relax are innately vulnerable to stress and the turbulence it creates.

Any turbulence buffets the walls of hard blood vessels, causing wear and tear (known as dysfunction). Turbulence is especially severe at points where blood must go round corners or divide to go in different directions. This is why these points break first and are most prone to atherosclerosis, the process of narrowing that leads to heart attacks and strokes. Turbulent blood is also harder to pump than smooth flowing blood, as it creates resistance for the heart. Blood pressure then becomes elevated in order to get blood to where it needs to go, making extra work for the heart.

Used up

 A toaster has a limited capacity to toast. After using it for a long time, eventually there will come a day when one of its parts will give way and it won't pop anymore. So if we want toast for breakfast, we'll have to get a new one. Our toaster is built to eventually die (at least after the warranty has expired), to be replaced by the next generation. The human heart may be the same.

During an average human lifespan, our heart will beat about 2 billion times. This is almost the same as a chicken. But as the average heart rate of a chicken is four times faster, unless they are cooked, fried or baked, this means the unfettered lifespan of a chicken should be four times shorter. Which it is.

This kind of fascinating coincidence has led to the widely held belief that if we only have about two billion heartbeats available to us, and, if we could reduce the stresses that increase our heart rate, literally slow down a bit, we would all take a lot longer to use these 2 billion beats up. In other words, we would live a lot longer.

Unfortunately, this thinking has scared many people away from intensive physical exercise, afraid to use up the limited resource of their heartbeats on something as trivial as running round the block. However, regular physical exercise and the physical fitness that comes from it, results in a lower heart rate during the times we are not exercising, which more than makes up for the times that we are.

A very significant shock can stop the heart from beating, although it is rare. We have all seen movies where someone dies of fright, drops dead during an argument or dies of a broken heart. It does happen in real life too. For example, some deaths following earthquakes are not due to any physical damage, but rather the heart-stopping shock of the quake.

This usually only happens to people with already damaged hearts, as they have less spare capacity. A damaged heart can more easily lose its rhythm and its (oxygen) balance when it is stressed, like when we are angry, running, having an intense dream or even making love.

As a result many people with heart problems are treated with medicines that specifically block the effect of stress on their heart. These are known as beta-blockers. These medications can reduce the risk of suddenly dropping dead by about one-third. However, beta-blockers are also banned in many sports, because by reducing the effects of stress, in some cases they can improve performance (or at the very least reduce the symptoms of performance anxiety).

Stressed fat

As discussed earlier in this book, a leading cause of illness and premature death today is having too much fat in all the wrong places in our body. Although we lay down fat every time we consume more energy than we expend during our physical activities and metabolism, there comes a point when our capacity to store it safely is exceeded. So it spills over into places where it shouldn't be, damaging our health as a result.

Stress also plays an important role in this balance. For many people, stress is one of the important reasons why they have got fat in the first place. For others, stress is the major reason they lose weight.

For example, when we are really stressed, we sometimes don't feel much like eating. This is because our brain is so focused on the stressful issues it doesn't want or need the distraction of having to find food as well. So it shuts down our appetite. And of course when we don't eat, some of us can lose weight (e.g. a student coming up to exams, a bride before a wedding, those who are depressed or recently bereaved).

But at the same time, some people just seem to progressively gain weight when they are stressed, even if they experience the very same stresses that cause other people to lose weight. We all know of brides whose wedding gown ultimately did not fit on their wedding day because they had put on weight, students who get fatter during exam time, or people who are anxious or depressed sadly stacking on the kilos. So it's not so much the stress that is the cause of weight loss or weight gain, but rather our response to the suffering that stress causes that is the issue for our waistline.

As discussed earlier in this chapter, when we are stressed and our brain is working hard to find the answer, it needs more fuel to cover its extra workload. Without any appreciable energy stored in our brain itself, a stressed brain sends out signals to get more food, like dialling out for pizza when working a stressful all-nighter.

However, our brain only runs on glucose (sugar). Typically, about half of the glucose used by our body is used by our brain. When we are stressed this proportion can increase dramatically, sometimes to over 90 per cent. To make this switch a number of things must occur.

Firstly, our heart should beat a little faster and harder to help fuel our brain with extra helpings of sugar-rich blood.

Secondly, a brain in crisis-mode must be greedy and look after its own needs. So it must prevent, or at least slow, sugar from being used elsewhere in the body or taken up for storage, so more is available for its own thinking purposes. Fortunately, the functions of most other tissues can run just as easily off fat or other fuels as they can with sugar. They can switch what fuel they burn to keep going, like switching from electric to petrol (gas) to keep a hybrid car seamlessly running. But the brain can't switch. It is top dog with very specific requirements. Stress normally makes the rest of the body bow down to the sugary needs of our stressed-out brain (trying to find the solutions to our sticky problems).

Thirdly, if it can't easily get from our body the extra sugar required to think its way out of our difficulties, the brain sometimes increases our appetite (known as **stress eating**), or at least changes our appetite in a way that encourages us to gravitate to sugar-rich 'comfort' food that our brain loves. This has essentially the same effect as diverting sugar energy to a stressing brain by fuel switching. But it has the opposite effect on our waistline.

When the brain's need for sugar drives our appetite, we are compelled to quench our brain's desires in much the same way we just have to scratch an itch (although we know we shouldn't).

Scratch that itch

 It seems counter-intuitive that something so painfully itchy should make us want to scratch it some more. Surely it would be best to leave it alone? But what is an itch for if not to make you scratch it? And if you don't want to scratch it, is it really an itch?

If we step onto a sharp stone, it hurts. We instinctively draw away from the thing hurting us. Ow! On the other hand, when something is itchy we just have to investigate it, find out what has caused the itch, such as a bug that has landed on our arm, so we can flick it off. When we scratch the itch, it triggers sensations through the same nerves that caused it, blotting out the sensation of itchiness, at least temporarily.

But scratching that itch also feels really good. This is more than just removing the itch. The pleasurable sense of relief we get is the brain's reward that we have done what it wants us to do. As Ogden Nash wrote, 'Happiness is having a scratch for every itch'.

Similarly, many people report that they feel compelled to eat sweet foods when they are stressed. This is partly to blot out the sensation of stress that they feel and receive the pleasurable reward that the brain dishes out, even for a moment, just like scratching an itch. For some people this reward can also become an incentive for overeating and a loophole through which cues for eating, such as advertisements or just food availability, can remind us of the benefits of eating (i.e. scratching that itch).

What makes a stressed brain feed itself by pilfering any stored energy (e.g. the anxious bride getting thinner) rather than simply eating more (e.g. the anxious bride getting fatter) is still unclear. One idea is that the body's fuel switching doesn't work so well in those people who tend to stress or comfort eat. For example, when our brain wants more food to fuel its thinking, the body doesn't hear the phone call or ignores the ringing. The food doesn't get delivered, i.e. the fuel switch that makes it possible never occurs. So instead the brain dials out for sugary comfort food. This turns people into **stress eaters.**

There are many possible reasons that the signal does not get through. For example, some get so used to living under habitual stress that the signals the brain sends become muted, and so the body doesn't hear them. This is known as **habituation**. These people (known as habituators) tend to get fatter and eat more during periods of stress to feed their brain.

By contrast, some people mount the same strong stress response to each stress, over and over, sending out the same signals to the body to send more sugar. Because the body delivers, these so-called non-habituators are generally the ones who lose weight when subjected to a prolonged period of stress in their lives.

Sometimes the signal for more sugar may be correctly sent out by our stressed brain but our fat and liver might not listen because they are stuffed full of fat and resistant to messages from the brain. Our muscles might not listen to the stressed brain because they have been inactive for so long. Consequently, on average, fat inactive people are more likely to get fatter with stress than thin active ones, who more often lose weight when they are stressed.

Overall, these are thought to be the main reasons why some people get fatter and some thinner when they are stressed. But it's never this simple. Different stresses, at different intensities and different settings can affect people and their appetites in very different ways. This is why it's never easy to say, yes the stress made me fatter. But it can. And increasingly in this overweight age, it does.

A real headache

Headaches are among the most common causes of ill health in all human beings. We all get headaches, women more than men, younger people more than older. At some time or another, we all get headaches. At least half of us experience episodic headaches every year. Fortunately, our headaches are usually mercifully infrequent, episodic, dull and short-lived, lasting from several hours up to a few days at a time, at most.

This kind of headache is widely known as a stress or tension headache, as stress has been long believed to be its root cause. So much so, that the word 'headache' is commonly used to describe something stressful; for example, 'work was such a headache' (i.e. it's stressful) or 'she's being a headache' (she's causing us stress).

Most people report that stress and mental tension are the most common precipitants of their headaches. Yet, despite this widely held belief, stress is not the cause. It is just the usual suspect, an obvious fall-guy that we recognize as disagreeable, to which it is easy to assign blame. But we are stressed so very often and most of the time we don't get a headache.

Even though it seems to, the pain of tension headaches doesn't actually come from taxing our brain with stress. In fact, the brain itself doesn't feel pain. It is actually possible to do surgery on the brain while the patient is still awake without them ever feeling someone poking around upstairs, let alone pain.

Instead, our brain relies on signals coming from pain receptors located throughout our body to know where it's hurting us and how bad it is. When the pain receptors are activated in and around our head, our brain tells us through the unpleasant sensation of headache.

Obviously if we walked into a door and hit our nose, or our sinuses were inflamed, or we went to the dentist to have a crown fixed, these traumas would directly activate pain receptors and our head would ache for a very good reason. So a headache can sometimes be 'secondary' to something else. But for most headaches there is usually nothing obvious to explain why we've got a headache today but not yesterday or tomorrow.

Our face is the most active as well as most sensitive part of our body. For our brain to accurately know what is happening, the signals it receives from the facial senses have to be spot on. Any distortion of the signal and the message can become lost in translation, or even result in the wrong message being received. One theory for headaches is that our brain confuses some of the innocuous signals that it gets, and calls them a headache.

Chinese Whispers

 There is an old game played by children called Chinese Whispers, Telephone or Gossip. One child whispers a message into the ear of another. They then turn and pass the message on to another, who then turns and passes the message on again, around the room. The game is hilarious, as the message gets progressively distorted so that in the end it barely resembles the original.

Before headphones and Google translate, an interpreter's job was to listen and simultaneously whisper the translated words into the ear of their master. This is known as chuchotage. It is arduous work and usually requires teams of interpreters, all working in turn.

It is thought that the transformation of English words into the incomprehensible (to Western ears) four-toned complexities of Mandarin, via whispering interpreters is the origin of the name for the game. In the 18th and 19th centuries (and even today to some extent) everything about China was confusing. So Chinese Whispers simply reflected the confusing correspondence with China, which was often the norm. Prior to this, the game may have been known as Russian Whispers for the same reasons.

It was originally thought that excessive tensing of the muscles in the face, which might occur when we look tense, could trigger tension-type headaches in some susceptible people. Certainly, these headaches often feel like a tense band of pain across the forehead, temple or back of the head. In addition, the muscles in our head often feel tender to touch when we have a headache. People with more tender facial muscles also have more headaches. But this is probably just because the associated nerves are very sensitive, not because the muscles are actually sore.

Some people get tension-type headaches not just occasionally, but at least every other day. This really debilitating condition probably stems from their brain, which as a result of repeated signals and repeated headaches becomes rewired and sensitized to pain.

Some people experience an altogether different kind of headache, known as a **migraine**. It is usually but not always on one side of the head and tends to have a throbbing or pulsating quality associated with an awful sick feeling. Often, people feel strangely different (irritable, depressed, euphoric, etc.) one to two days before the migraine comes on, meaning that habitual sufferers can sometimes predict a migraine is about to happen.

Stress is also often implicated as the trigger factor in most migraine sufferers. However, feeling stressed may simply be the warning symptom of a migraine coming. Many other things can set off migraines in some sufferers, including lack of sleep, changing hormone levels, the weather, wine, fasting and even certain smells.

But in each case it needs the right mix of brain wiring to make a migraine happen, and most people experiencing stress or drinking wine do not get migraines.

Migraines are thought to happen because the parts of our brain that receive pain signals suddenly become hypersensitive, so that any little thing can set them off and make us feel as if we have been clonked on the head with a frying pan. This is a bit like the feedback in a microphone when the amplifier is turned up too high. Everything is fine until we start to speak into it. Then a painfully high-pitched screech blasts out from the speakers, is relayed directly into the microphone and then relayed back to the speakers again in a vicious circle. And we all go, 'AAAAH! &@#$!'

Burn out

Our bodies have many defence and healing mechanisms that are designed to turn on quickly when confronted by a potential threat, such as poisons, injury or infection, and deal with it before it can harm us. This defence is coordinated by our immune system. Like any security force, our immune system is composed of many different specialized components.

These defence forces can be broadly divided into two arms. First, there is an immediate, aggressive but generic security system. When this is tripped by anything getting into our territory, the alarm goes off and the police get called to come to a particular location and deal with the problem. This is known as **innate immunity**, and our white blood cells are the police, the chief defence against toxic invaders. The recruitment and accumulation of white cells into an area of our body is called **inflammation**.

The word inflammation originally came about as a practical way to describe that red-hot sensation experienced when a part of the body is inflamed. For example, when joints are inflamed (e.g. arthritis), skin is inflamed (e.g. dermatitis) or sinuses are inflamed (e.g. sinusitis) things feel uncomfortably hot, red and swollen, just as if we have been burnt by a flame.

We all need inflammation at certain times to fight infection or heal wounds. However, if left unchecked, inflammation can also lead to collateral damage as friendly fire causes scars and casualties for the home team. In fact, many so-called diseases are largely the result of collateral damage we have caused to ourselves from inopportune inflammation. For example, damage in areas of chronic inflammation can make cancers more common.

Like any conflict, it is not just the conflict zone that is affected. Inflammation can also lead to widespread changes affecting other tissues, even if they are not inflamed themselves. This occurs due to the release of signalling molecules (known as cytokines), which not only augment inflammation but also communicate the extent of the conflict to all corners of our body.

The big problem with this is that if inflammation is also going on elsewhere, there is a domino effect. This means that, for example, chronic joint inflammation may kindle the inflammation that causes heart disease and strokes, and vice versa.

Stress is one way we stoke the fire of inflammation, making it burn stronger or longer and causing more damage than it otherwise would. This is because when we are feeling stressed, facing an adversary, we need all our weapons not only available but supercharged so they can deal with it. Our ability to become inflamed and stay inflamed is boosted by stress.

Of course, in the short term this can be a good thing, like turning back an invader or recovering from an injury. But a long-term conflict without end is costly and damaging, not just where it is being fought, but in the home countries as well. The same goes for inflammation. Heightened and chronic inflammation is perhaps the main reason why most doctors point to stress as a bad thing for our health.

Unlike an alarm system that can be set off by anything, and cause the security team to get called, the other arm of our security system is smarter and more selective. This is known as the **adaptive immune system**. It is a programmable system designed to only recognize specific villains. This is something like the facial-recognition software used by passport control and security agencies to quickly identify potential threats, and trigger the rapid mobilization of targeted defences against them. The success of this defensive system is perhaps best demonstrated by immunization.

Immunization

 Viruses are toxic invaders, and the cause of many nasty illnesses and the deaths of countless children and young adults. Immunization largely prevents these deaths from happening.

When we get immunized we get a peek at what a specific dangerous virus looks like. We don't meet the live virus itself in the flesh. Rather we get to know the details of its profile by being injected with a dead or dummy version of the real thing. This primes our adaptive immune system to instantly recognize the virus. If it attempts to cross our borders, alarms will go off and our immune system will respond specifically against it.

When lots of people are immunized, even if one person gets sick the virus has nowhere to spread, as its next potential host most likely has been vaccinated. This drives down infection rates and makes it less likely for any unvaccinated people, or those in whom the vaccine has only been partly effective, to meet the virus themselves. This is known as herd immunity and is just as important in protecting a population from illness as it is for people to receive the vaccination individually. This is why government-supported vaccination programs are for the greater good as much as they are for individual health. In the case of smallpox, it allowed for the complete eradication of a disease that once killed hundreds of millions of people.

Stress can influence our susceptibility and resistance to undesirable bugs by suppressing the defences associated with adaptive immunity. For example, people who feel that they are under higher levels of stress are more likely to get a cold when they are confronted by a cold-causing virus. The bacteria that cause stomach ulcers are also enhanced when we are stressed. And of course the bacteria on our skin that cause acne (which are normally kept under control by our immune system) are often let loose when we are stressed.

Equally, the protective response to a vaccine is reduced by chronic stress. For example, people looking after parents with Alzheimer's who go and get their flu vaccine can often have a blunted response, compared to other people who are not under this high level of stress. It is thought that chronic stress interferes with the ability of the body to display the image of an invader to the appropriate authorities, so infections are harder to recognize, or are only recognized too late once they have got a foothold.

Sleepless and stressed in Seattle

The third of our life we spend fast asleep can significantly affect the two-thirds we spend awake. We all need a good quantity and good quality of sleep to keep brains and bodies working in peak condition.

The reason we need to regularly get some sleep has nothing to do with conserving energy for daylight activities. If this were all that sleep was good for, it would be far more practical for us to stay awake and eat just one extra banana a day to make up for the extra calories saved by laying down our tools and going to sleep.

Sleep is more important than just physical rest. In fact, sleep serves a number of essential functions we simply can't do without. One of the most important of these is dealing with the stress of life.

One common message for people dealing with stressful situations is to 'have a good night's sleep and it will all feel better in the morning'. Obviously sleep is harder to come by and is more broken when people are under stress. Again this is because our stressed brain is busy working on dealing with the stress and stubbornly refuses to let anything get in its way. This includes sleep. Having a good night's sleep would be easy *if we weren't so stressed!*

Moreover, not getting enough sleep is a significant source of stress itself, partly amplifying the effects of other stressors. So anyone not getting enough quality sleep (like those who are stressed) who then fortuitously get a good night's sleep will actually feel better in the morning. *As if this weren't so blindingly obvious!*

But before we jump at the next person who suggests we just need to get some rest, it turns out that they could be right in many more ways than they realized.

Our body may not be doing anything while we are dozing, but our brain is. It is making use of the time that sleep provides to process the events of the day, but without the visceral charge of sensation and immediacy. Without these nasty sharp edges, events can be stripped back to what happened in the brain during daylight hours and then safely evaluated without needing to stress over them. Deep sleep is therefore the time when our brain rewires the circuits that connect events, sensations and other information, to ensure all newly gained knowledge is organized and safely stored for future use. Some of these changes lead to learning and memory. Some of these also lead to forgetting the unimportant bits.

It's not that we don't learn things on the spot during the day. But rather, some of the same brain cells that get used during our busy day get fired up again at night to consolidate their interconnections. This is how getting more quality sleep really does help us remember, process and understand things better. This is also why an active (stressed) brain demands more sleep.

During other parts of the night, our brain plays back some of our memories to see how well any new ones work and if old ones still fit, like an enormous wardrobe full of thousands of dresses. Every night we take some out to look them over. Without anyone looking over our shoulder we can get creative, mixing and matching to find the best combinations for different occasions. We are more likely to check out the ones we have recently purchased. But often we also go back to the old faithful ones. Sometimes we even check out the really old ones to consider what we were really thinking at the time, and whether they might be better given away.

This is how we dream. Unlike during deep sleep when our emotions and stress are suppressed for the sake of clarity, when we dream these restrictions are turned off. This means we can look at events again and discover how we really feel about them, without being limited by what others might think or other consequences in real life. Although most dreams are quite mundane, some dreams can therefore be highly emotionally charged, including erotic fantasies as well as nightmares.

Nightmares

 We all have bad dreams from time to time. The really bad ones are called **nightmares**. This is because in times past, it was thought that nightmares were caused by demons, known as 'mares'.

These evil elves would quietly enter your bedroom through the keyhole at night. While you were sleeping they would climb onto your bed, sit on your chest to immobilize you or even try to strangle you. Not surprisingly, these antics would cause you to wake in fright, short of breath and covered in sweat.

These demons were also notorious for tangling your hair up during the night, resulting in 'mare-locks'. Today, we just know this as morning hair or bed-head.

Today, it is recognized that all dreams, bad and good, are just the mirror of our memories, with our brain responding in much the same way as it does when we look into a mirror or watch TV (another kind of mirror). Like our cupboards and our TV viewing, the visions revealed in most dreams are filled with recent acquisitions and new shows. But there are favoured dreams we go back to again and again, just like re-watching a favourite movie or re-wearing a favourite dress.

We know dreams are made from memories and experiences because people who are blind from birth do not have visual dreams. Equally, people from the thirties and forties who only watched black and white TV and film, actually dreamt in black and white at least a quarter of the time. In the era of the colour TV, hardly anyone dreams in black and white. However, our dreams never really look like our memories and experiences, even though they are made from them. Dreams are more fanciful, creative imaginings. It is just like trying on an outfit made up of different pieces of clothing purchased at different times and seeing if they work together. Often we don't actually see the outfit, but imagine ourselves wearing it in different settings, like a wedding or a date. In the same way we look over our memories, and imagine them in different settings or situations. Sometimes these places are strange, illogical and impossible. But this allows us to make better sense of them.

Like our outfits, dreaming is the time we can test out memories, get a little creative, mix and match, find out what goes with what, refine and improve them to achieve a better balance. Dreaming is also a time when we can take another look at how we really feel about things and decide to throw away the bad buy or move it into the back of the wardrobe away from the light of day.

Some dreams are recurring. This is like when we can't quite make up our minds and keep trying it on again and again. There is something about it that isn't quite right but we just don't know exactly what. In the same way, most people believe that recurring dreams stem from unresolved memories that are not easily bought or discarded.

Remember the dream

 Dreams peek at our memories in the mirror. But while memories are real, dreams are only the reflection, so they usually don't enter our long-term memory. In fact it is quite uncommon to remember our dreams for more than a few minutes, if at all. Most dreams are like that word on the tip of your tongue that is impossibly out of reach, but still so naggingly close to remembrance that we can almost feel it there.

Some people are in the habit of writing down their dreams (or at least their impression of them) as soon as they wake. Often there is a notion that by recording and interpreting our dreams we may reveal some hidden truths about ourselves. Indeed, some major discoveries have been attributed to visions remembered from dreams, including (famously) the periodic table listing the known elements, which came to Russian chemist Dmitri Mendeleev in a dream. Keith Richards famously dreamt the riff to *Jumping Jack Flash* and wrote it down as soon as he woke up. Some dream!

Dream recall is more likely with broken sleep patterns, or when waking suddenly in the middle of a dream rather than naturally at the end. This may also be one reason why nightmares, erotic fantasies and really vivid dreams seem to be more memorable than other everyday dreams.

At least six years of every life is spent dreaming. Given the importance of dreaming to brain management and psychological wellbeing, there is no shortage of ways recommended for having bigger, badder and therefore more memorable dreams. The most popular include eating dairy products (especially cheese), cucumbers, meat, kiwifruit, tart cherry juice or even just too much food right before bed. There is no good evidence that any of these things makes the slightest difference, although individuals will swear that one or other food makes a big difference to them. This may be more due to their memories and associations than the food itself.

Dreams are certainly more vivid after a night out drinking. But this is because alcohol is a sedative that suppresses dreaming during the early part of the night, meaning that when our brain emerges from the sedating effects of the booze, it tries to catch up and packs more dreaming into the few hours remaining before daylight. The same goes when we miss out on sleep for other reasons, like getting up for a child during the night, making our last dream much more intense.

Our deep, dark whole

When we are suffering, being pulled one way or another by our fears and desires, our brain tries to find a solution. It tries to help us cope. This is what our brain is for. There are many ways our brain tries to help us fight or protect us in our flight. One way is through our emotions.

Let's say we are walking to our friend's house over the hill, but are running late. We really wanted to be there on time, but it's not looking likely now. How do we feel? Or rather, what does our brain make us feel?

Sometimes we respond by getting angry and frustrated. Anger is generally considered a very negative emotion, associated as it is with the fight response — fighting is usually considered in a negative light. However, anger can be extremely useful; in the context of a conflict or a negotiation it can make us appear and feel more powerful. When we are angry, our desire for the thing that is making us angry is heightened, so we work even harder to get over the hill and get there on time.

But anger plays out in many different ways. Some people become overtly aggressive, while others fight back in a different way through denial and disbelief, acting as if something never happened. Some angry people play out their anger by becoming secretive or evasive, making bad decisions (asking for trouble) and attributing blame.

The opposite of anger is sorrow. Again, we are walking to our friend's house over the hill and we're running late. We really wanted to be there on time, but it's not going to happen. We feel sad.

Like anger, sorrow is also a coping reaction to stress and leads to many different behaviours. Some sad people become withdrawn and feel negative, resigned, hopeless or fearful. This is why sorrow is also generally viewed as a 'bad' or negative emotion. But also like anger, feeling sorrow can be part of the resolution process, as a step between distress and acceptance.

Many people cope with sadness by nurturing themselves and their children and getting together with others. This is often known as the 'tend-and-befriend' response (the opposite to the fight-or-flight response to threats). Things like going to a spa, getting a facial or a haircut become an important avenue to nurture and tend ourselves in times of stress. Sometimes, we try to resist unwanted change by creating a sense of permanence and focusing on controlling aspects of our lives, especially when everything seems out of control. Like tend and befriend, this response serves to bolster our self-esteem and confidence in time of crisis.

All these different reactions are often called defence or **coping mechanisms.** They are a normal part of coming to terms with any stress. Part of coping will inevitably involve experiencing many different emotional responses. Which ones we use depends a lot on the kind of stress we are under, our personality and factors such as our gender. For example, men are, on average, more likely to become angry or withdrawn when they are stressed. In contrast, women are more likely to have a tend-and-befriend response.

These emotions usually help us cope with stress. However, sometimes we can become stuck in these emotions. For example, when dealing with chronic stress we can become persistently grumpy for long periods of times, or persistently resigned, fearful or despondent. For many of us it feels like we have entered a deep, dark hole. It can be hard to get out of the hole. But we usually do, eventually.

Sometimes our mind becomes really stuck in the hole and the results can be disastrous. The best known example is **depression.** Depression is a very common illness. At least one in every six adults will experience depression during their lifetime.

Depression is also a very serious problem. It is not just a brief period of feeling sad or an understandable sorrow in response to adversity. Depression is a disproportionate and pervasive black cloud that interferes with our ability to function as a whole. It can affect our relationships, our work, our sleep, and many other aspects of our health and wellbeing, including our very survival.

Under the same circumstances and adversity, depression will not happen to everyone, or be as severe and recalcitrant to the same extent. Those who remain strong in the face of adversity somehow don't allow their losses to capture, encumber and confine them. In other words, they don't get easily stuck. We often think of these people as having resilience, like a tree bent by the wind that can spring back, or fortitude (literally an attitude built like a fort to keep adversaries at bay).

Resilience

 There are certain patterns in the way people think that make them more or less susceptible to being broken by adversity, to becoming depressed, angry, fearful or lost in times of stress. These distinct thinking patterns make up our individual character.

The resilience of our character is determined by the four walls that surround it:

- our self-esteem
- our sense of optimism
- our confidence that we have the resources to cope
- our sense of calm.

Some losses are so traumatic that anyone can have their walls knocked down. But in general, people who have high self-esteem, are optimistic, confident and calm, are more resilient. It is not that they do not ever encounter loss or ignore it when it occurs. Rather, they can deal with it more easily because stress doesn't contaminate their character and change who they are.

On the other hand, some people have low self-esteem, are pessimistic, lack confidence and/or are inherently tense and fearful. In these people adversity can more easily penetrate their fortress walls because they are not as strong. Think of the gloomy character Eeyore, the grey donkey in *Winnie the Pooh*. He is always expecting the worst. So when anything bad happens he readily goes into a funk.

Some people are less resilient than others. This is just the way of things. It does not imply they are inherently weak of mind or will. In fact, many great minds and strong characters, Winston Churchill for example, suffered from episodes of severe depression. But often, the greater the expectations we have of ourselves, the greater the stress we put our walls under, and sometimes they just give.

What makes our walls strong or weak is partly determined by the genes we inherit from our parents. A big component is also moulded by our social environment and experiences, particularly during the formative years of growing up. For example, experiencing trauma during our childhood can alter our sensitivity to stress and particularly our response to adversity. And this may predispose some people to depression in later life.

By the time we are about thirty, almost all of our character and its relative resilience is set in place. We become pretty much set in our ways. This is often referred to as our personality. It's not that we can't change it — there are many ways to become more optimistic, improve our self-esteem or our sense of calm — it's just that, after thirty, we seldom take the opportunity.

Depression is not the only mental hole people find themselves in. Some people become beset by fears and paranoia (known as anxiety disorders). Some people seemed filled with irrational anger and rage. Some people strike irrational bargains and become addictive risk takers. Each of these people is seriously ill from being emotionally 'stuck in a hole', as stress and suffering takes over their personality. The longer they are stuck there, the darker and darker it gets for them.

Stress management

As stress can be a cause of physical as well as mental illness, it is not surprising that avoiding or eliminating stress from our lives is high on our health checklist.

The problem is that every time we think about taking it easy, we also think how impossible this would be. Without stress we wouldn't get anything done. Most people think of stress as a motive force (motivation) that makes us act toward desired outcomes or away from undesirable ones, like the tension on the strings of a puppet that both keep it upright and moving in the right directions.

Stress is a common motivation, it's true. But a world without stress is not a world where we'd be unable to do anything. This is a common fallacy. It is also why stress is such a pervasive problem. We can act without strings. The problem is that we are so attached to them.

All stress management focuses on disentangling ourselves from our attachments to outcomes, and from our desires and our fears that pull unrelentingly on our strings. This can be done in many different ways. The success or relevance of each technique really depends on what it is that we are so attached to.

Some techniques concentrate on bringing an inner stress into the light, outside of the immediate emotion of being stressed, so that it can be studied and better understood. This includes techniques such as disclosure, guided visualization, mindfulness and other behavioural interventions.

Worry dolls

 Sometimes the best way to deal with our worries is to describe them honestly to others. Talking is an easy way we can catch our thoughts in a manner that is almost impossible inside our heads. Talking about our fears and desires tests their reality and often makes them more amenable to change.

All religions include the sharing of our burdens with a god or gods, whether embodied in a priest, a prayer, an idol or other object. In the Central American country of Guatemala, the same end is achieved with worry dolls.

Worry dolls are tiny figures made out of wool and wire. Children are told to tell their worries to the doll and then place them under their pillow. The more worries, the more dolls that are used. However, in the morning the worries will be gone.

These worry dolls have become extremely popular, not just in Guatemala but globally. There may be many reasons for their success. For one thing they take the space left by evening prayer. They are adorable (who can feel worried when looking at a cute little doll?), partly because they are a reminder that maybe we don't have it so bad, and partly because they actually work. Studies in children troubled by anxiety have shown that talking to a non-judgemental, non-parent friend really helps them. And a tiny doll fits perfectly under a pillow.

Some techniques aim to address the stress itself. The most common things we stress about are work, money and relationships. So undertaking practical things like time-management skills, financial planning, and relationship counselling are obvious and direct ways to resolve these common causes of stress. Another practical technique involves walling off stress so it does not become all pervasive.

Some stress-management techniques provide additional support to improve our resilience to stress, so we are less likely to get stuck in a hole. This includes things like cultivating optimism, building confidence, marital, family and social support. Religion and faith are also important supports for many people.

There are also techniques that allow the mind to function free of attachments for a while, so that it can have breathing space to reorganize. The most obvious one we use all the time is to go on vacation and try to leave our stress behind. But this only works for a short while. Usually within a couple of weeks we are back to our usual stressed selves. Many other techniques provide the same chance to release the pull of stress on a regular and frequent basis, including relaxation techniques, breathing techniques, biofeedback, prayer, self-hypnosis, yoga, meditation (relaxation with focused attention), posture, massage, acupuncture, micro-breaks, physical exercise, gardening, music, art, knitting and many other creative activities. Each to their own.

The bottom line

Stress causes suffering. Suffering shortens lives. The same protective defence mechanisms that make our stress response a lifesaver (fight or flight), when relentlessly repeated or made chronic, commit us into an unwinnable war, with local and collateral damage to our health.

Sometimes we can stay resilient, optimistic, confident and calm. We can cope. This is how to live. At other times, stress can get the best of us, and penetrates our very character. This is how we can become physically and mentally ill when stressed. It is sometimes also how we die young.

To live long we all have to find our own way to deal with the stresses we inevitably encounter. The trick is to call out stress for what it is: only the pull of our attachments, our fears and our desires. Knowing where our stress is coming from is the first step to make it go away.

Do I really have to ...

#17

Find love?

Q: Why does being in love feel so good?
A: Rose-tinted glasses.

Q: Won't having children kill me?
A: It only seems that way, sometimes.

Q: Does it matter who or what I love?
A: Only if it matters to you.

Q: Why is being lonely so bad?
A: We all need somewhere to belong.

Q: How do I find my perfect partner?
A: Fate, karma and luck.

Q: Is there an elixir of love?
A: Only in *Harry Potter*.

All we need is love. We may want for many other things, but love is all we need. Even if it weren't such a catchy mantra, there are very many reasons for believing it to be absolutely true. Not least of which is the significantly better health and longevity experienced by those people in supportive long-term, loving relationships.

But really, how could love make us live longer? It's very hard to know, partly as there is no easy way to work out who is lovingly coupled and who is not. One possible indicator of this kind of relationship is marriage. Obviously, not a perfect indicator. But still, if long-term love existed in the past, it was often but not always associated with marriage.

And it turns out that people who get hitched have, on average, better health and a longer life expectancy than those who live alone and never marry. Despite its obvious limitations, marriage remains one of society's most useful health-giving institutions, chiefly through its capacity to enhance and sustain relationships. Simply as public health strategy alone, marriage deserves to be more widely available.

Equally, it is abundantly clear that those people who, for whatever reason, have few social connections are not only isolated, lonely people (like Eleanor Rigby) but their health also suffers from their loneliness.

The magnitude of this burden is probably as significant for their survival as being a smoker, being overweight or a couch potato. For example, lonely hearts have twice as many heart attacks and are four times less likely to survive them, even after adjusting for higher blood pressure, cholesterol and rates of smoking. Cancer, stroke and other diseases are also more common. At every stage of our adult lives, it seems that those people in a stable relationship are less likely to die than those who are out on their own.

How this actually works is mostly still a mystery. Much like love itself.

Happy thoughts

One possible reason for this longevity is that, no matter their composition, people in happy relationships behave and think differently from those who are not. We have all seen the change in couples when they get together. Often their lifestyle choices tend to be healthier. Not always, but most of the time. Of course we can do many things about our health without love. But then, what's the point?

Rose-tinted glasses

 When compared to singles, many couples are more optimistic and see life through rose-tinted glasses. Of course, almost no one wears red lenses in their glasses today. But this phrase comes from a time when it was very popular.

In the 16th century, during the plague of Black Death sweeping through Europe, doctors wore elaborate masks incorporating ruby-red glass eyes, ostensibly to make them less susceptible to evil. Rubies were thought to magically change colour, becoming dark and cloudy when danger was near. This is possibly because when we look through ruby/rose-tinted glasses anything dark-red looks black in colour. And this includes blood. Not so scary now?

A good example of how less scary life is through rose-tinted glasses can be found in chickens. Chickens get all riled up and also fight more when they see the sight of red blood. This can be fixed by putting a hood with red lenses on the chicken. No more red blood means no more aggression and stress for a livid chicken, so a life viewed through rose-tinted glasses is much more rosy.

There are many social and emotional pressures to fall in love and share this bond with others, whether in a family, a couple, a band, a team or even a community. There are also biological pressures that pull us towards others.

As discussed in Chapter 16, when we are pulled by the pressures of expectation, we are stressed and suffer as a result. When the stress of our loneliness is superimposed on other life stresses, the cumulative burden can be even greater.

But it's not only what we have but what we do with it that counts. Our relationships can sometimes be stressful too, and bad relationships can be a significant source of bad health. Relationships are a frequent cause of conflicts, worries and demands in our lives and these stresses are associated with a shortened life expectancy when compared to those people whose relationships are habitually free of these problems. But more often, our relationships also have the capacity to bolster our physical, mental and spiritual resources when we need them.

At different times in our lives, different kinds of relationships are important for us. For example, in our teens and twenties it is all about quantity — girls in groups and boys in packs. In our thirties, it is more about quality, with fewer but closer relationships.

But while special close relationships are beneficial to us, they are not essential. Many people make up for quality with quantity. Extra friends, extra commitments, even extra wives seem to be beneficial to health, in the absence of one true love.

In each case, the sum of our loves is an important determinant of our present and future wellbeing, providing ready resources we need, as well as preparing us for the next steps in our lives. It could be one person or it could be many. It could even be a pet.

Children and small animals

It is a well-known show business superstition that actors should never work with children or animals. Any parent or pet owner will easily understand that despite their best attempts at training, their charges are essentially unpredictable. But an actor's biggest fear is that the cute faces of the little monkeys will simply steal the show, confining the actor to dramatic obscurity and shortening their future career on the stage. Or even worse, if it goes well, they will have to do it again!

The same is not true on the stage of life. It may feel as if our children take years off our life, steal the show and ultimately are going to be the death of us. But this doesn't usually happen. If anything, childless couples don't live as long on average as those who are parents.

Of course, this probably has nothing to do with the kids. For one thing, there is no dose-response. If kids were that good for our health then adding more would be even better. But it doesn't work that way.

An obvious reason that being a parent is good for our health is that it changes the way we live our lives. Many parents tend to take their health and lifestyle choices seriously, for the sake of their children. If we imagine a life without our children, think of the things we might have got up to. Would we have travelled more, eaten out more often or drunk more alcohol? Would fewer of our choices have been healthy ones?

Parents also have more access to a whole range of other parents though their children that they would never have met or worked with in other circumstances. Mothers' groups, school groups, sports groups and the like provide a valuable social network.

Nuns and monks seldom have children, but outlive most parents. However, they have the benefit of a different social network and an altogether different kind of marriage with their maker.

But it's not just children who change our lives. Taking care of animals makes us feel needed, co-dependent, responsible and valued unconditionally. Pets are easy to please, which brings its own satisfactions including pleasure, relaxation and stress reduction. Dogs in particular are great exercise partners. Pets provide an important source of physical intimacy (touching and stroking our human partner may be less readily achieved and doesn't work every time). Pets can also be a catalyst for social networking with others (e.g. meeting other people while out walking the dog).

As payback, pet owners can enjoy a better quality of life on average. This is known as the 'pet effect'. So much so that pets are used as part of the care of those with physical and mental illness. Again it has nothing to do with the pet, but rather the sense of emotional belonging that comes with it. Even robotic dogs can improve the health of people when a (surrogate) bond is forged.

One obvious reason is that, in the absence of social connections, anxious and lonely people are more likely to attribute human-like traits to their pets. In return they can fulfil the human-like need of belonging in a relationship. People in a loving, supportive relationship don't do this as often, possibly because (while in love) they have all they need.

Cat people

 About half of all homes have a pet of one kind or another. About half of the rest would like to have a pet one day.

Some people have birds, fish or other, more exotic, companions. But mostly there are dog people and there are cat people. These separations seem obvious, given the antipathy of cats and dogs. Having a foot in both camps (so called bi-pet-uals) seldom really works around the home or in relationships.

Some people argue that it's our personality that determines if we prefer dogs over cats. Like goes with like. In other words, dog owners tend to be a bit more outgoing, social and obedient, like their dogs. By contrast, cat owners are cool and curious but also a bit more sensitive, just like their cats. It is debatable whether cat owners are any more intelligent, but they usually think so. Certainly more women prefer cats than men do.

The differences are not huge, and there is substantial overlap. There are as many extroverted cat owners as antisocial dog lovers, but on average cat owners and dog owners are as different as George Harrison and Paul McCartney.

Whether it is the owner's personality that chooses the pet or the pet that transforms the owner's personality is still debated. One of the characteristics of rapport in a relationship is when we mirror the behaviours of others, running and panting with our dog, socially interacting with other dog owners or giving our cat what it wants. Some of these habits bleed through into our daily life and make us subconsciously reflect our pet's behaviours.

A far more important factor than personality is the pets we grew up with. Our memories of the pets in our family influence the kind of pets we prefer and ultimately own. For example, growing up with cats makes it far more likely we will get cats ourselves, and very unlikely we will become a dog person, without any other inducement.

A place to be

It is not just people and small furry animals we fall in love with. We also forge a relationship with our environment. We put down roots and fall in love with the spirit of place and find ourselves drawn inexorably back to where we belong. For some people there's no place like home. For others, it may be our connections to other places (an easy chair, a neighbourhood, a community, a local pub, the church, that beach, that holiday, the sports ground and our local team) that capture our soul.

It is not just the people or the social interaction we receive from a place, but the environment and its spirit we are somehow connected to. Even when there is no one else there, home is still home. When we are there, we feel as though we are where we are meant to be, giving us the easy sense of stress-free satisfaction. When we are far away, we can become homesick.

Belonging is one of the most important needs of being human. Belonging can come from our acceptance of social interactions with people or their surrogates (e.g. pets, dolls, robots and any other things we want or need to make a little human) and the value we place in them. But our physical environment also matters. Part of who we are is where we are.

This is more than just familiarity. It's nice to be in a place where we know where to find the fridge and the toilet. It's disorienting otherwise. Lost in space. But just because we know our way around a place doesn't mean we love it there.

Our connection with a place is also more than what it means to be there, or what being there will allow us to do. For example, 'I'm home' means 'I'm not at work' or 'I'm here to interact with you'.

The third element is the sense of belonging. This is the difference between a space and a place, a house and a home. In fact, we often use the phrase 'feel at home' to describe a place where we are in our element, as though we belong.

Spirit of place

 Some places have a certain energy, a charm, a soul or a spirit. In times past these special places were thought to be enchanted. The Romans actually thought of them as a specific supernatural deity, which they worshipped as the genius loci (the local genie).

Qi (pronounced chee) is a similar concept in the mystical Eastern philosophy of Feng Shui, which aims to take advantage of the positive energy of Qi for good health and prosperity.

One of the great challenges of the modern mass-produced globalized world is that we end up in so many (valueless) spaces, but not nearly enough places (with a value). It's just a shop. It's just a house. It's just a city. It's a non-place. The tragedy for our health is that we have killed off the spirit of place, and with it our healthy sense of belonging.

Love and other drugs

The composition of our relationships is not as critical to our health as our **fidelity** — being faithful and committed supporters of the team. Spouses, friends, family, neighbours, religion and even the love of specific sports teams make life feel worthwhile and better as a result, even if the team isn't winning. We just have to stick with them wholeheartedly. But to call it love we have to be truly addicted.

In many ways love is similar to addiction. Our relationships are inherently rewarding, or at least we anticipate we will get a boost when we interact with the object of our affection. And best of all, it feels easy. We receive pleasure without too much effort because we know where we need to be and who or what we need to be with. We have learnt this because we have received significant pleasure in the past and link the two together in our mind. This reconfigures the connections and transforms simply liking something or someone into desiring them.

Of course our interactions aren't always as rewarding or exciting every time. But it is hard to unlearn the connections we make in our brain that tell us where the good things are, even if they don't deliver every time. Remember that time when our football team won the competition? They haven't won since, but we remember when they did and still barrack for another success.

In fact, the anticipation of future success is one of the things that keeps us interested. If our football team won every year without fail it wouldn't be as interesting. We'd become tolerant of the rush when they won or more prone to feel disappointed if they actually lost. But while there is still the allure of potential success, while there is still hope, then there is love.

Like an addiction, it is almost impossible for another person to truly understand the strength of our feelings unless they share them or have their own secret addiction they can relate to. We think of the love-struck and the addict as equally mad or, at the very least, hedonistic.

Hedonism

 We all enjoy pleasure. We all dislike pain. It is not unreasonable to live our lives gravitating towards our likes and avoiding our dislikes. Simplifying our lives to just a choice of like over dislike, pleasure over pain, is known as hedonism.

Hedonism is an idea that was first conceptualized in Ancient Greece. The hedonists argued that the only important thing in life was to cultivate pleasure for ourselves and others, but without harming anyone or anything in the process.

This was not a new idea. In fact, the search for reward with less effort (the quick fix) is the central theme of all human development and discovery.

We may look at hedonism as self-indulgent pleasure seeking, but the world would not be what it is today without our human desire to make our lives easier, pleasurable and less painful. Agriculture, society, music, art and even the wheel have all come about from a desire to make our journey more comfortable and the road less bumpy. This is probably also the reason we fall in love.

Like any addiction, we miss it when it's gone. Addiction is not all about feeling good when we have got what we want. It's also about doing those things to avoid the stress and suffering when we haven't. This is one of the things that reinforces addictions and draws us back in, or alternatively, drives us to look for a substitute (e.g. such as being 'on the rebound') to fill the void.

Although our infatuations, lusts and addictions have much in common, including much of the brain chemistry involved in their origin, what often separates them is their potential for adverse consequences. If getting our fix will mostly lead to pleasure and good health, what's the harm? But when it causes pain or ruins our mental or physical health then we are prepared to call it some kind of addiction or clearly a mental disorder, and go into rehab to find a solution. It's not as though we never get caught up with the wrong person, the wrong crowd or barrack for the wrong team. It's just that it usually, but not always, turns out all right in the end.

There's the passively addicted state of infatuation, helplessly under the spell of love. And then there's love. Most couples are infatuated or addicted to some degree. But love is much more than this because of the active level of commitment that love implies — to realistically stick with them wholeheartedly and remain faithful and committed supporters of the team.

Intimacy

There is something special about romantic love that sets it apart from other kinds of love. It could be that intimacy draws partners closer to each other than in other kinds of relationships, or at the very least, makes it less easy to fall apart. Think of how holding hands or just a simple hug can make us feel warm, successful, needed and loved; how it makes us feel connected and wanting to stay that way forever.

Several websites have reported that men who kiss their wives every morning live five years longer than men who don't. There may be something to it?

Physical intimacy is mostly a tasty bait to get us well and truly hooked on love. It is not the only attraction and may not even be required, but it is a hook nonetheless. Each pleasurable reward our infatuated brain receives from intimacy makes us believe more and more that this is where we are meant to be. That it's easy.

Chemical bonding

 Between lovers there is real chemistry. The best example of this is the chemistry that helps create the love bond between a mother and her infant child. For example, during breastfeeding, the hormone oxytocin is released from the mother's brain. Oxytocin has many effects, but one in particular is to actually help rewire the brain of both mother and infant.

Remember, the brain's circuits are plastic. This means not only can our brain make new connections, but it can also amplify or silence signals running through established connections, making them seem more or less salient or worth our attention. This programming allows us to immediately recognize what is important to us. Oxytocin is thought to increase the sensitivity of its reward circuits to social signals.

The release of oxytocin during breastfeeding reinforces positive interactions between mother and infant, contributing to bonding. But oxytocin is a two-edged sword. It also has the effect of reinforcing negative social signals as well and can intensify bad memories as much as the good ones.

Oxytocin is also released into the brains of women when rocking their cervix during intercourse or by playing with their breasts. In men, physical intimacy is also associated with the release of chemicals into their brain, including oxytocin and vasopressin (which is 90 per cent identical to oxytocin and plays a similar role). So not only is intimacy pleasurable, but its chemistry helps us create a bond that makes us want to stick together.

Oxytocin is also released when we cuddle, kiss or bond socially. Even playing with our dog can cause a little oxytocin release. However, neither of these releases as much oxytocin as during sex. Consequently our intimate bonds are generally more intense.

It is often said that having regular sex keeps us alive. Studies have actually shown that, at least in men, those who have intercourse at least twice a week had something near half the chance of dying over a ten-year period when compared to those who had sex less than monthly. Similarly, the frequency of sex in a particular country is significantly correlated with the average life-expectancy in the same country. This appears to be more than just having the kind of relationship or youthful vigour that makes both good health and frequent sex possible. It is not enough to assume causality, but it is a reason to live.

The perfect partner

Most of what we find attractive in a potential partner is contained in their behaviour and appearance. We all have our likes and dislikes that are highly personal. However, when presented in a line-up, heterosexual women will generally revert to stereotype, and favour characteristics in potential partners that signal a man has the status and the resources to, at the very least, satisfy their needs and preferably give them a lift up the social ladder. These status characteristics are more often seen in men who are older than the women and, by and large, women prefer older men. Interestingly, in doing so, women married to older men get a bonus of living longer than women married to younger men.

Possibly because they can afford to be more choosy or simply have access in the social circles in which they move, highly affluent women with plenty of resources tend, on average, to favour even older men than those women with less financial independence.

It's not the only thing women want. Another key characteristic in a prospective partner is their potential for fidelity. Romance is a long game and what good are a man's financial resources if they ultimately leave with him? Male behaviours that appear exploitative, self-interested, exaggerated or frankly narcissistic, are all predictors of future infidelity, are not a good basis for a successful long-term relationship, and so are usually considered a turn-off.

The idea that women always go for bad boys and that nice guys finish last is simply a fallacy cooked up by the selfish ego of the narcissists. Women generally prefer nice guys. In particular, those men who recognize and understand a woman's feelings and needs (i.e. show empathy) are not only are being nice, they are also showing the potential for fidelity and this is therefore desirable. One simple way to judge a man's potential for fidelity may be by his ability to tell a good story. In general, women find charming storytellers far more attractive than poor storytellers and flirts.

And because of this clear female preference to (usually but not always) invest wisely, in general, men are more preoccupied with displays of wealth, strength and bravado, alongside pledges of undying fidelity. Because this is what men imagine women want: prince plus charming. Status plus empathy.

Men, on the other hand, generally find sexual vitality and youth more desirable than power status or a good story. These vital statistics are more often seen in women who are younger than they are, so generally, older men prefer younger women. Although there are limits. Going out with a woman who is half their age plus seven is generally viewed as socially unacceptable or 'cradle snatching'.

Interestingly, there is also a payback. Men married to younger women tend to live longer than men married to older women. And unlike women, the more affluent men become the more they prefer younger and even more attractive women, possibly because they too can afford to be choosy.

Because of this obvious male preference, (generally but not always) women are more preoccupied with the appearance of youth and sexiness. Because this is what women imagine that men want: Sleeping Beauty.

Of course, this is all a very, very crude generalization. Nothing is ever so base as gold diggers and trophy wives. These are obvious stereotypes. It may have worked this way in the past, but it never happens this way in an erudite modern society. Or does it?

In fact, in tests where men and women are confronted with hypothetical scenarios in which they have to choose one image of a potential partner over another, the statistics don't lie about what we ideally prefer. Prince Charming's attractive status and empathy works for women. Sleeping Beauty's youthful and attractive appearance works for men.

There's nothing wrong with having ideals. When we have limited information and are forced to make a decision, all we can use are stereotypes. But we are never that impulsive in real life. If we followed through with our perfect ideals, with freedom to choose and with no limitations, the age difference in couples would be, on average, a decade between the older man and the younger woman. In reality the difference is more like three years, on average, with lots of variability either way. In at least half of all couples who live together, the man is at least a year older than the woman, but usually no more than five years. It is probable that we take what we can get, as most people in our social circle are of similar age to us.

In about a third of couples, their ages are no more than a year apart. This figure seems pretty high, until we consider the fact that couples of a similar age have an exceedingly low divorce rate on average. By contrast, relationships with bigger age differences, while not doomed to failure, don't last as well and so bring the average down.

In the remaining couples, in about one in seven the woman is older, but again usually not by much. It seems the idea of cougars is one of those many sexual myths invented by male teenagers who paradoxically find older women more attractive, bucking the trend.

Interestingly, in gay and lesbian relationships, the age gap between partners is on average twice that seen in heterosexual relationships, much closer to the imaginary ideal when studying the perceived attractiveness of hypothetical partners.

The elixir of love

Given the desirability of being desired, it is not surprising that, if we were wizards instead of muggles, the one spell we would really want to know would be *amortentia*, the most powerful love potion in existence. It would be dangerous, sure — just think of 'love potion number 9'. But would that really stop us?

Love potions have been the stuff of legends for as long as there have been legends. This is their appeal, but it does not mean they actually work. If they do, it's usually by accident, like the famous story of Nemorino.

L'elisir d'amore

 Nemorino loves Adina. Adina thinks he is a fool. Nemorino is only a poor peasant, but she is rich and could have a different lover every day if she so desired.

Her indifference drives poor Nemorino crazy, and in desperation he spends his last dime on a bogus love potion (in reality a cheap bottle of wine). Nonetheless (or possibly because of the booze) he feels liberated and at last declares his undying love for Adina. To punish him, she immediately responds by agreeing to marry someone else.

Not dissuaded by the first disaster, Nemorino needs a more powerful potion. But he now has no money. Desperate for a remedy, he sells himself to the army and in return receives a wad of cash. Another bottle of cheap wine is dully delivered. At the same time, after seeing his money, other women start closing in on Nemorino. The elixir must be working, he thinks.

Adina, on the other hand, is rightly miffed and wants an explanation. She is told that Nemorino has spent all his money on a love potion to win the affection of some cold-hearted b****. Recognizing that it was her that he loved, and moved by his desperation, she falls into his arms.

While the love potion is merely a liberating mechanism for allowing the lovers to realize their true love, it is still a great money spinner. The story ends with everyone cueing up for the great elixir of love.

Many of the most famous aphrodisiacs acquired their fallacious reputation simply by being exclusive or expensive. Chocolate, oysters, rhino horn, Lamborghinis and diamonds have all in their time been seen as the way into a woman's arms. Not because they were actually aphrodisiacs at all. But because of what they said about the lengths the suitor had gone to win a woman's affection. Expensive diamonds! He must really mean it! And then there is the fact he can actually afford these things.

The original love potions were probably just toxic herbs, like deadly nightshade. This plant is also known as *belladonna* (an Italian word which translates as 'pretty woman'), as it was used by women to dilate the dark pupils of their eyes. These big round pupils created the facial appearance of wide-eyed arousal or excitement in otherwise bored women of the Italian court. The other thing that belladonna eye-drops did was make it hard to see things clearly in the light, as dilated pupils let too sunshine much in. So not only did these women appear aroused, but they were able to look this way without having to see their suitor in the harsh light of day.

The modern equivalent is probably alcohol, which causes both arousal and a degree of blindness when it comes to sexual attraction. But like most aphrodisiacs this is mostly from a sense of anticipation, rather than any magic chemistry of alcohol in our brain. For example, in one carefully controlled study, men showed more sexual arousal to images when they were led to believe their drink contained alcohol, even if it didn't! The same is true for Viagra, which only works for male erections and has no direct effect on the male brain. But through anticipation and very obvious association, it nonetheless has profound effects on sexual behaviour.

However, given enough alcohol, the effects can also be incapacitating, particularly on our emotions. Like belladonna, excess alcohol is not a love potion. As with Nemorino, the cheap wine itself was not able to make Adina fall in love with him. Rather, his subsequent irresponsible actions (spending his last dollars on another bottle and then joining the army) and her biased perception of what this meant was enough to bring them together. This is just what alcohol can accidentally do.

In more recent times, illicit drugs have also been used including roofies, GHB (aka liquid ecstasy) and ketamine (aka Special K) to alter our perceptions and incapacitate control over our emotions and their boundaries. These may be taken deliberately by those wanting to enhance their sociability or unknowingly spiked into drinks for nefarious purposes.

But if there ever was an *amortentia* love potion the active ingredient would probably be pheromones, the special chemical signals made by the body that send a message by smell and taste. In the animal kingdom, pheromones are a very important determinant of attractiveness. For example, female mice prefer male mice that smell distinctly different to themselves, reflecting subtle differences from their prospective mate and consequently the prospects for greater diversity in their offspring. Similar experiments in women suggest that, they too, prefer the smell of dissimilar men, which creates not only the potential for diversity but may also improve the chances for having healthy children in the future.

The definitive existence of any human pheromone remains to be established. But it is true that certain smells can unconsciously affect a women's desire for sex. For example, one study showed that the smell of a breastfeeding mother unconsciously increased the libido of other (clucky) women smelling it. Men unknowingly exposed to pheromones emitted by fertile women (in and around the time of their ovulation) behave and think differently when compared to other times in the women's menstrual cycle, especially with regards to sex. For example, when asked to judge a woman's sexual arousal, adding the undetectable scent of a fertile woman produced a higher estimation of her desirability. Consistent with this, men tip more money to lap dancers when they are fertile. In another study, men were asked to sit next to a woman. Some of these women had the smell of fertile women sprayed onto their T-shirt; the man sat closer to that woman, on average. Interestingly, when offered an alcoholic drink, these men also unconsciously drank more.

The bottom line

When we look back on our life, the things we most treasure are our loves: when we felt like we belonged, were connected, when we were part of something bigger than ourselves, when we were a member of the team or the band. Even though we may have broken up and gone our separate ways (or even on to solo careers), the bonds we have made continue to define us in so many ways. Just one of these is our health and longevity.

Our loves give us pleasure, for sure. But more than just a good time, belonging in any kind of positive relationship gives us access to more things to value than ourselves. Maybe this means we look after ourselves a little better. Maybe this means we have a more rosy view of the world, and don't get as easily riled up or stressed in the face of adversity. Maybe it rewires our brain or gives us other resources we need to prosper. Who knows? Love is an enigma, but it's hardly a mystery why we should want some.

Of course, it's easier said than done. For all the potions, fragrances and body odour, for all the good looks and all the money, attraction is an unpredictable coincidence. Given its allure, we are more than willing to try our luck. But there is more than only one kind of love. What matters to our health is that we find belonging, somewhere to put ourselves into context, a place to be (ourselves). Every day there are new opportunities to fall a little in love with people, with pets, with enchanting places. And after all, in the end, it's the love we make that counts.

Read more about ...

Chapter 1. The chocolate

Buitrago-Lopez, A, et al., 'Chocolate consumption and cardiometabolic disorders: Systematic review and meta-analysis', *British Medical Journal* (2011).

Coe, Sophie D. & Coe, Michael D., *The True History of Chocolate* (2013).

Dillinger, Teresa L., 'Food of the gods: Cure for humanity? A cultural history of the medicinal and ritual use of chocolate', *Journal of Nutrition* (2000).

Golomb, B.A., Koperski, S., & White, H.L., 'Association between more frequent chocolate consumption and lower body mass index', *Archives of Intern Medicine* (2012).

Kwok, C.S., et al., 'Habitual chocolate consumption and risk of cardiovascular disease among healthy men and women', *Heart* (2015).

Lemery, Louise, *A Treatise of All Sorts of Foods* (1764).

Macht, M. & Mueller, J., 'Immediate effects of chocolate on experimentally induced mood states', *Appetite* (2007).

Messerli, Franz H., M.D. 'Chocolate consumption, cognitive function, and Nobel Laureates', *New England Journal of Medicine* (2012).

Salonia, A., et al., 'Chocolate and women's sexual health: An intriguing correlation', *Journal of Sex Medicine* (2006).

Chapter 2. The booze

Knott, C.S., et al., 'All-cause mortality and the case for age specific alcohol consumption guidelines: Pooled analyses of up to 10 population based cohorts', *British Medical Journal* (2015).

Leong, D.P., et al., 'Patterns of alcohol consumption and myocardial infarction risk. Observations from 52 countries in the INTERHEART case-control study', *Circulation* (2014).

Rehm, J., et al., 'Global burden of disease and injury and economic cost attributable to alcohol use and alcohol-use disorders', *Lancet* (2009).

Chapter 3. The caffeine

Bhatti, S.K., O'Keefe, J.H. & Lavie, C.J., 'Coffee and tea: Perks for health and longevity?', *Current Opinion in Clinical Nutrition Metabolic Care* (2013).

De Balzac, Honoré, *The Pleasures and Pains of Coffee* (1832).

Freedman, N.D., et al., 'Association of coffee drinking with total and cause-specific mortality', *New England Journal of Medicine* (2012).

García-Blanco, T., Dávalo, A. & Visioli, F., 'Tea, cocoa, coffee, and affective disorders: Vicious or virtuous cycle?', *Journal of Affective Disorders* (2016).

Sheng, J., et al., 'Coffee, tea, and the risk of hip fracture: a meta-analysis', *Osteoporosis Int.* (2014).

Sho, H., 'History and characteristics of Okinawan longevity food', *Asia Pacific Journal of Clinical Nutrition* (2001).

Chapter 4. The waist

Bray, G.A., 'Medical consequences of obesity', *Journal of Clinical Endocrinology and Metabolism* (2004).

Mathieu, P., et al., 'Ectopic visceral fat: A clinical and molecular perspective on the cardiometabolic risk,' *Reviews in Endocrine and Metabolic Disorders* (2014).

Mattson, M.P., et al., 'Impact of intermittent fasting on health and disease processes', *Ageing Research Reviews* (2016).

Tchernof, A., et al., 'Pathophysiology of human visceral obesity: an update', *Physiological Reviews* (2013).

Chapter 5. The couch

Andersen, L.B., Mota, J., Di Pietro, L., 'Update on the global pandemic of physical inactivity', *Lancet* (2016).

Berbesque, J.C., et al., 'Hunter-gatherers have less famine than agriculturalists', *Biology Letters* (2014).

Després, J.P., 'Physical activity, sedentary behaviours, and cardiovascular health: When will cardiorespiratory fitness become a vital sign?', *Can J Cardiol.* (2016).

Ekelund, U., et al., 'Does physical activity attenuate, or even eliminate, the detrimental association of sitting time with mortality? A harmonised meta-analysis of data from more than 1 million men and women', *Lancet* (2016).

Neufer, P.D., et al., 'Understanding the cellular and molecular mechanisms of physical activity-induced health benefits', *Cell Metabolism* (2015).

Paffenbarger, R.S., et al., 'A history of physical activity, cardiovascular health and longevity: The scientific contributions of Jeremy N. Morris, DSc, DPH, FRCP', *International Journal of Epidemiology* (2001).

Rogerson, M.C., et al., 'Television viewing time and 13 year mortality in adults with cardiovascular disease: Data from the Australian Diabetes, Obesity and Lifestyle Study (AusDiab)', *Heart, Lung and Circulation* (2016).

Wasfy, M.M., et al., 'Exercise dose in clinical Practice', *Circulation* (2016).

Chapter 6. The fat

De Souza, R.J., et al., 'Intake of saturated and trans unsaturated fatty acids and risk of all cause mortality, cardiovascular disease, and type 2 diabetes: Systematic review and meta-analysis of observational studies', *British Medical Journal* (2015).

Estruch, R., et al., 'Primary prevention of cardiovascular disease with a Mediterranean diet', *New England Journal of Medicine* (2013).

Fodor, J.G., et al., '"Fishing" for the origins of the "Eskimos and heart disease" story: facts or wishful thinking?', *Canadian Journal of Cardiology* (2014).

Foster, R. & Lunn, J., '40th Anniversary Briefing Paper: Food availability and our changing diet', *Nutrition Bulletin* (2007).

Ramsden, C.E., et al., 'Re-evaluation of the traditional diet-heart hypothesis: Analysis of recovered data from Minnesota Coronary Experiment (1968–73)', *British Medical Journal* (2016).

Chapter 7. The added sugar

'Sugar by half' see http://www.sugarbyhalf.com/

2015–2020 Dietary Guidelines for Americans (2015).

Erickson J & Slavin J., 'Are restrictive guidelines for added sugars science based?', *Nutrition Journal* (2015).

World Health Organization Sugars intake for adults and children (2015).

Chapter 8. The starch

Aller, E.E., et al., 'Starches, sugars and obesity', *Nutrients* (2011).

Brand-Miller, J., Foster-Powell, K., & McMillan-Price, J., *The Low GI Diet Revolution: The definitive science-based weight loss plan*, Marlowe and Co, USA (2004).

Brinkworth, G. & Taylor, P., *The CSIRO Low-Carb Diet*, CSIRO Publishing (2017).

De Giorgio, R., Volta, U., & Gibson, P.R., 'Sensitivity to wheat, gluten and FODMAPs in IBS: Facts or fiction?', *Gut* (2016).

Keenan, M.J., et al., 'Role of resistant starch in improving gut health, adiposity, and insulin resistance', *Advances in Nutrition* (2015).

Khan, T.A. & Sievenpiper, J.L., 'Controversies about sugars: Results from systematic reviews and meta-analyses on obesity, cardiometabolic disease and diabetes', *European Journal of Nutrition* (2016).

Chapter 9. The fruit and vegetables

Crowe, F.L., et al., 'Dietary fibre intake and ischaemic heart disease mortality: The European Prospective Investigation into Cancer and Nutrition-Heart study', *European Journal of Clinical Nutrition* (2012).

Key, T.J., et al., 'Dietary habits and mortality in 11,000 vegetarians and health conscious people: Results of a 17-year follow up', *British Medical Journal* (1996).

Mihrshahi, S., et al., 'Vegetarian diet and all-cause mortality: Evidence from a large population-based Australian cohort — the 45 and Up Study', *Preventative Medicine* (2016).

Produce for Better Health Foundation, State of the Plate, 2015 Study on America's Consumption of Fruit and Vegetables, Produce for Better Health Foundation (2015), http://www.PBHFoundation.org.

Wang, X., et al., 'Fruit and vegetable consumption and mortality from all causes, cardiovascular disease, and cancer: Systematic

review and dose-response meta-analysis of prospective
cohort studies', *British Medical Journal* (2014).

Chapter 10. The cholesterol
Cholesterol Treatment Trialists' (CTT) Collaboration, et al.,
'Efficacy and safety of LDL-lowering therapy among men
and women: Meta-analysis of individual data from 174,000
participants in 27 randomised trials', *Lancet* (2015).
Endo, A., 'A gift from nature: The birth of the
statins', *Nature Medicine* (2008).
Varbo, A. & Nordestgaard, B.G., 'Remnant Cholesterol and Triglyceride-
rich lipoproteins in atherosclerosis progression and cardiovascular
disease', *Arteriosclerosis, Thrombosis, and Vascular Biology* (2016).

Chapter 11. The blood pressure
James, Paul A., et al., 'Evidence-based guideline for the management of
high blood pressure in adults report from the panel members appointed
to the Eighth Joint National Committee', (JNC 8) *JAMA* (2014).
Johnson, N.B., et al., CDC National Health Report: Leading
causes of morbidity and mortality and associated behavioral
risk and protective factors: United States, 2005–2013,
Morbidity and Mortality Weekly Report, Suppl. (2014).
Mohammad, H., et al., 'Global burden of hypertension and systolic blood
pressure of at least 110 to 115 mm Hg, 1990–2015', *JAMA* (2017).
World Health Organization, 'Global burden of disease', http://www.who.int/
healthinfo/global_burden_disease/GlobalHealthRisks_report_part2.pdf

Chapter 12. The fresh air
Acuff, L., et al., 'Third-hand smoke: Old smoke, new
concerns', *Journal of Community Health* (2016).
Couraud, S., et al 'Lung cancer in never smokers — A
review', *European Journal of Cancer* (2012).
Li C, et al., 'Long-term exposure to ozone and life expectancy
in the United States, 2002 to 2008', *Medicine* (2016).
Royal College of Physicians, 'Every breath we take: The
lifelong impact of air pollution. Report of a working
party, London', Royal College of Physicians (2016).

Chapter 13. The sunshine
Chua, J. & Wong, T.Y., 'Myopia: The silent epidemic that
should not be ignored' *JAMA Ophthalmololgy* (2016).
Doblhammer, G. & Vaupel, J.W., 'Lifespan depends on month of birth',
Proceedings of the National Academy of Sciences, USA (2001).
Holick, M.F., 'Sunlight, ultraviolet radiation, vitamin D and
skin cancer: How much sunlight do we need?' *Advances
in Experimental Medicine of Biology* (2014).

Sánchez, G., et al., 'Sun protection for preventing basal cell and squamous cell skin cancers', Cochrane Database of Systematic Reviews (2016).

Tosini, G, et al., 'Effects of blue light on the circadian system and eye physiology', *Molecular Vision* (2016).

Chapter 14. The common cold

Ackerman, J., *Ah-Choo! The Uncommon Life of Your Common Cold*, Twelve (2010).

Eccles, R. & Weber, O., *Common Cold*, Birkhäuser (2009).

Hendrie, C.A. & Brewe, G., 'Kissing as an evolutionary adaptation to protect against human cytomegalovirus-like teratogenesis', *Medical Hypotheses* (2010).

Chapter 15. By accident

Kim, E., et al., 'Vision zero: A toolkit for road safety in the modern era', *Injury Epidemiology* (2017).

Martin, T.L., et al., 'A review of alcohol-impaired driving: The role of blood alcohol concentration and complexity of the driving task', *Journal of Forensic Science* (2013).

Moyer, V.A., et al., 'U.S. Preventive Services Task Force recommendation statement vitamin D and calcium supplementation to prevent fractures in adults', *Annuals of Internal Medicine* (2013).

Robertson, M.C. & Gillespie, L.D., 'Fall prevention in community-dwelling older adults', *JAMA* (2013).

Chapter 16. The stress

Grandner, M.A., *Sleep, Health, and Society*, Sleep Medicine Clinics (2017).

Pedersen, C.B., et al., 'A comprehensive nationwide study of the incidence rate and lifetime risk for treated mental disorders', *JAMA Psychiatry* (2014).

Peters, A. & McEwen, B.S., 'Stress habituation, body shape and cardiovascular mortality', *Neuroscience and Biobehavioural Reviews* (2015).

Steptoe, A. & Kivimäki, M., 'Stress and cardiovascular disease', *Nature Reviews Cardiology* (2012).

Tawakol, A., et al., 'Relation between resting amygdalar activity and cardiovascular events: A longitudinal and cohort study', *Lancet* (2017).

Chapter 17. The love

Alexander, B. & Youn, L., *The Chemistry Between Us: Love, sex and the science of attraction*, Penguin (2012).

Casey, E.S., *The Fate of Place*, University of California Press (1997).

Gardner, J. & Oswald, A., 'How is mortality affected by money, marriage, and stress?' *Journal of Health Economics* (2004).

Sifferlin, A., 'Do married people really live longer?' *Time* (2015).

Index